Essential Medical Disorders of the Stomach and Small Intestine

Brian E. Lacy PhD, MD
John K. DiBaise MD, FRCPC
Mark Pimentel MD, FRCP(C)
Alexander C. Ford MBChB,
MD, FRCP
Editors

Essential Medical Disorders of the Stomach and Small Intestine

A Clinical Casebook

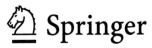 Springer

Editors
Brian E. Lacy
Mayo Clinic
Jacksonville, FL
USA

John K. DiBaise
Mayo Clinic
Scottsdale, AZ
USA

Mark Pimentel
Cedars-Sinai Medical Center
Los Angeles, CA
USA

Alexander C. Ford
Leeds Teaching Hospitals
NHS Trust
Leeds Gastroenterology Institute
Leeds
UK

ISBN 978-3-030-01116-1   ISBN 978-3-030-01117-8   (eBook)
https://doi.org/10.1007/978-3-030-01117-8

Library of Congress Control Number: 2018964576

This Springer imprint is published by the registered company Springer Nature Switzerland AG
The registered company address is: Gewerbestrasse 11, 6330 Cham, Switzerland

Finally, we would all like to thank our families for their unwavering support during this project.

Preface

Medical disorders of the stomach and small intestine are quite common in the general population. Community-based surveys consistently demonstrate that up to 20% of the Western population suffers from symptoms of dyspepsia, while 10% report symptoms of recurrent nausea and vomiting, and more than 30% suffer from chronic symptoms of gas and bloating. These symptoms are, unfortunately, persistent for the majority of patients who, after failing dietary modifications and over-the-counter agents, turn to their primary care providers for assistance and advice.

Despite the high prevalence of these disorders, a concise, up-to-date, and easy-to-use reference source describing these essential medical conditions of the stomach and small intestine is not available. This book is designed to fill that educational gap. Using a case-based approach, a panel of international experts has reviewed the 21 most common and vital medical disorders of the stomach and small intestine.

The book is divided into five parts: nausea and vomiting, dyspepsia and other disorders of neuromuscular function, chronic abdominal pain, demystifying the challenging postoperative patient, and small bowel disorders. Each of the five parts has been edited by experts in the field. Within each part, chapters begin with a typical case study illustrating a specific condition along with a list of learning objectives. The epidemiology and pathophysiology of each condition are then summarized, followed by a concise review of the diagnosis and treatment. Chapters will conclude with a follow-up of the case study, after testing has been performed and treatment initiated, and a list of key "clinical pearls" to highlight the most important teaching points. Each chapter also contains a series of test questions designed to emphasize important clinical care issues surrounding each case. Answers to the questions are provided at the end of the book, so that the reader can track their knowledge about each disorder.

We would like to dedicate this book to two groups of people. First, to our co-authors, who willingly, enthusiastically, and cheerfully found time in their very busy lives to write a state-of-the-art chapter on one of their specialties in gastro-enterology. Your tireless efforts in support of this educational endeavor are truly appreciated. Second, on behalf of all of the editors and authors, this book is dedicated to our patients. Thank you for letting us work with you and learn from you. We hope that the information in this book will provide help-ful educational information to health-care providers, so that they will be able to provide exceptional care to their patients.

Lastly, writing and editing a book requires the combined efforts of many people who work behind the scenes, often without credit. We would like to thank our Developmental Editor, Lorraine Coffey, for all of her hard work helping to coordinate this project. We would also like to thank Andy Kwan at Springer who was instrumental in bringing this proj-ect to fruition. Finally, we would all like to thank our families for their unwavering support during this project.

Jacksonville, FL, USA   Brian E. Lacy, PhD, MD
Scottsdale, AZ, USA   John K. DiBaise, MD, FRCPC
Los Angeles, CA, USA   Mark Pimentel, MD, FRCP(C)
Leeds, UK   Alexander C. Ford, MBChB,
                                           MD, FRCP

Contents

Contributors

Imran Aziz Department of Internal Medicine and Clinical Nutrition, Institute of Medicine, Sahlgrenska Academy, University of Gothenburg, Gothenburg, Sweden

Neelima Bonthi Division of Gastroenterology and Hepatology, Mayo Clinic, Rochester, MN, USA

Steven P. Bowers Mayo Clinic Florida, Jacksonville, FL, USA

Michael Camilleri Clinical Enteric Neuroscience Translational and Epidemiological Research (CENTER), Division of Gastroenterology and Hepatology, Mayo Clinic, Rochester, MN, USA

Amanda K. Cartee Mayo Clinic, Rochester, MN, USA

Dane R. Cook Global Research, The University of Newcastle, New Lambton, NSW, Australia

Andrew P. Copland Division of Gastroenterology and Hepatology, University of Virginia Health System, Charlottesville, VA, USA

Enrico Stefano Corazziari Department of Gastroenterology, Clinical Institute Humanitas, Rozzano, Italy

Brooke Corning Division of Gastroenterology and Hepatology, University of Virginia Health System, Charlottesville, VA, USA

Sheila Eileen Crowe Division of Gastroenterology, Department of Medicine, University of California in San Diego, La Jolla, CA, USA

Apaar Dadlani Department of Gastroenterology, Tufts Medical Center, Boston, MA, USA

Scott L. Gabbard Digestive Disease Institute, Cleveland Clinic, Cleveland, OH, USA

Magnus Halland Division of Gastroenterology and Hepatology, Mayo Clinic, Rochester, MN, USA

Kimberly Harer Division of Gastroenterology, University of Michigan Health System, Ann Arbor, MI, USA

William L. Hasler Division of Gastroenterology, University of Michigan Health System, Ann Arbor, MI, USA

Colin W. Howden Division of Gastroenterology, University of Tennessee Health Science Center, Memphis, TN, USA

Isabel A. Hujoel Division of Internal Medicine, Mayo Clinic, Rochester, MN, USA

Amrit K. Kamboj Department of Internal Medicine, Mayo Clinic, Rochester, MN, USA

David A. Katzka Division of Gastroenterology and Hepatology, Mayo Clinic, Rochester, MN, USA

Muhammad Ali Khan Division of Gastroenterology, University of Tennessee Health Science Center, Memphis, TN, USA

Michael J. Kingsley Department of Medicine, Division of Gastroenterology, Hepatology, and Nutrition, University of Pittsburgh Medical Center, Pittsburgh, PA, USA

Department of Medicine, VA Pittsburgh Healthcare System, Pittsburgh, PA, USA

Sobia N. Laique Internal Medicine, Cleveland Clinic, Cleveland, OH, USA

John Leung Center for Food Related Diseases at Tufts Medical Center, Boston, MA, USA

Food Allergy Center at Floating Hospital of Tufts Medical Center, Boston, MA, USA

Department of Gastroenterology and Department of Pediatric Allergy and Immunology, Tufts Medical Center, Boston, MA, USA

David J. Levinthal Department of Medicine, Division of Gastroenterology, Hepatology, and Nutrition, University of Pittsburgh Medical Center, Pittsburgh, PA, USA

Carolina Malagelada Digestive System Research Unit, University Hospital Vall d'Hebron, Barcelona, Spain

Centro de Investigación Biomédica en Red de Enfermedades Hepáticas y Digestivas (Ciberehd), Barcelona, Spain

Juan R. Malagelada Digestive System Research Unit, University Hospital Vall d'Hebron, Barcelona, Spain

Centro de Investigación Biomédica en Red de Enfermedades Hepáticas y Digestivas (Ciberehd), Barcelona, Spain

Zubair Malik Gastroenterology Section, Department of Medicine, Temple University School of Medicine, Philadelphia, PA, USA

Amar Mandalia Division of Gastroenterology and Hepatology, University of Michigan, Ann Arbor, MI, USA

Joseph A. Murray Mayo Clinic, Rochester, MN, USA

Amy S. Oxentenko Division of Gastroenterology and Hepatology, Department of Internal Medicine, Mayo Clinic, Rochester, MN, USA

Nadia Pallotta Department of Internal Medicine and Medical Specialties, Department of Gastroenterology A, University La Sapienza, Rome, Italy

Henry P. Parkman Gastroenterology Section, Department of Medicine, Temple University School of Medicine, Philadelphia, PA, USA

Eamonn M. M. Quigley Division of Gastroenterology, Houston Methodist Hospital, Houston, TX, USA

Alberto Rubio-Tapia Division of Gastroenterology and Hepatology, Mayo Clinic, Rochester, MN, USA

Gregory S. Sayuk Division of Gastroenterology, Washington University School of Medicine, St. Louis, MO, USA

Department of Psychiatry, Washington University School of Medicine, St. Louis, MO, USA

Gastroenterology Section, St. Louis Veterans Affairs Medical Center, St. Louis, MO, USA

Allison R. Schulman Division of Gastroenterology and Hepatology, University of Michigan, Ann Arbor, MI, USA

Magnus Simrén Department of Internal Medicine and Clinical Nutrition, Institute of Medicine, Sahlgrenska Academy, University of Gothenburg, Gothenburg, Sweden

Center for Functional Gastrointestinal and Motility Disorders, University of North Carolina, Chapel Hill, NC, USA

Nicholas J. Talley Global Research, The University of Newcastle, New Lambton, NSW, Australia

David A. Tendler Duke University, Durham, NC, USA

Hans Törnblom Department of Internal Medicine and Clinical Nutrition, Institute of Medicine, Sahlgrenska Academy, University of Gothenburg, Gothenburg, Sweden

Priya Vijayvargiya Clinical Enteric Neuroscience Translational and Epidemiological Research (CENTER), Division of Gastroenterology and Hepatology, Mayo Clinic, Rochester, MN, USA

Ted Walker Division of Gastroenterology, Washington University School of Medicine, St. Louis, MO, USA

Part I

Nausea and Vomiting

Chapter 1
Approach to Nausea and Vomiting

Zubair Malik and Henry P. Parkman

Case Study

A 47-year-old female presents with complaints of fullness, early satiety, nausea, and vomiting for the past 2 months. She feels nauseous throughout the day, although it is generally worse in the morning. She vomits occasionally after meals, usually 20–30 min after completing the meal. The vomitus consists of partially digested food and some bile, without blood or undigested food. She has not traveled recently and denies sick contacts or the use of illicit drugs. She has no significant past history other than being in a car accident 4 months ago in which she had a femur fracture; she is currently being prescribed nonsteroidal anti-inflammatory agents (NSAIDs) for her pain. She has lost 3 pounds over this time period. Her physical examination was normal. Laboratory tests, including a complete blood count (CBC), complete metabolic profile (CMP), thyroid stimulating hormone (TSH), and urine pregnancy test, were all normal. A CT scan of her abdomen, with both oral and intravenous

Z. Malik (✉) · H. P. Parkman
Gastroenterology Section, Department of Medicine, Temple University School of Medicine, Philadelphia, PA, USA
e-mail: zubair.malik@tuhs.temple.edu; henryp@temple.edu

© Springer Nature Switzerland AG 2019
B. E. Lacy et al. (eds.), *Essential Medical Disorders of the Stomach and Small Intestine*,
https://doi.org/10.1007/978-3-030-01117-8_1

3

contrast, was normal. Due to persistent symptoms, an upper endoscopy was performed. This revealed mild gastritis but was otherwise normal. She was found to be *H. pylori* negative on biopsies.

Objectives

- Understand the etiology of nausea and vomiting
- Gain an overview of the pathophysiology of nausea and vomiting
- Recognize the broad differential diagnosis for nausea and vomiting
- Review the different treatment options for patients with nausea and vomiting

Epidemiology

Nausea is a subjective symptom defined as a vague unpleasant feeling of unease with the sensation that vomiting might occur. Vomiting is an objective finding of the rapid and forceful ejection of gastric contents from the mouth [1]. Nausea and vomiting are important defense mechanisms to protect the body from the ingestion, and absorption, of potentially harmful substances [2]. Acute nausea and vomiting is defined by symptom duration of 7 days or less, while chronic nausea and vomiting is defined by symptoms of 4 weeks or longer. The epidemiology of chronic nausea and vomiting is not well understood. A survey of 21,128 adults found that 7% of the respondents experienced nausea and vomiting within the past 3 months. The study also revealed that vomiting led to a mean of 4.4 workdays, and 5.7 leisure days, missed over the preceding 3 months [3]. The epidemiology of several distinct disease states associated with chronic nausea and vomiting, such as gastroparesis, chemotherapy, and pregnancy, has been more carefully studied. For example, the Rochester Epidemiology Project estimated a prevalence rate of diagnosed gastroparesis of 9.6 per 100,000 in men and 37.8 per

100,000 in women. This rate is lower than an estimated prevalence of gastroparesis of 1.8%, which was calculated based on symptoms suggestive of gastroparesis, suggesting that there are many undiagnosed patients with gastroparesis.

Pathophysiology

The vomiting center (aka emetic center) is located in the dorsal lateral reticular formation of the medulla. Many neuroanatomical pathways converge on the emetic center, and stimulation of this area can lead to nausea and vomiting. Different afferent signaling pathways from the gastrointestinal (GI) tract, vestibular system, musculoskeletal system, heart, and the oropharynx converge at this center, along with signals from the chemoreceptor trigger zone and cerebral cortex. Efferent pathways from the emetic center to the GI tract, diaphragm, abdominal wall muscles, and oropharynx are responsible for coordinating the complex act of vomiting. Several key neurotransmitters are involved in this process including histamine, dopamine, serotonin, norepinephrine, acetylcholine, substance P, cortisol, beta-endorphin, and vasopressin. Vomiting is associated with cessation of antral contractions and relaxation of the stomach, increased pyloric tone, relaxation of the lower esophageal sphincter, and contraction of the abdominal wall, with the end result that gastric contents are propelled upward toward the mouth. The final step is a brief pause in respiration with closure of the glottis and vocal cords and elevation of the soft palate. This final step is important to prevent aspiration [4, 5].

Etiology

The etiologies of nausea and vomiting are vast and include a broad range of pathologic and physiologic conditions affecting the GI tract, the peritoneal cavity, central nervous system (CNS), as well as the endocrine system

(Table 1.1) [1]. These causes can be divided into several broad categories including medication and toxins, infections, GI motility disorders, GI obstruction, CNS causes, psychiatric disorders, endocrine and metabolic causes, and postoperative and other causes (both within and outside of the GI tract). A host of medications can cause nausea and vomiting; some of the most common include chemotherapeutic agents, digitalis, opiates, anticholinergic agents, antibiotics, and marijuana. Infectious causes can be either viral or bacterial in origin and typically involve the GI tract (e.g., a viral gastroenteritis), but infections in other areas of the body (e.g., otitis media) can also cause nausea and vomiting. Motility disorders of the GI tract such as gastroparesis, cyclic vomiting syndrome, pseudoobstruction, and mechanical obstruction involving the stomach (e.g., gastric outlet obstruction), small intestine (e.g., strictures), or colon (e.g., tumors, ischemia) can all lead to chronic nausea and vomiting. Gastrointestinal malignancies (e.g., adenocarcinoma of the pancreas, hepatocellular carcinoma), inflammatory bowel disease, ischemia, and hepatitis can also lead to symptoms. A number of central nervous system causes are associated with chronic nausea and vomiting. Some of the most common include migraine headaches, increased intracranial pressure (e.g., tumors, pseudotumor cerebri), and seizure disorders.

Pregnancy is a common cause of nausea and vomiting, and up to 50–75% of pregnant women report symptoms. One study reported that approximately 8.5 million working days per year are missed due to nausea and vomiting of pregnancy, and a mean of 62 h of work are missed during pregnancy in those that are severely affected [6].

Diagnostic Evaluation

The approach to patients with chronic nausea and vomiting needs to be methodical given the diverse causes. Determining the underlying cause of the nausea and vomiting is one of the most important aspects of patient care, because treating the

TABLE 1.1 Differential diagnosis of nausea and vomiting, divided into major categories

Medications and toxins*

(see Table 1.2)

Infectious causes

GI infections

   Viral

   Bacterial

Non-GI infections

GI motility disorders

Gastroparesis

Gastroparesis like syndrome

Chronic intestinal pseudoobstruction

Irritable bowel syndrome

Severe constipation

Functional dyspepsia

Achalasia

GI obstruction

Gastric outlet obstruction

Small bowel obstruction

Extrinsic compression of the GI tract

Ischemic stenosis

Other GI causes

Cyclic vomiting syndrome

Crohn's disease

Cannabinoid hyperemesis syndrome

Chronic nausea and vomiting syndrome

Pancreatic adenocarcinoma

(continued)

TABLE 1.1 (continued)

Inflammatory intraperitoneal disease

Peptic ulcer disease

Pancreatitis

Cholecystitis or cholangitis

Mesenteric ischemia

Mucosal metastasis

Retroperitoneal fibrosis

Hepatitis

Infiltrative biliary disease

Partial biliary obstruction

Zenker's diverticulum

Psychiatric

Anxiety

Depression

Conversion disorder

Eating disorders

   Anorexia

   Bulimia

Psychogenic vomiting

Pain

Learned behaviors

CNS disorders

Migraine

Parkinson's

Seizure disorders

Increased intracranial pressure

TABLE 1.1 (continued)

Malignancy

Hemorrhage

Hydrocephalus

Congenital malformation

Meningitis

Abscess

Infarction

Congenital malformation

Vestibular disorders

Labyrinthitis

Tumors

Meniere's disease

Motion sickness

Chronic otitis media

Endocrine and metabolic

Pregnancy

Diabetic ketoacidosis

Uremia

Hypo–/hyperparathyroid

Hyperthyroid

Addison's disease

Acute intermittent porphyria

Postoperative

Ileus

Post vagotomy

Other

(continued)

TABLE 1.1 (continued)

Alcohol abuse

Cardiac

   Ischemia

   Congestive heart failure

   Radiofrequency ablation

Renal and urologic

   Renal insufficiency

   Nephrolithiasis

   Obstruction

Connective tissue disorders

   Scleroderma

   SLE

Vascular disorders

   Median arcuate ligament syndrome

   SMA syndrome

   Chronic ischemia

Starvation

Food allergies or intolerances

Paraneoplastic syndromes

Radiation induced

Angioedema

Glaucoma

Mitochondrial disorders

Ion channel disorders

---

underlying disease will generally improve symptoms. A good clinical history can usually elicit the underlying cause of nausea and vomiting. It is important to first evaluate the patients' medications, and this should include an evaluation of over-the-counter agents, herbal products, complementary products, weight loss agents, and supplements (Table 1.2). If a careful history uncovers an offending agent (e.g., a medication or supplement), then the first step is to discontinue that agent, if possible. In an older patient, the possibility of polypharmacy causing nausea should not be overlooked.

Determining the chronicity of the symptoms during the initial interview helps to narrow the broad differential diagnosis. Patients with the acute onset of symptoms need to be evaluated for serious and life-threatening disorders including bowel obstruction, perforation, or peritonitis. If identified the patient should be admitted to the hospital for further evaluation and management [7] (Fig. 1.1). The patient should also be assessed for incapacitating symptoms, dehydration, and/or electrolyte imbalances, and if found these should be corrected with intravenous fluids and electrolyte repletion. In the absence of life-threatening emergencies (e.g., bowel perforation), most acute cases of nausea and vomiting are infectious in nature (usually viral), and supportive care is the mainstay of therapy as these cases are usually self-limited. If an underlying bacterial infection is suspected, treatment with the appropriate antibiotic will often resolve the symptoms.

Chronic symptoms usually warrant a diagnostic evaluation although some providers favor an empiric approach (Fig. 1.2). For example, empiric acid suppression can be given, especially in those cases where reflux or an ulcer is thought to be the etiology. An upper endoscopy can help identify severe erosive esophagitis, peptic ulcer disease, or an obstructive cause for the symptoms. An upper GI series, including a small bowel follow-through, can also be used to identify obstructive causes.

Evaluating characteristics of the vomiting is another useful step in determining the underlying etiology. Questions should

TABLE 1.2 Medications and toxins that can cause nausea and vomiting

Analgesics

    Opiates

    NSAIDs

    Antigout drugs

    Auranofin

Antibiotics

    Erythromycin

    Tetracycline

    Sulfonamides

    Acyclovir

    Antituberculosis drugs

Cardiovascular medications

    Digoxin

    Calcium channel blockers

    Beta blockers

    Diuretics

    Antiarrhythmics

Chemotherapy

    Cisplatinum

    Dacarbazine

    Nitrogen mustard

    Busulfan

    Cyclophosphamide

    Doxorubicin

    Epirubicin

    Ifosfamide

TABLE 1.2 (continued)

Streptozocin

Procarbazine

Vismodegib

Temozolomide

Etoposide

Methotrexate

Carboplatin

Interferon alfa

Oxaliplatin

Cytarabine

Fluorouracil

Vinblastine

Tamoxifen

GI medications

Sulfasalazine

Azathioprine

CNS drugs

L-Dopa

Bromocriptine

Antiparkinsonian drugs

Anticonvulsants

Oral contraceptives

Estrogens

Oral antidiabetics

Radiation therapy

Ethanol abuse

Jamaican vomiting sickness

Hypervitaminosis

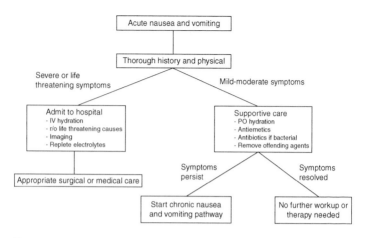

FIGURE 1.1 Approach to patients with acute nausea and/or vomiting

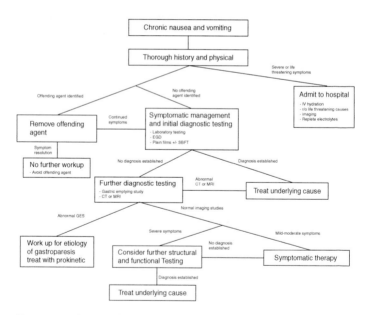

FIGURE 1.2 Approach to chronic nausea and vomiting

be asked regarding the frequency of vomiting, the amount of vomiting, whether the vomitus is digested or undigested food, whether the vomitus is projectile or not, and the relationship of vomiting to meal ingestion and the time of the day. Vomiting of pregnancy is often worse in the morning, along with vomiting related to uremia, alcohol ingestion, and increased intracranial pressure. Patients with increased intracranial pressure often have projectile vomiting without preceding nausea. Vomiting of undigested food can occur with achalasia, a Zenker's diverticulum, or an esophageal stricture, whereas vomiting partially digested food without bile is common in patients with gastric outlet obstruction. Feculent vomiting may be reported by patients with a small bowel obstruction [8]. Esophageal disorders causing nausea and vomiting usually produce symptoms within 10–15 min after eating, while gastric causes produce symptoms 2–3 h later, and small bowel causes produce symptoms 4–5 h after meal ingestion.

A careful physical examination may uncover the etiology of symptoms as well as to help determine the severity of symptoms. Providers should carefully assess the patient to look for jaundice, lymphadenopathy, ascites, abdominal masses, and blood in the stool. Cranial nerve defects are often found in association with CNS tumors, and as such a neurologic exam is necessary in these patients. A brief assessment of the patient's psychological status is important to identify disorders that may causes chronic nausea and vomiting (e.g., psychogenic vomiting). Examination of the skin and extremities may identify a variety of rheumatologic disorders that can involve the GI tract and cause nausea and vomiting (e.g., scleroderma, systemic lupus erythematosus). Dry palms, absence of axillary sweat, loss of saliva, and tachycardia are signs of dehydration. A brief dental exam identifying loss of enamel may identify patients with bulimia. A succussion splash detected on auscultation while palpating the abdomen suggests excessive fluid in the stomach from gastroparesis or gastric outlet obstruction. An abdominal bruit may be evidence of an ischemic process.

Laboratory testing in patients with chronic nausea and vomiting can be useful for several reasons. First, it may determine whether there are significant electrolyte imbalances present or if there is evidence of dehydration. Second, laboratory testing can identify an underlying etiology at times. For example, an elevated hemoglobin A1c may lead to a diagnosis of diabetes- and diabetic-related gastroparesis. An abnormal CBC may indicate a malignancy or an infectious etiology. Inflammatory markers (e.g., elevated CRP) may point to an underlying disease such as IBD or malignancy. Electrolyte abnormalities could indicate Addison's disease. A pregnancy test should always be performed in women of child-bearing age, especially before diagnostic tests (e.g., CT scan or upper endoscopy) are performed or empiric medications are provided.

Diagnostic testing should be guided by the history and physical examination. If no alarm symptoms are present, an empiric trial of an antiemetic or a gastric acid suppressive medication could be performed, although no validated data is available to support this approach. In those with symptoms of obstruction, an abdominal series should be promptly performed, often followed by urgent or emergent CT scan imaging. Upper endoscopy can be performed to rule out an upper (e.g., esophagus, stomach, duodenal) obstructive process, mass, tumor, or ulcer. Retained food in the stomach is suggestive of gastroparesis if no obstructive etiology is seen. A scintigraphic gastric emptying scan can assess motor function of the stomach; this should be a 4-h study using a solid-phase meal (liquid meals and scans less than 4 h are not useful). Two alternatives to scintigraphy exist to measure gastric emptying: the wireless motility capsule and isotope breath testing. The wireless capsule motility provides additional information as it also measures small bowel and colonic transit. Isotope breath testing can be performed in the office rather than the nuclear medicine department. Esophageal manometry and/or barium esophagram can be useful to assess esophageal motility and to rule out achalasia or a Zenker's diverticulum. An upper GI series with small bowel follow-through can visualize the small bowel and determine if there is a mass or high-grade obstruction, but this may fail to detect low-grade obstructions and smaller mucosal lesions. For patients with persistent symptoms and no identifiable cause, specialized testing may be required (e.g., antroduodenal manometry, electrogastrography, and whole gut transit scintigraphy), although these tests are usually only available at dedicated motility centers. If symptoms are thought to be due to ischemia, a mesenteric duplex is a good initial study, followed by either MR or CT angiogram, if necessary. If a central disorder is suspected, CT or MRI of the brain should be performed. Finally, psychological screening for eating disorders or other psychiatric disorders is an important tool, especially for patients with ongoing symptoms, normal diagnostic tests, and failure to respond to empiric therapy [8].

Treatment

The treatment of nausea and vomiting can be accomplished in three steps. The first step is to correct any consequences or complications from nausea and vomiting (e.g., electrolyte disturbances, treatment of a Mallory-Weiss tear). The second step is to identify the underlying cause and select appropriate targeted therapy. The final step is to improve or eliminate symptoms [1]. Ideally, treatment would be based on the underlying etiology of the nausea and vomiting. Offending agents or toxins should be withdrawn if at all possible. Infection should be treated appropriately. Glycemic control should be maintained, as acute hyperglycemia can slow gastric emptying [9]. Diet and oral nutrition should be maintained, and if symptoms prevent maintaining a reasonable weight, then enteral or even parenteral nutrition may be required.

A number of different antiemetic therapies are now available to provide symptomatic relief of nausea and vomiting. Unfortunately, no validated treatment algorithm exists; thus the art of treatment rests on understanding the array of treatment options available and recognizing their benefits, costs, and potential side effects. Dopamine receptor antagonists (metoclopramide and domperidone) and motilin receptor agonists (azithromycin, erythromycin) are prokinetic agents that increase gastric motility which may improve symptoms of nausea and vomiting in some patients [10]. In addition to its prokinetic effects, metoclopramide has central antiemetic effects, which would appear to make it a first choice for therapy. However, metoclopramide is associated with many side effects including tremor, difficulty sleeping, gynecomastia, a worsening of anxiety, alterations in mood, and changes in libido and menstrual cycles. The worst possible side effect is tardive dyskinesia, which may be irreversible; the precise risk of this is unclear although it is thought to be less than 1% of all treated patients. Current recommendations are that metoclopramide should only be used for up to 12 weeks. Domperidone is not FDA approved in the United States but can be prescribed under an FDA treatment protocol; the primary concern is that of cardiac arrhythmias from a prolonged QTc. Patients treated with domperidone should have a baseline EKG checked. Erythromycin improves gastric emptying but does not have antiemetic qualities; tachyphylaxis occurs with this agent within a few weeks. Azithromycin also improves gastric motility but does not have antiemetic qualities; in clinical practice it has little utility. Prucalopride, a $5HT_4$ receptor agonist, treats symptoms of chronic constipation and is available in Europe. It may become available in the United States in 2019 and has the potential to improve symptoms of nausea and vomiting in some patients with an underlying disorder of GI motility [8, 11].

Antiemetic agents without prokinetic properties are usually the first choice of primary care providers for the treatment of chronic nausea and vomiting. Phenothiazines (prochlorperazine), antihistamines, $5-HT_3$ receptor antagonists (ondansetron, granisetron), transdermal scopolamine, cannabinoids, and neurokinin-1 receptor antagonists (aprepitant) are some of the agents available [10]. Unfortunately, data from large, randomized, placebo-controlled studies evaluating these agents are not available. Many of these agents can be safely used in combination (e.g., ondansetron and prochlorperazine), and providers should feel confident trying various combinations of antiemetics (always starting with a low dose of one agent and then slowly add in the second agent, all the while monitoring the patient carefully for potential side effects). Many patients with chronic nausea and vomiting also suffer from chronic visceral pain (e.g., gastroparesis patients). Opiates should be avoided as they will delay stomach emptying and also impair esophageal, small bowel, and colonic function. Tricyclic antidepressants (TCAs), mirtazapine, and gabapentin have been used to improve visceral pain with some success; the occasional patient notes an improvement in nausea and vomiting when pain improves or resolves. Focusing just on the gastroparesis patient, interventions that relieve pylorospasm (e.g., botulinum toxin, gastric per oral endoscopic myotomy (G-POEM), or pyloroplasty or pyloromyotomy) or which modulate the enteric nervous system (gastric electrical stimulation) may prove useful in the occasional patient, although these therapies are only available at specialized motility centers [12].

Many patients prefer to use alternative therapies due to perceived benefits in terms of cost, availability, and safety. Commonly used alternative therapies include ginger, acupuncture, electroacupuncture, iberogast, caraway oil, peppermint oil, and hypnotherapy. Though there is limited data for all of these lines of treatment, small studies suggest benefit, and side effects are minimal [8].

Clinical Case Study Follow-Up

Upon a more detailed review of the patient's history, the patient revealed that she was taking oxycodone that had been given to her by a friend. She had started taking the medication several days prior to the onset of her symptoms and had been taking it consistently twice a day throughout the last 10 weeks, as it had been helping her pain. She was advised to discontinue the medication, and upon doing so her symptoms of nausea and vomiting resolved. A more detailed initial history could have potentially avoided unnecessary testing with a CT scan and upper endoscopy.

Clinical Pearls

- Symptoms of nausea and vomiting can occur due a broad range of conditions and diseases including medication side effects, infections, GI disorders, and CNS disorders.
- A detailed clinical history and physical exam is important as it frequently identifies the underlying etiology of chronic nausea and vomiting.
- Life-threatening acute etiologies of nausea and vomiting should be ruled out first, and then further testing should be driven by findings from the history and physical.
- Treatment is ideally directed at the underlying cause of symptoms.

Self-Test

Question 1. Where is the vomiting center located?

A. Posterior lateral reticular formation of the medulla
B. Dorsal lateral reticular formation of the medulla
C. Posterior lateral reticular formation of the somatosensory cortex
D. Doral lateral reticular formation of the somatosensory cortex

Question 2. All of the following are causes of nausea and vomiting except for:

A. Cisplatinum
B. Metoprolol
C. Tetracycline
D. Aprepitant
E. Sulfasalazine

Question 3. In a patient with symptoms of nausea and vomiting, after ruling out a life threatening illness, what is the next step in the approach?

A. Remove offending agents
B. Check blood work
C. Check obstruction series
D. Treat with antiemetics

References

1. Quigley EMM, Hasler WL, Parkman HP. AGA technical review on nausea and vomiting. Gastroenterology. 2001;120(1):263–86.
2. Sharkey KA, Darmani NA, Parker LA. Regulation of nausea and vomiting by cannabinoids and the endocannabinoid system. Eur J Pharmacol. 2014;722:134–46.
3. Camilleri M, Dubois D, Coulie B, Jones M, Kahrilas PJ, Rentz AM, et al. Prevalence and socioeconomic impact of upper gastrointestinal disorders in the United States: results of the US upper gastrointestinal study. Clin Gastroenterol Hepatol. 2005;3(6):543–52.
4. Hornby PJ. Central neurocircuitry associated with emesis. Am J Med. 2001;111(Suppl 8A):112S.
5. Lang IM, Sarna SK, Dodds WJ. Pharyngeal, esophageal, and proximal gastric responses associated with vomiting. Am J Phys. 1993;265(5 Pt 1):963.
6. Gadsby R. Pregnancy sickness and symptoms: your questions answered. Prof Care Mother Child. 1994;4(1):16–7.
7. Hasler WL, Chey WD. Nausea and vomiting. Gastroenterology. 2003;125(6):1860–7.
8. Lacy BE, Parkman HP, Camilleri M. Chronic nausea and vomiting: evaluation and treatment. Am J Gastroenterol. 2018;113:647.
9. Bharucha AE, Camilleri M, Forstrom LA, Zinsmeister AR. Relationship between clinical features and gastric emptying disturbances in diabetes mellitus. Clin Endocrinol. 2009;70(3):415–20.
10. Hasler WL. Newest drugs for chronic unexplained nausea and vomiting. Curr Treat Options Gastroenterol. 2016;14(4):371–85.
11. Camilleri M. Novel diet, drugs, and gastric interventions for gastroparesis. Clin Gastroenterol Hepatol. 2016;14(8):1072–80.
12. Tack J, Carbone F. Functional dyspepsia and gastroparesis. Curr Opin Gastroenterol. 2017;33(6):446–54.

Essential Reading

Quigley EMM, Hasler WL, Parkman HP. AGA technical review on nausea and vomiting. Gastroenterology. 2001;120(1):263–86. This article provides an overview on nausea and vomiting and sets the framework for other papers

Lacy BE, Parkman HP, Camilleri M. Chronic nausea and vomiting: evaluation and treatment. Am J Gastroenterol. 2018. This article provides a recent update on nausea and vomiting with up-to-date diagnostic and treatment strategies.;113:647.

Hasler WL. Newest drugs for chronic unexplained nausea and vomiting. Curr Treat Options Gastroenterol. 2016;14(4):371–85. This article provides insight on the newer drugs for treatment of nausea and vomiting.

Chapter 2
Gastroparesis

Priya Vijayvargiya and Michael Camilleri

Case Study

Mrs. G is a 62-year-old female with a past medical history of insulin-requiring type 2 diabetes mellitus for ~30 years, complicated by retinopathy and nephropathy. She presents with progressive nausea, early satiety, fullness, bloating, loss of appetite, and weight loss of 7 pounds over the past 8 months. Her blood glucose control has been erratic in recent months. Vital signs demonstrated a heart rate of 64/min, supine blood pressure of 123/76 mmHg, standing blood pressure of 95/60 mmHg, respiratory rate of 12/min, and 92% oxygen saturation. Physical exam was unremarkable other than background diabetic retinopathy and BMI of 37.5 kg/m^2. Previous evaluations included normal complete blood count, electrolyte panel, INR, liver function test, upper gastrointestinal endoscopy, and abdominal CT scan. HbA1c has ranged from

P. Vijayvargiya · M. Camilleri (✉)
Clinical Enteric Neuroscience Translational and Epidemiological
Research (CENTER), Division of Gastroenterology and
Hepatology, Mayo Clinic, Rochester, MN, USA
e-mail: camilleri.michael@mayo.edu

© Springer Nature Switzerland AG 2019   23
B. E. Lacy et al. (eds.), *Essential Medical Disorders*
of the Stomach and Small Intestine,
https://doi.org/10.1007/978-3-030-01117-8_2

8% to 9% in the last year. Gastric emptying scan, based on a 1-h radiolabeled liquid (5% glucose drink) meal, showed $T_{1/2}$ of 40 min. She was started on liquid formula metoclopramide, 5 mg TID, 15 min before meals, without improvement in symptoms, and she developed uncontrollable movements of her head, neck, and arms, which resolved upon discontinuation of the metoclopramide. She had three main questions: (1) What is the diagnosis? (2) What are future management options? and (3) Is there anything that can improve my appetite?

Objectives

1. Understand the pathophysiology of gastroparesis.
2. Review diagnostic strategies for patients with upper gastrointestinal symptoms suggestive of gastroparesis.
3. Understand principles of dietary treatment.
4. Review pharmacological, device, and endoscopic options for gastroparesis.

Epidemiology

Gastroparesis is defined as the presence of delayed gastric emptying in association with upper gastrointestinal symptoms, without the presence of mechanical obstruction. This condition is at best uncommon, and the prevalence depends on a number of factors such as the underlying cause. Gastroparesis is more prevalent in females, and the most common cause of, or association with, gastroparesis is diabetes mellitus or idiopathic. Reports from tertiary care referral centers suggest that the prevalence of gastroparesis is 40% among patients with type 1 diabetes attending a secondary referral clinic [1]; however, a population-based, US cohort study showed a lower prevalence. Thus, the cumulative proportion of patients with type 1 diabetes who developed gastroparesis over a 10-year period was 5.2% compared to a prevalence of 1% in patients with type 2 diabetes and 0.2% in the general population [2]. Age-adjusted prevalence and incidence per 100,000 person years were about 4 times higher for women (37.8 and 9.8, respectively) than for men (9.6 and 2.4, respectively) [3]. Despite the low prevalence of gastroparesis, this condition has a tremendous impact on patients who suffer from it, and it is a significant healthcare burden.

Etiology/Pathophysiology   The stomach's primary motor functions are relaxation upon food entry into the stomach and antral trituration of food in order to control the size of food particles that pass into the duodenum, thereby facilitating enzymatic digestion in the small bowel. The process of trituration involves liquid shearing forces set up by the antral contractions and initial contraction of the pylorus to retropel food into the body for further enzymatic and mechanical digestion. The resistance to flow of solids provided by the pyloric sphincter ensures that the size of solid food particles emptied from stomach is 1–2 mm. These functions depend on a combination of extrinsic and intrinsic neuromuscular functions, including neurons that generate and transmit electrical signals, pacemaker cells [such as the interstitial cells of Cajal (ICCs) and PDGFRα-positive fibroblast-like cells], and smooth muscles. Extrinsic nerves include the vagus nerve, and intrinsic neurons include nitrergic and cholinergic neurons. Alterations or abnormalities in any of these components can result in delayed gastric emptying.

The most common causes of gastroparesis are idiopathic, diabetes, postsurgical, post-viral, and iatrogenic (related to medication), as shown in Table 2.1. A single-center report has demonstrated that ~36% of 146 consecutive patients with gastroparesis were idiopathic, 29% were diabetic, and 13% developed symptoms after gastric surgery [4].

TABLE 2.1 Gastroparesis etiologies with associated mechanisms

Mechanism	Common causes	Uncommon causes
Idiopathic	Idiopathic	
Extrinsic neuropathy	Postsurgical (surgery for peptic ulcer disease and fundoplication), diabetes mellitus	Multiple sclerosis, brainstem stroke or tumor, amyloid neuropathy, AIDS, Parkinsonism, paraneoplastic syndrome
Intrinsic neuropathy	Diabetes mellitus	Paraneoplastic syndrome (most commonly seen with small-cell lung cancer)
Infectious	Post-viral (EBV, CMV, Norwalk, rotavirus, VZV)	
Medications	Clonidine Tricyclic antidepressants Calcium channel blockers Dopamine agonists Muscarinic cholinergic receptor Antagonists Octreotide GLP-1 agonists (liraglutide or exenatide) Cyclosporine Narcotics	
Myopathy		Scleroderma (typically has clinical disease affecting skin, lungs, and/or esophagus) Polymyositis
Ischemia		Mesenteric ischemia (reversible)

Individuals with type 1 diabetes are more likely to develop gastroparesis compared to those with type 2 diabetes [2, 3]; however, given that the prevalence of type 2 diabetes is much greater than type 1, recent studies (e.g., clinical trials) of patients with gastroparesis have shown almost equal numbers of persons with types 1 and 2 diabetes. Among the diabetic complications of autonomic neuropathy, retinopathy, and nephropathy, it was found that only retinopathy significantly predicted the development of gastroparesis. Additionally, baseline HbA1c, duration of diabetes over 30 years, and average HbA1c were markers that were significant predictors of delayed gastric emptying [5]. Biopsies from the stomach have demonstrated a decrease in ICCs, nitrergic neurons, and CD206 macrophages, particularly among patients with diabetes and gastroparesis [5, 6]. Multiple molecular mechanisms have been proposed as potential causes of delayed gastric emptying, including hyperglycemia, insulin resistance-induced glycation end products, reactive oxygen species, and protein kinase C [7].

Postsurgical gastroparesis results from vagal nerve injury or resection of the antrum, both of which decrease the stomach's ability to triturate and empty solid food. The most common surgeries resulting in postsurgical gastroparesis are fundoplication, Billroth II gastrectomy, and lung or heart transplantation [8]. There are reports of vagal injury following variceal sclerotherapy and botulinum toxin injection for achalasia [9–11]. Rarely, vagal injury may result from radiofrequency ablation of the heart for atrial fibrillation; this injury may be reversible over months [12].

Post-viral gastroparesis is typically preceded by a viral prodrome. Typical viruses include Norwalk virus, rotavirus, cytomegalovirus (CMV), Epstein-Barr virus (EBV), and varicella zoster virus (VZV). Typically, the symptoms resolve within 1 year [13] except when dysautonomia accompanies the viral gastroparesis. Thus, the presence of extraintestinal autonomic dysfunction is associated with a poorer prognosis, especially when it occurs with CMV, EBV, and VZV [14, 15].

Several medications (Table 2.1) can delay gastric emptying. The most common medication classes that can delay gastric emptying are narcotics, which result in increased pylorus contractions and decreased antral contractility, and GLP-1 or amylin agonists or analogs used for the treatment of type 2 diabetes.

Symptoms

Common presenting symptoms of gastroparesis include nausea, vomiting, early satiety, fullness, bloating, weight loss, and abdominal pain (Table 2.2). Population studies have reported that the rates of nausea, vomiting, and dyspepsia among individuals with diabetes are similar to those in community, nondiabetic controls. However, there are higher rates of symptoms in patients with type 1 compared to type 2 diabetes [16], and there was a slightly higher prevalence of upper GI symptoms in patients with diabetes than controls in an Australian population-based study [17].

Few data are available regarding symptoms that are more characteristic of a specific cause of gastroparesis, except for the general principle that patients with idiopathic gastroparesis present more commonly with abdominal pain or discomfort and less vomiting or early satiety as compared to patients with diabetic gastroparesis [18]. Unfortunately, many of the studies that evaluated upper

TABLE 2.2   Common upper gastrointestinal symptoms associated with gastroparesis

Nausea
Vomiting
Abdominal pain
Bloating
Early satiety/fullness
Heartburn

gastrointestinal symptoms (UGI Sx) and gastric emptying were complicated by medication confounders, which included narcotics, tricyclic antidepressants, and anxiolytics [19]. Experienced clinicians have learned the dictum, "If the predominant symptom is pain, think again!" The diagnosis of predominant pain may be central sensitization or functional abdominal pain, the most common etiology being functional dyspepsia.

A recent comprehensive meta-analysis demonstrated significant association of delayed gastric emptying with UGI Sx. Thus, patients who presented with UGI Sx and objectively delayed gastric emptying were more likely to present with nausea, vomiting, bloating, and early satiety/fullness, and were less likely to present with abdominal pain. Moreover, patients with diabetes with delayed gastric emptying were most likely to present with early satiety and fullness [20].

Diagnostic Evaluation

A number of tools are available to diagnose and assess patients with suspected gastroparesis. The validated symptom assessment scales are Patient Assessment of Gastrointestinal Symptoms (PAGI-SYM) and Gastroparesis Cardinal Symptom Index (GCSI) by daily diary [21]. Both assess symptom subgroups such as nausea/vomiting, early satiety/fullness, and bloating. GCSI scores in patients with delayed gastric emptying are higher compared to normal gastric emptying providing validity of the GCSI-DD as a patient-reported outcome [22]. However, these tools are principally used for determining outcomes in clinical trials.

Physical exam can provide key clues to initiate further evaluation of delayed gastric emptying in patients with UGI Sx, for example, Raynaud phenomenon (in patients with systemic sclerosis), or peripheral neuropathy and signs of autonomic dysfunction such as orthostatic hypotension in patients with diabetes. However, none of these are diagnostic for gastroparesis.

Figure 2.1 shows an algorithm for the evaluation of patients with UGI Sx. In addition to abnormal gastric emptying, impaired accommodation and hypersensitivity are commonly encountered and may even occur in combination [23]. Vagal injury can impair gastric accommodation and cause nausea and vomiting. There was a higher prevalence of vomiting in patients with abnormal gastric emptying and gastric accommodation compared to patients with normal and impaired gastric accommodation [23]. Additionally, patients

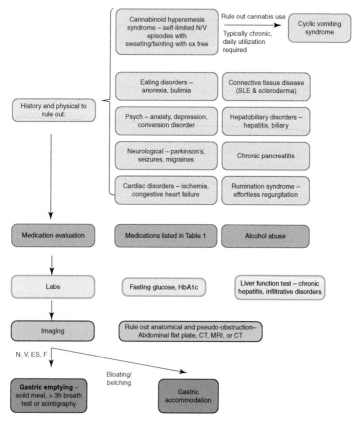

FIGURE 2.1 Proposed diagnostic algorithm for the most common causes of upper gastrointestinal symptoms

with diabetes may present with rapid, normal, or delayed gastric emptying. In one study, 42% of patients with diabetes had normal gastric emptying, 36% delayed gastric emptying, and 22% rapid gastric emptying [24]. Therefore, an accurate gastric emptying test is required to help guide therapy.

Three components of gastric emptying tests need to be carefully assessed before analyzing the results: test modality, meal composition, and duration of the gastric emptying study. Table 2.3 details the diverse gastric emptying methods and their advantages/disadvantages. The gold standard tests are scintigraphy using a radiolabeled solid meal and ^{13}C-spirulina breath tests. The teat meal composition, either solid versus liquid and fat content, significantly alters the rate of gastric emptying, as detailed in Fig. 2.2 for meals of different compositions and caloric contents. Gastric emptying of solids correlates significantly with UGI Sx in contrast to liquid emptying [26]. The higher fat content of a meal represents a greater "burden," and meals with little to no fat (e.g., 2% fat associated with egg-substitute meals) may not effectively assess the ability to empty a typical meal in contrast to meals such as real eggs (30% fat calories).

The duration of gastric emptying tests can range from 1 to 6 h, with the gold standard study length being ≥3 h for both scintigraphy and breath test. There is a high correlation between gastric emptying test results at 3 and 4 h, but the association is not as robust with the result at 2 h. Additionally, there is greater correlation with UGI Sx for the amount emptied at 4 h compared to 1 and 2 h [27].

Treatment

Symptom Management

Dietary adjustments include small, frequent, low-fat, blenderized meals to improve stomach emptying and UGI Sx. The benefit of a small particle meal has been demonstrated in a randomized, controlled trial [28]. A variety of

TABLE 2.3 Gastric emptying tests with respective advantages and disadvantages

Test	Test method	Advantages	Disadvantages
Gastric scintigraphy	Radiolabeled (^{99m}Tc) egg-based meal is ingested and followed through the stomach for >3 h to determine emptying time	Gold standard Direct visualization of gastric emptying Solid meal	Requires gamma camera Radiation exposure
Breath test	Stable carbon isotope ($^{13/14}$C) is placed in the meal. Upon digestion within the duodenum, the radiolabeled carbon is converted to CO_2 and then exhaled and measured in the breath. The rate-limiting step is gastric emptying	No radiation Simple equipment	Cannot be used in patients with severe liver or lung disease
Ultrasound	Gastric emptying is the time it takes for the stomach to return to fasting volume	No radiation Simple equipment	Can only utilize liquid meals Requires skilled technician Requires lower abdominal weight
Magnetic resonance imaging (MRI)	Gastric emptying is the time it takes for the stomach to return to fasting volume	No radiation	Only can utilize liquid meals More expensive Supine position

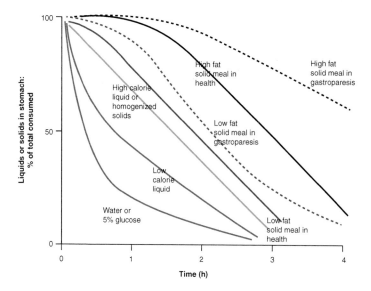

FIGURE 2.2 Pattern of gastric emptying with various types of meals. Starting from the left, liquid meals empty the stomach at a faster rate than solid meals. High-fat or high-nutrient meals take longer to empty from the stomach compared to low-fat or water-based meals. (Reproduced from Camilleri and Shin [25])

antiemetics have been found to be effective in patients with gastroparesis, including phenothiazines, antihistamines (e.g., promethazine), 5-HT$_3$ receptor antagonists (e.g., ondansetron), and neurokinin-1 receptor antagonists (e.g., aprepitant) [29]. Medications such as scopolamine (which has anticholinergic activity) and cannabinoids (which retard gastric emptying) [30] should be avoided as they can exacerbate delay in gastric emptying and nausea/vomiting. Figure 2.3 depicts a proposed treatment algorithm [31].

Prokinetics

The four major classes of medications approved or under development for the treatment of gastroparesis are

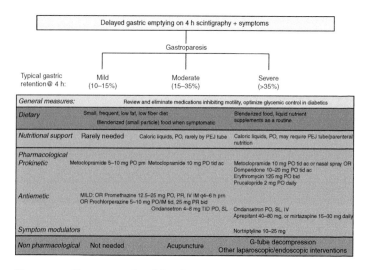

FIGURE 2.3 Treatment algorithm for gastroparesis, including dietary, pharmacological, and non-pharmacological interventions. (Reproduced from Lacy et al. [31])

summarized in Table 2.4. Motilin receptor agonists (off-label) and metoclopramide, a D_2 receptor antagonist (black box warning), are the only prokinetics that are FDA-approved in the United States.

1. Motilin receptor agonists, such as erythromycin and azithromycin, were the most effective prokinetics with improvement in UGI Sx when compared to $5HT_3$ and D_2 antagonists [32]. However, tachyphylaxis occurs within a 14-day period [61], and their greatest use should be for short-duration treatment to control symptoms and prevent hospitalizations.

2. Dopamine-D2 receptor antagonists include metoclopramide and domperidone. Although effective, metoclopramide use can be complicated by reversible involuntary movements and, rarely (<1%), by irreversible tardive dyskinesia [62]. Guidelines recommend starting at the lowest dose (5 mg TID) and titrating up to a maximum dose of 10 mg TID with close follow-up. If no improvement is noted within 12 weeks, metoclopramide should be discontinued [63].

TABLE 2.4 Available prokinetics for treatment of gastroparesis. Included are the patient population on which the medication was tested, doses reported in the literature, effectiveness of improvement of gastric emptying (GE) and upper gastrointestinal symptoms (UGI Sx), and adverse effects

Medications (reference[b])	Patients	Dose/ formulation	% GE improvement from baseline	% UGI Sx improvement from baseline	Adverse effects
Macrolides – motilin receptor agonists					
Erythromycin[a] [32]	GP	40–250 mg TID before meals, liquid	44 ± 11.28%	25%	1. Tachyphylaxis - ↑ doses and duration >4 wks 2. QT prolongation when taking other medication that inhibit CYP3A4
Azithromycin[a] [33]	GP	250–500 mg IV	Similar to erythromycin in increasing antral activity and motility index		1. QT prolongation but less than erythromycin 2. ↓ GI side effects

(continued)

Table 2.4 (continued)

Medications (reference[b])	Patients	Dose/formulation	% GE improvement from baseline	% UGI Sx improvement from baseline	Adverse effects
Dopamine 2 receptor antagonists					
Metoclopramide [34, 35]	**DM GP**	**5–10 mg QID with meals and before bed, liquid**	**20% improvement**	**~50% improvement**	**1. Neurological motor dysfunction, including irreversible tardive dyskinesia**
[36]	DM GP	10 mg intranasal QID with meals and before bed		~40% improvement from baseline in women	1. Dysgeusia 2. Headaches
Domperidone[b] [37–39]	DM GP	10–20 mg TID and at bedtime if necessary	17% improvement compared to controls	65% improvement compared to controls	1. Prolonged QTc → cardiac arrhythmias (>450 ms M, >470 ms F) 2. Hyperprolactinemia

Itopride [40, 41]	DM GP	200 mg TID	None	None	1. Abdominal pain/diarrhea 2. Leukopenia
5HT3 agonists					
Mirtazapine[a] [42, 43]	GP, paraneoplastic GP	15 mg qhs	None	19–29% improvement	10–33% · 1. Somnolence 2. Xerostomia 3. Constipation 4. Agranulocytosis 5. Depression exacerbation
Cisapride [44–48]	GP	10–20 mg QID with meals and before bed	$21.1 \pm 13.3\%$	$50.6 \pm 14.6\%$	1. QTc prolongation $\mapsto$ cardiac arrhythmias and sudden cardiac death 2. Abdominal discomfort/diarrhea
Cinitapride [49]	GP	1 mg TID	None	None	1. Headache (no changes in ECG)

(continued)

TABLE 2.4 (continued)

Medications (reference[b])	Patients	Dose/ formulation	% GE improvement from baseline	% UGI Sx improvement from baseline	Adverse effects
Mosapride [50]	FD	5 mg TID		10% improvement from baseline	1. Abdominal pain 2. Dizziness 3. Headache (no effect on hERG channels)
Revexepride [51]	FD	0.02–0.5 mg TID	None	45–52% improvement from baseline	1. Diarrhea 2. Headache 3. Abdominal pain 4. Nausea
Renzapride [52]	FD	0.5–2.0 mg daily	None		1. Abdominal pain 2. Headache 3. Diarrhea
Ghrelin agonists					
TZP 101 [53, 54]	DM GP	80–600 µg/kg (iv)	~20% improvement from baseline	0–62.7% improvement from baseline	1. Abdominal pain 2. Diarrhea 3. Headache 4. Bradycardia (no changes in ECG)

TZP 102 [55, 56]	DM GP	10–40 mg daily	4–14% improvement from baseline	29–40% improvement from baseline	1. Nausea 2. Vomiting 3. Constipation 4. Hyperglycemia 5. Abdominal pain (no changes in ECG)
Relamorelin[b] [57–60]	DM GP	20–200 mg subQ	3–11%	13–43% improvement	1. GI disorders 2. Diarrhea 3. Hyperglycemia 4. UTI 5. LFT abnormalities 6. DKA

Bolded medications are FDA-approved for the indication of gastroparesis

DKA diabetic ketoacidosis, *DM* diabetes mellitus, *ECG* electrocardiogram, *F* females, *FD* functional dyspepsia, *GP* gastroparesis, *LFT* liver function test, *M* males, *UTI* urinary tract infection

[a]indicates medications that are FDA-approved, but not for gastroparesis

[b]Medications that are currently undergoing further investigational studies for FDA approval

Domperidone has similar efficacy to metoclopramide, but it does not cross the blood-brain barrier or cause the neurological complications seen with metoclopramide. However, there have been reports of prolongation of QTc, arrhythmias, and sudden cardiac death. FDA has not approved this medication but is allowing further investigational studies.

Prokinetics in Development

1. 5-HT$_4$ receptor agonists improve both gastric emptying and UGI Sx. The most effective 5-HT$_4$ agonist to date was cisapride. Unfortunately, earlier 5-HT$_4$ receptor agonists also stimulated the HERG channel in the heart and may be associated with arrhythmias and QTc prolongation leading to torsades de pointes [64]. New molecular entities such as prucalopride are selective 5-HT$_4$ agonists that do not activate the hERG channel [65]. Investigational studies of prucalopride in gastroparesis are being conducted in Canada (ClinicalTrials.gov Identifier: NCT02031081).
2. Ghrelin agonists – Ghrelin is known as the "hunger hormone." Among its many roles, ghrelin accelerates gastric emptying and promotes hunger and increased food intake. A pentapeptide ghrelin agonist, relamorelin, administered by subcutaneous injections, improved gastric emptying and UGI Sx in phase 2A and 2B trials.

Pyloric Interventions

Pyloric interventions aim to remove the resistance to flow by decreasing the pyloric sphincter tone either via botulinum toxin injection or pyloromyotomy, surgical or endoscopic. To date, these studies have been open-label and have demonstrated improvement in both gastric emptying and UGI Sx. Lacy et al. proposed an algorithm for pursuing pyloric interventions which relies on identifying patients who have pylorospasm via antroduodenal manometry or Endoflip® (Crospon Co., Galway, Ireland) (Fig. 2.4). Alternatively, patients responding to pyloric injection of botulinum toxin might be good candidates for peroral or surgical pyloromyotomy [31].

Gastric Electrical Stimulation

Gastric electrical stimulation (GES) involves an implantable device that was initially designed to restore normal electrical activity within the stomach by stimulating normal gastric slow waves. However, this was not found to significantly improve UGI Sx in clinical trials. Stimulation parameters were reprogrammed to induce low-energy, high-frequency waves intended to modulate gastric sensory nerve activity. Open-label studies and only one controlled study have demonstrated significant improvement in UGI Sx [66]. A meta-analysis showed that open-label studies documented significant improvement in total UGI Sx. However, further analysis identified a significant difference in baseline UGI Sx in patients undergoing GES compared to patients receiving medical therapies, indicating that regression to the mean may explain the benefit observed with GES in open-label studies [67].

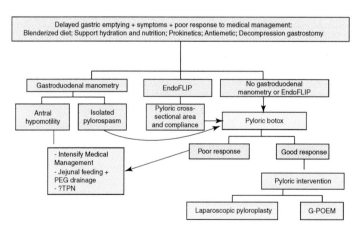

FIGURE 2.4 Proposed algorithm for pyloric interventions for gastroparesis unresponsive to medical treatment. (Reproduced from Lacy et al. [31])

Case Study: Follow-Up

The 4-h gastric emptying scintigraphy test was repeated utilizing a solid meal (320 kcal, 30% fat meal) and demonstrated moderate delay in gastric emptying of solids: 161 min, 2-h retention of 80%, and 4-h retention of 60%. Mrs. G was counseled on dietary changes, including a blenderized, low-fat, low-fiber diet. Since she had developed neurological complications with metoclopramide, that medication was not retried. Mirtazapine, 15 mg/day, was prescribed since it is a good alternative to improve gastric emptying [42], nausea, and vomiting symptom control and increases nutrient tolerance and appetite [68]. Additionally, ondansetron, 4 mg, was introduced as needed to help control nausea.

Clinical Pearls

- Gastroparesis diagnosis requires gastric scintigraphy or breath test conducted over a 4-h period along with a solid meal having sufficient proportion of fat.
- Patients with diabetes may present with rapid, normal, or delayed gastric emptying. Those with delayed gastric emptying present with early satiety and fullness. Accurate diagnosis with scintigraphy or breath test is required before starting any treatment in patients with diabetes who present with UGI Sx.
- Gastroparesis management should include dietary interventions: blenderized foods and low-fat, low-fiber diet.
- Only open-label studies have demonstrated an improvement in UGI Sx with pylorus interventions and gastric electrical stimulation.

Acknowledgment The authors thank Mrs. Cindy Stanislav for excellent secretarial assistance.

Self-Test

Question 1. A 52-year-old male with past medical history significant for medically complicated obesity, type 2 diabetes for 5 years on oral medications and HbA1c 7.4% without any end-organ complications, GERD refractory to oral proton-pump inhibitors, and s/p Nissen fundoplication 2 weeks prior presents with nausea, early satiety, and fullness. He suffered from an upper gastrointestinal viral infection 1 year ago. He managed his symptoms with oral hydration. He did not develop postural orthostasis requiring IV fluid hydration. Four-hour breath test demonstrated moderate gastroparesis. Upon placement of anti-nausea medications and gastroparesis diet, his symptoms significantly improved. What was the most likely etiology for his gastroparesis?

A. Postsurgical
B. Idiopathic
C. Diabetic
D. Viral

Question 2. What is the gold standard test to quantify gastric emptying?

A. Scintigraphy, 2 h, liquid meal
B. Breath test, 4 h, solid meal
C. Ultrasound, 4 h, solid meal
D. MRI, 3 h, liquid meal
E. Wireless motility capsule, 6 h, solid meal

Question 3. Which of the following is the only FDA-approved medication for the treatment of gastroparesis?

A. Cisapride
B. Erythromycin
C. Domperidone
D. Metoclopramide
E. Relamorelin

References

1. Iber FL, Parveen S, Vandrunen M, Sood KB, Reza F, Serlovsky R, et al. Relation of symptoms to impaired stomach, small bowel, and colon motility in long-standing diabetes. Dig Dis Sci. 1993;38(1):45–50.

2. Choung RS, Locke GR 3rd, Schleck CD, Zinsmeister AR, Melton LJ 3rd, Talley NJ. Risk of gastroparesis in subjects with type 1 and 2 diabetes in the general population. Am J Gastroenterol. 2012;107(1):82–8.

3. Jung HK, Choung RS, Locke GR 3rd, Schleck CD, Zinsmeister AR, Szarka LA, et al. The incidence, prevalence, and outcomes of patients with gastroparesis in Olmsted County, Minnesota, from 1996 to 2006. Gastroenterology. 2009;136(4):1225–33.

4. Soykan I, Sivri B, Sarosiek I, Kiernan B, McCallum RW. Demography, clinical characteristics, psychological and abuse profiles, treatment, and long-term follow-up of patients with gastroparesis. Dig Dis Sci. 1998;43(11):2398–404.

5. Bharucha AE, Batey-Schaefer B, Cleary PA, Murray JA, Cowie C, Lorenzi G, et al. Delayed gastric emptying is associated with early and long-term hyperglycemia in type 1 diabetes mellitus. Gastroenterology. 2015;149(2):330–9.

6. Bernard CE, Gibbons SJ, Mann IS, Froschauer L, Parkman HP, Harbison S, et al. Association of low numbers of CD206-positive cells with loss of ICC in the gastric body of patients with diabetic gastroparesis. Neurogastroenterol Motil. 2014;26(9):1275–84.

7. Ördög T, Hayashi Y, Gibbons SJ. Cellular pathogenesis of diabetic gastroenteropathy. Minerva Gastroenterol Dietol. 2009;55(3):315–43.

8. Fich A, Neri M, Camilleri M, Kelly KA, Phillips SF. Stasis syndromes following gastric surgery: clinical and motility features of 60 symptomatic patients. J Clin Gastroenterol. 1990;12(5):505–12.

9. Davion T, Delamarre J, Reix N, Lambert A, Capron JP. Gastric bezoar: another side effect of endoscopic variceal sclerotherapy. Scand J Gastroenterol. 1989;24(7):818–20.

10. Masclee AA, Lamers CB. Effect of endoscopic sclerotherapy of esophageal varices on vagus nerve integrity. J Hepatol. 1994;21(5):724–9.

11. Radaelli F, Paggi S, Terreni N, Toldi A, Terruzzi V. Acute reversible gastroparesis and megaduodenum after botulinum toxin injection for achalasia. Gastrointest Endosc. 2010;71(7):1326–7.

12. Park SY, Camilleri M, Packer D, Monahan K. Upper gastrointestinal complications following ablation therapy for atrial fibrillation. Neurogastroenterol Motil. 2017;29(11):e13109.
13. Naftali T, Yishai R, Zangen T, Levine A. Post-infectious gastroparesis: clinical and electerogastrographic aspects. J Gastroenterol Hepatol. 2007;22(9):1423–8.
14. Vassallo M, Camilleri M, Caron BL, Low PA. Gastrointestinal motor dysfunction in acquired selective cholinergic dysautonomia associated with infectious mononucleosis. Gastroenterology. 1991;100(1):252–8.
15. Lobrano A, Blanchard K, Abell TL, Minocha A, Boone W, Wyatt-Ashmead J, et al. Postinfectious gastroparesis related to autonomic failure: a case report. Neurogastroenterol Motil. 2006;18(2):162–7.
16. Maleki D, Locke GR 3rd, Camilleri M, Zinsmeister AR, Yawn BP, Leibson C, et al. Gastrointestinal tract symptoms among persons with diabetes mellitus in the community. Arch Intern Med. 2000;160(18):2808–16.
17. Bytzer P, Talley NJ, Leemon M, Young LJ, Jones MP, Horowitz M. Prevalence of gastrointestinal symptoms associated with diabetes mellitus: a population-based survey of 15,000 adults. Arch Intern Med. 2001;161(16):1989–96.
18. Parkman HP, Yates K, Hasler WL, Nguyen L, Pasricha PJ, Snape WJ, et al. Similarities and differences between diabetic and idiopathic gastroparesis. Clin Gastroenterol Hepatol. 2011;9(12):1056–64. quiz e133-4
19. Pasricha PJ, Colvin R, Yates K, Hasler WL, Abell TL, Unalp-Arida A, et al. Characteristics of patients with chronic unexplained nausea and vomiting and normal gastric emptying. Clin Gastroenterol Hepatol. 2011;9(7):567–76.e1-4.
20. Vijayvargiya P, Jameie-Oskooei S, Camilleri M, Chedid V, Erwin P, Murad M. Association between delayed gastric emptying and upper gastrointestinal symptoms: a systematic review and meta-analysis. Gut. 2018;in press.
21. Revicki DA, Camilleri M, Kuo B, Norton NJ, Murray L, Palsgrove A, et al. Development and content validity of a gastroparesis cardinal symptom index daily diary. Aliment Pharmacol Ther. 2009;30(6):670–80.
22. Khayyam U, Sachdeva P, Gomez J, Ramzan Z, Smith MS, Maurer AH, et al. Assessment of symptoms during gastric emptying scintigraphy to correlate symptoms to delayed gastric emptying. Neurogastroenterol Motil. 2010;22(5):539–45.

23. Park SY, Acosta A, Camilleri M, Burton D, Harmsen WS, Fox J, et al. Gastric motor dysfunction in patients with functional gastro-duodenal symptoms. Am J Gastroenterol. 2017;112(11):1689–99.

24. Bharucha AE, Camilleri M, Forstrom LA, Zinsmeister AR. Relationship between clinical features and gastric emptying disturbances in diabetes mellitus. Clin Endocrinol. 2009;70(3):415–20.

25. Camilleri M, Shin A. Novel and validated approaches for gastric emptying scintigraphy in patients with suspected gastroparesis. Dig Dis Sci. 2013;58(7):1813–5.

26. Sachdeva P, Malhotra N, Pathikonda M, Khayyam U, Fisher RS, Maurer AH, et al. Gastric emptying of solids and liquids for evaluation for gastroparesis. Dig Dis Sci. 2011;56(4):1138–46.

27. Pathikonda M, Sachdeva P, Malhotra N, Fisher RS, Maurer AH, Parkman HP. Gastric emptying scintigraphy: is four hours necessary? J Clin Gastroenterol. 2012;46(3):209–15.

28. Olausson EA, Storsrud S, Grundin H, Isaksson M, Attvall S, Simren M. A small particle size diet reduces upper gastrointesti-nal symptoms in patients with diabetic gastroparesis: a random-ized controlled trial. Am J Gastroenterol. 2014;109(3):375–85.

29. Pasricha PJ, Yates KP, Sarosiek I, McCallum RW, Abell TL, Koch KL, et al. Aprepitant has mixed effects on nausea and reduces other symptoms in patients with gastroparesis and related disor-ders. Gastroenterology. 2018;154(1):65–76.e11.

30. Esfandyari T, Camilleri M, Ferber I, Burton D, Baxter K, Zinsmeister AR. Effect of a cannabinoid agonist on gastrointes-tinal transit and postprandial satiation in healthy human subjects: a randomized, placebo-controlled study. Neurogastroenterol Motil. 2006;18(9):831–8.

31. Lacy BE, Parkman HP, Camilleri M. Chronic nausea and vomiting: evaluation and treatment. Am J Gastroenterol. 2018;113(5):647–59.

32. Sturm A, Holtmann G, Goebell H, Gerken G. Prokinetics in patients with gastroparesis: a systematic analysis. Digestion. 1999;60(5):422–7.

33. Moshiree B, McDonald R, Hou W, Toskes PP. Comparison of the effect of azithromycin versus erythromycin on antroduodenal pressure profiles of patients with chronic functional gastrointes-tinal pain and gastroparesis. Dig Dis Sci. 2010;55(3):675–83.

34. McCallum RW, Ricci DA, Rakatansky H, Behar J, Rhodes JB, Salen G, et al. A multicenter placebo-controlled clinical trial of

oral metoclopramide in diabetic gastroparesis. Diabetes Care. 1983;6(5):463–7.

35. Ricci DA, Saltzman MB, Meyer C, Callachan C, McCallum RW. Effect of metoclopramide in diabetic gastroparesis. J Clin Gastroenterol. 1985;7(1):25–32.

36. Parkman HP, Carlson MR, Gonyer D. Metoclopramide nasal spray reduces symptoms of gastroparesis in women, but not men, with diabetes: results of a phase 2B randomized study. Clin Gastroenterol Hepatol. 2015;13(7):1256-63.e1.

37. Sahamoto Y, Kato S, Sehino Y, Sakai E, Uchiyama T, Iida H, et al. Effects of Domperidone on gastric emptying: a crossover study using a continuous real-time C-13 breath test (BreathID system). Hepato-Gastroenterology. 2011;58(106):637–41.

38. Heer M, Muller-Duysing W, Benes I, Weitzel M, Pirovino M, Altorfer J, et al. Diabetic gastroparesis: treatment with domperidone--a double-blind, placebo-controlled trial. Digestion. 1983;27(4):214–7.

39. Horowitz M, Harding PE, Chatterton BE, Collins PJ, Shearman DJ. Acute and chronic effects of domperidone on gastric emptying in diabetic autonomic neuropathy. Dig Dis Sci. 1985;30(1):1–9.

40. Stevens JE, Russo A, Maddox AF, Rayner CK, Phillips L, Talley NJ, et al. Effect of itopride on gastric emptying in longstanding diabetes mellitus. Neurogastroenterol Motil. 2008;20(5):456–63.

41. Venkatesh V, Kulkarni KP. Itopride and pantoprazole outcomes in diabetic gastroparesis trial (IPOD trial). J Indian Med Assoc. 2008;106(12):814–5.

42. Kumar N, Barai S, Gambhir S, Rastogi N. Effect of mirtazapine on gastric emptying in patients with cancer-associated anorexia. Indian J Palliat Care. 2017;23(3):335–7.

43. Malamood M, Roberts A, Kataria R, Parkman HP, Schey R. Mirtazapine for symptom control in refractory gastroparesis. Drug Des Devel Ther. 2017;11:1035–41.

44. Lehmann R, Honegger RA, Feinle C, Fried M, Spinas GA, Schwizer W. Glucose control is not improved by accelerating gastric emptying in patients with type 1 diabetes mellitus and gastroparesis. A pilot study with cisapride as a model drug. Exp Clin Endocrinol Diabetes. 2003;111(5):255–61.

45. Braden B, Enghofer M, Schaub M, Usadel KH, Caspary WF, Lembcke B. Long-term cisapride treatment improves diabetic gastroparesis but not glycaemic control. Aliment Pharmacol Ther. 2002;16(7):1341–6.

46. Borovicka J, Lehmann R, Kunz P, Fraser R, Kreiss C, Crelier G, et al. Evaluation of gastric emptying and motility in diabetic gastroparesis with magnetic resonance imaging: effects of cisapride. Am J Gastroenterol. 1999;94(10):2866–73.

47. Camilleri M, Malagelada JR, Abell TL, Brown ML, Hench V, Zinsmeister AR. Effect of six weeks of treatment with cisapride in gastroparesis and intestinal pseudoobstruction. Gastroenterology. 1989;96(3):704–12.

48. Isobe H, Sakai H, Nawata H. Effects of CISAPRIDE on gastric-emptying and gastrointestinal symptoms in patients with liver-cirrhosis - a pilot-study. Curr Ther Res Clin Exp. 1995;56(2):129–33.

49. Portincasa P, Mearin F, Robert M, Plazas MJ, Mas M, Heras J. Efficacy and tolerability of cinitapride in the treatment of functional dyspepsia and delayed gastric emptying. Gastroenterol Hepatol. 2009;32(10):669–76.

50. Hongo M, Harasawa S, Mine T, Sasaki I, Matsueda K, Kusano M, et al. Large-scale randomized clinical study on functional dyspepsia treatment with mosapride or teprenone: Japan Mosapride mega-study (JMMS). J Gastroenterol Hepatol. 2012;27(1):62–8.

51. Tack J, Rotondo A, Meulemans A, Thielemans L, Cools M. Randomized clinical trial: a controlled pilot trial of the 5-HT4 receptor agonist revexepride in patients with symptoms suggestive of gastroparesis. Neurogastroenterol Motil. 2016;28(4):487–97.

52. Mackie AD, Ferrington C, Cowan S, Merrick MV, Baird JD, Palmer KR. The effects of renzapride, a novel prokinetic agent, in diabetic gastroparesis. Aliment Pharmacol Ther. 1991;5(2):135–42.

53. Ejskjaer N, Dimcevski G, Wo J, Hellstrom PM, Gormsen LC, Sarosiek I, et al. Safety and efficacy of ghrelin agonist TZP-101 in relieving symptoms in patients with diabetic gastroparesis: a randomized, placebo-controlled study. Neurogastroenterol Motil. 2010;22(10):1069–e281.

54. Ejskjaer N, Vestergaard ET, Hellstrom PM, Gormsen LC, Madsbad S, Madsen JL, et al. Ghrelin receptor agonist (TZP-101) accelerates gastric emptying in adults with diabetes and symptomatic gastroparesis. Aliment Pharmacol Ther. 2009;29(11):1179–87.

55. McCallum RW, Lembo A, Esfandyari T, Bhandari BR, Ejskjaer N, Cosentino C, et al. Phase 2b, randomized, double-blind 12-week

studies of TZP-102, a ghrelin receptor agonist for diabetic gastroparesis. Neurogastroenterol Motil. 2013;25(11):e705–17.

56. Ejskjaer N, Wo JM, Esfandyari T, Mazen Jamal M, Dimcevski G, Tarnow L, et al. A phase 2a, randomized, double-blind 28-day study of TZP-102 a ghrelin receptor agonist for diabetic gastroparesis. Neurogastroenterol Motil. 2013;25(2):e140–50.

57. Camilleri M, McCallum RW, Tack J, Spence SC, Gottesdiener K, Fiedorek FT. Relamorelin in patients with diabetic gastroparesis: efficacy and safety results from a phase 2b randomised, double-blind, placebo controlled, 12-week study (RM-131-009). United European Gastroenterol J. 2017;5(5 Supplement 1):A55–A6.

58. Shin A, Camilleri M, Busciglio I, Burton D, Smith SA, Vella A, et al. The ghrelin agonist RM-131 accelerates gastric emptying of solids and reduces symptoms in patients with type 1 diabetes mellitus. Clin Gastroenterol Hepatol. 2013;11(11):1453–9.e4.

59. Shin A, Camilleri M, Busciglio I, Burton D, Stoner E, Noonan P, et al. Randomized controlled phase Ib study of ghrelin agonist, RM-131, in type 2 diabetic women with delayed gastric emptying: pharmacokinetics and pharmacodynamics. Diabetes Care. 2013;36(1):41–8.

60. Lembo A, Camilleri M, McCallum R, Sastre R, Breton C, Spence S, et al. Relamorelin reduces vomiting frequency and severity and accelerates gastric emptying in adults with diabetic gastroparesis. Gastroenterology. 2016;151(1):87–96.e6.

61. Thielemans L, Depoortere I, Perret J, Robberecht P, Liu Y, Thijs T, et al. Desensitization of the human motilin receptor by motilides. J Pharmacol Exp Ther. 2005;313(3):1397–405.

62. Rao AS, Camilleri M. Review article: metoclopramide and tardive dyskinesia. Aliment Pharmacol Ther. 2010;31(1):11–9.

63. Camilleri M, Parkman HP, Shafi MA, Abell TL, Gerson L. Clinical guideline: management of gastroparesis. Am J Gastroenterol. 2013;108(1):18–37. quiz 8.

64. Giudicessi JR, Ackerman MJ, Camilleri M. Cardiovascular safety of prokinetic agents: a focus on drug-induced arrhythmias. Neurogastroenterol Motil. 2018;30:e13302.

65. De Maeyer JH, Lefebvre RA, Schuurkes JA. 5-HT4 receptor agonists: similar but not the same. Neurogastroenterol Motil. 2008;20(2):99–112.

66. O'Grady G, Egbuji JU, Du P, Cheng LK, Pullan AJ, Windsor JA. High-frequency gastric electrical stimulation for the treatment of gastroparesis: a meta-analysis. World J Surg. 2009;33(8):1693–701.

67. Levinthal DJ, Bielefeldt K. Systematic review and meta-analysis: gastric electrical stimulation for gastroparesis. Auton Neurosci. 2017;202:45–55.
68. Carbone F, Vanuytsel T, Tack J. The effect of mirtazapine on gastric accommodation, gastric sensitivity to distention, and nutrient tolerance in healthy subjects. Neurogastroenterol Motil. 2017;29(12)

Essential Reading

Camilleri M, Parkman HP, Shafi MA, Abell TL, Gerson L. American College of Gastroenterology. Clinical guideline: management of gastroparesis. Am J Gastroenterol. 2013;108:18–37.
Lacy BE, Parkman HP, Camilleri M. Chronic nausea and vomiting: evaluation and treatment. Am J Gastroenterol. 2018; https://doi.org/10.1038/s41395-018-0039-2. [Epub ahead of print].
Camilleri M. Novel diet, drugs, and gastric interventions for gastroparesis. Clin Gastroenterol Hepatol. 2016;14:1072–80.
Vijayvargiya P, Jameie-Oskooei S, Camilleri M, et al. Association between delayed gastric emptying and upper gastrointestinal symptoms: a systematic review and meta-analysis. Gut. 2018, in press.

Chapter 3
Nausea and Vomiting of Pregnancy and Postoperative Nausea and Vomiting

Ted Walker and Gregory S. Sayuk

Case Study 1

A 26-year-old G1P0 female with no significant past medical history presents to the office for a well woman exam at 8-weeks' gestation. She complains of a 1-week history of daily nausea with occasional non-bloody, non-bilious emesis. Her symptoms usually are worse during the morning but are present throughout the day. She has been avoiding exposures

T. Walker
Division of Gastroenterology, Washington University School of Medicine, St. Louis, MO, USA
e-mail: twalker24@wustl.edu

G. S. Sayuk (✉)
Division of Gastroenterology, Washington University School of Medicine, St. Louis, MO, USA

Department of Psychiatry, Washington University School of Medicine, St. Louis, MO, USA

Gastroenterology Section, St. Louis Veterans Affairs Medical Center, St. Louis, MO, USA
e-mail: gsayuk@wustl.edu

© Springer Nature Switzerland AG 2019   51
B. E. Lacy et al. (eds.), *Essential Medical Disorders of the Stomach and Small Intestine*,
https://doi.org/10.1007/978-3-030-01117-8_3

which exacerbate her symptoms, such as greasy or spicy foods and strong odors. She is not on any prescription medications but continues to take a daily prenatal vitamin she started prior to becoming pregnant. She also initiated over-the-counter vitamin B6 after a friend recommended it as helpful for nausea.

Case Study 2

A 45-year-old female with a past medical history of obesity, type 2 diabetes mellitus, hypertension, and migraine head-aches is recovering in the postanesthesia care unit (PACU) after a laparoscopic cholecystectomy. Her cholecystectomy was performed without difficulty, and there were no reported complications. Twelve hours following her surgery, she devel-ops the acute onset of nausea and reports two episodes of non-bloody, non-bilious emesis. She is unable to tolerate oral intake. Her preoperative labs including a complete blood count, metabolic panel, and coagulation studies all were within normal limits. She is currently hemodynamically stable and afebrile.

Objectives

1. Describe the etiology, pathophysiology, and risk factors of nausea and vomiting in pregnancy.
2. Describe the differential diagnosis and exam findings of nausea and vomiting in pregnancy.
3. Discuss strategies and treatment options for nausea and vomiting of pregnancy.
4. Understand the etiology, pathophysiology, and risk factors for postoperative nausea and vomiting.
5. Develop prophylactic strategies and treatment plans for postoperative nausea and vomiting based on a recognition of modifiable risk factors.

Nausea and Vomiting of Pregnancy

Epidemiology

Nausea and vomiting of pregnancy is very common, with nausea affecting between 50% and 80% and vomiting affecting up to 50% of pregnant women; 15–81% of affected women experience recurrent symptoms in subsequent pregnancies [1]. Symptoms of nausea and vomiting usually begin early in pregnancy, between 6 and 8 weeks' gestation, with symptoms peaking before the end of the first trimester and resolving by 20 weeks [2].

Symptoms can range from mild and self-limiting to severe and profoundly debilitating. Hyperemesis gravidarum (HG) represents the most severe form, occurring in 0.3–3% of pregnancies [3]. Hyperemesis gravidarum is characterized by intractable vomiting, dehydration, electrolyte imbalances, ketosis, and weight loss. While milder cases of nausea and vomiting in pregnancy infrequently are associated with miscarriage, more severe forms can have a significant effect on both the mother and fetus; HG can be associated with preterm delivery, low birth weights, and fetal loss [1]. Other complications of severe and prolonged symptoms are rarer but can include splenic avulsion, esophageal rupture, pneumothorax, and acute tubular necrosis [4]. Even in milder cases, women who suffer from nausea and vomiting of pregnancy report lower quality of life, particularly if symptoms impact work capacity, household activities, and interactions with their other children [3].

Etiology/Pathophysiology

The etiology of nausea and vomiting in pregnancy is not fully understood but is believed to be related to genetic and hormonal factors [3]. A hereditary role to the development of HG is supported by several observations: (1) HG is more likely to occur in siblings of affected women. (2) Symptom concordance has been demonstrated among monozygotic twins. (3) HG occurs in secondary pregnancies in 15.2% of women who experienced symptoms in prior pregnancy compared to 0.7% of women who did not. (4) HG is increased threefold in daughters of women with a history of HG during pregnancy [5].

The role of endocrine factors is supported by observations that higher levels of human chorionic gonadotropin (HCG) and estradiol are associated with nausea and vomiting and HG. The placental hormone HCG is thought to function as an emetogenic stimulus, with peak HCG levels correlating with symptoms of nausea and vomiting. Higher levels of HCG also are found in pregnant women with HG [3]. Further, nausea and vomiting of pregnancy and HG are more common in advanced molar gestation and multiple gestations [6].

Multiple risk factors have been linked to the development of nausea and vomiting of pregnancy including a history of motion sickness, migraines, gastroesophageal reflux, sensitivity to estrogen therapy, family history, and prior self-history of symptoms [6]. Women with *Helicobacter pylori* infection are three times more likely to have nausea and vomiting of pregnancy than uninfected women [7]. Female gender of the fetus has also been reported to be associated with more severe symptoms. Tobacco may be protective against symptoms, as smoking is related with lower levels of both HCG and estradiol.

Diagnosis

Nausea and vomiting of pregnancy remains a diagnosis of exclusion. It is important to consider the timing of onset of symptoms when making the diagnosis. Symptoms typically arise early in pregnancy, between 6 and 8 weeks' gestation. In cases of symptom onset beyond 9 weeks, an alternative diagnosis should be considered. Although there are no established criteria for the diagnosis of HG, it is usually characterized by persistent vomiting, often with objective data of starvation (ketonuria), weight loss (5% of prepregnancy weight), and electrolyte or liver chemistry abnormalities [1].

The physical examination of women with nausea and vomiting of pregnancy should be largely benign. Exam findings that point to an alternative diagnosis include significant abdominal pain or tenderness, suprapubic tenderness, peritoneal signs, abdominal distension, or neurological abnormalities, including nystagmus. In the presence of these findings, or with severe and persistent symptoms, it is important to exclude other causes of nausea and vomiting. Several other gastrointestinal disorders, urinary tract infections, metabolic and endocrine disorders, medication or drug effects, psychological disorders, and pregnancy-related conditions such as molar pregnancy should be considered in the differential diagnosis of nausea and vomiting of pregnancy (see Table 3.1) [3].

Mild nausea and vomiting of pregnancy may not require further laboratory testing or imaging. In HG, laboratory testing may reveal elevated liver enzymes (<300 U/L), elevated

TABLE 3.1 Differential diagnosis of hyperemesis gravidarum

Gastrointestinal conditions
Gastroenteritis
Gastroparesis
Achalasia
Biliary tract disease
Hepatitis
Intestinal obstruction
Peptic ulcer disease
Pancreatitis
Appendicitis
Conditions of the genitourinary tract

(continued)

TABLE 3.1 (continued)

Pyelonephritis

Uremia

Ovarian torsion

Kidney stones

Degenerating uterine leiomyoma

Metabolic conditions

Diabetic ketoacidosis

Porphyria

Addison's disease

Hyperthyroidism

Hyperparathyroidism

Neurologic disorders

Pseudotumor cerebri

Vestibular lesions

Migraine headaches

Tumors of the central nervous system

Lymphocytic hypophysitis

Miscellaneous conditions

Drug toxicity or intolerance

Psychologic conditions

Pregnancy-related conditions

Acute fatty liver of pregnancy

Preeclampsia

Reprinted from Goodwin [6], with permission from Elsevier

bilirubin (< 4 mg/dL), or a mild increase in amylase and lipase (<5 times upper limit of normal). In patients where an alternative diagnosis is suspected, the diagnostic testing should be conducted based on clinical history and exam findings. A pelvic ultrasound can be obtained to rule out pregnancy-associated conditions such as molar pregnancy or multiple gestations.

Treatment

Approaches to the management of nausea and vomiting of pregnancy should take into account the severity of symptoms, impact on the patient's well-being, and the potential effect of treatment on both the patient and the fetus. An essential aspect of treatment focuses on the prevention of symptoms. Some evidence suggests that treatment of symptoms early in the course may successfully prevent progression to HG [1]. The American College of Obstetricians and Gynecologists (ACOG) recommends that prenatal vitamins be taken for at least 1 month prior to fertilization, as this approach is associated with a lower incidence of nausea and vomiting and HG, perhaps via optimization of nutrients and/or increased levels of B6 (pyridoxine).

For women with persistent, regular symptoms, the treatment of nausea and vomiting of pregnancy and HG can be separated into three tiers, with treatment escalation based on persistent symptoms (Fig. 3.1) [2]. Common medications, doses, and adverse effects can be found in Table 3.2.

First-Line Therapy

First-line treatments start with lifestyle modifications to prevent symptoms. This includes eating smaller and more frequent meals and avoiding dietary triggers such as spicy, odorous, or fatty foods. Unnecessary medications or supplements, such as iron, should be stopped. Initial therapeutic

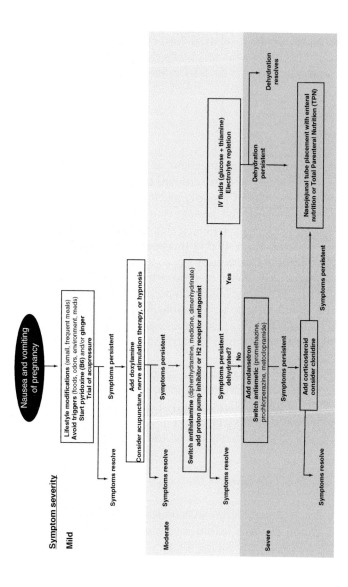

FIGURE 3.1 Treatment algorithm for the management of nausea and vomiting in pregnancy. Therapeutic approaches are tailored based on severity of symptoms. Escalation of therapy is guided by persistence of symptoms and the presence

TABLE 3.2 Common dose and adverse effects for medications used in nausea and vomiting of pregnancy

Medication	Dose	Adverse effects
First line		
Ginger	1–1.5 g divided over 24 h (250 mg four times daily)	Reflux
Vitamin B6 (pyridoxine)	10–25 mg every 6–8 h	Drowsiness, headache, neuropathy, paresthesia, ataxia
Second line		
Combination antihistamine/ vitamin B6 (doxylamine/ pyridoxine)	10 mg/10 mg. Initially two tablets at bedtime (maximum 4 tablets daily)	Drowsiness, dizziness, headache, dry mucous membranes, urinary retention
Metoclopramide	10 mg four times daily	Drowsiness, dystonic reaction, restlessness, fatigue, headache, dizziness
Prochlorperazine	5–10 mg four times daily 25 mg rectal suppository twice daily	Sedation, dizziness, rare extrapyramidal or dystonic reaction, QT prolongation
Promethazine	6.25–12.5 mg three times daily 25 mg rectal suppository twice daily	Agitation, sedation, rare QT prolongation, Parkinsonian symptoms
Ondansetron	4–8 mg every 8 h	Headache, fatigue, malaise, constipation

(continued)

TABLE 3.2 (continued)

Medication	Dose	Adverse effects
Third line		
Corticosteroids	Hydrocortisone 100 mg intravenously twice daily Prednisone 40–50 mg daily	Increased risk of infection and increased risk of gestational diabetes

approaches include over-the-counter interventions that do not require a physician prescription, such as ginger, vitamin B6, and acupressure. Ginger is available in several preparations including fresh root, tablets, capsules, and syrup. Several studies have shown improvement in symptoms compared to placebo, and it has also been shown to have similar efficacy to vitamin B6. Vitamin B6 has also demonstrated symptom improvement compared to placebo. There is modest evidence to support the use of acupressure. There has also been interest in using acupuncture, hypnosis, or nerve stimulation therapy. However, evidence for these therapies remains inconclusive.

Second-Line Treatment

For women with persistent symptoms despite lifestyle modifications and over-the-counter therapy, the next step involves antiemetic medications. There are multiple options that have proved efficacious. These include the combination of antihistamines, vitamin B6, dopamine antagonists, and serotonin receptor antagonists. Symptoms of dyspepsia can also be treated with histamine type-2 receptor antagonists or a proton pump inhibitor (PPI). Antihistamines are the most widely used medication, and the ACOG recommends that the combination of vitamin B6 and doxylamine be used first line given its efficacy and low-risk profile. This combination has demonstrated improvement in symptoms compared to placebo. It is more effective when used as a preventative measure rather than after onset of symptoms. Dopamine antagonists such as metoclopramide have also been shown to improve symptoms compared to placebo. The serotonin receptor antagonist (5-HT$_3$) ondansetron is effective in all stages of nausea and vomiting in pregnancy and HG and is often used. There is insufficient data to assess fetal safety of this medication. A few studies have demonstrated an increased incidence of cleft palate associated with ondansetron use, and women should be counseled on its use prior to 10 weeks of gestation.

Third-Line Treatment

When women have severe and persistent symptoms despite the use of antiemetic medications, then third-line treatment must be considered. It is important to monitor for signs of dehydration and lab abnormalities. Women in this category typically require inpatient admission for treatment with intravenous (i.v.) medications and fluid resuscitation. Studies have shown that fluids containing dextrose may be more efficacious compared to normal saline. Caution should be used when giving dextrose, with thiamine given beforehand, to prevent the complication of Wernicke's encephalopathy. Although there is no rigorous data, corticosteroids can be considered for severe and persistent symptoms. Studies have shown greater efficacy compared to promethazine and metoclopramide and have also shown it to be beneficial in HG. However, the use of corticosteroids has been associated with oral clefts, and its use should be avoided in the first 10 weeks of gestation. The benefit of this therapy must be weighed against the risk of adverse effect associated with steroids. Transdermal clonidine patch has also been studied in this setting; however, evidence for its effectiveness is lacking.

Apart from i.v. fluids and medications, it is important to maintain adequate nutrition in patients with persistent symptoms. For women that cannot tolerate oral intake and/or are losing weight, enteral tube feeding should be pursued. This requires placement of a nasojejunal tube. For women who cannot tolerate enteral feeding, total parenteral nutrition (TPN) should be initiated. However, TPN should be regarded as a last resort as peripherally inserted central catheters can be associated with considerable infectious and metabolic complications.

Postoperative Nausea and Vomiting

Epidemiology

Nausea and vomiting is frequently associated with recovery from anesthesia. Symptoms are distressing to patients and negatively impact quality of life. Postoperative nausea and vomiting (PONV) refers to nausea and vomiting that occur during the first 24–48 h following surgery. The prevalence of PONV is estimated to be between 11% and 73% but may be as high as 80% in higher-risk individuals [8]. Although PONV uniformly resolves, and thus can be treated without long-term sequela, its development leads to prolonged recovery time, unanticipated hospital admissions, and increased health-care costs [9].

Pathophysiology

The pathophysiology of PONV is multifactorial and believed to be related to activation of multiple receptors linked to nausea and emesis including the vestibular system, the area postrema, and the nucleus tractus solitarius [10]. Numerous ion channels and neurotransmitters have been associated with nausea and vomiting symptoms, including the gamma-aminobutyric acid (GABA), N-methyl-D-aspartic acid (NMDA), opioid, acetylcholine, dopamine D2, and 5-hydroxytryptamine (5-HT_3) receptors. Treatment of nausea and vomiting generally modulates these neurotransmitters.

Opioids are thought to induce nausea and emesis through action on the μ-opioid receptors in the area postrema and chemoreceptor trigger zone, as well as stimulation of the vestibulocochlear apparatus. Inhaled anesthetics interact with multiple ion channels such as GABA, NMDA, and acetylcholine in the CNS. Apart from the central effect of opioids and anesthetics, the peripheral effects of gastric dysrhythmia following surgery also lead to worsening symptoms.

Etiology

There are several known risk factors that lead to increased incidence of PONV. These factors are divided into patient, anesthesia, and surgical factors (Table 3.3a). Patient factors include female sex, prior history of PONV, nonsmoking status, history of motion sickness, and younger age (<50 years old) [9]. Women are three times as likely to experience PONV compared to men, and younger patients are two times more likely than older patients to experience PONV symptoms. The anesthesia factors that increase risk of PONV include the use of volatile anesthesia, longer duration of general anesthesia, postoperative opioid use, and the use of nitrous oxide. Lastly, particular surgical procedures including cholecystectomy, gynecological surgery, or laparoscopic surgery have all been associated with increased incidence of PONV compared to other types of procedures.

Diagnosis

The diagnosis of PONV is made in any patient who experiences acute onset of nausea and emesis during recovery from anesthesia. It is important to assess the patient risk of PONV prior to surgery as this can help guide medical management and prophylactic therapy. A commonly used tool to assess risk factor is the Apfel simplified risk score [11]. This score is calculated using four variables: female sex, history of PONV,

Table 3.3 (**a**) Risk factors associated with increased risk for PONV divided into patient, anesthesia, and surgical factors. (**b**) Apfel simplified risk score. The risk of developing PONV by number of risk factors

(**a**) *Patient factors*
Female sex
History of PONV
Nonsmoking status
History of motion sickness
Young age (<50)
Anesthesia factors
Volatile anesthesia
General anesthesia
Postoperative opioid use
Nitrous oxide
Surgical procedure
Cholecystectomy
Gynecological
Laparoscopic (abdominal)

(**b**) Apfel simplified risk score

Variables[a]	Risk of PONV %
0	10
1	20
2	40
3	60
4	80

Abbreviations: *PONV* postoperative nausea and vomiting
[a]Variables included in the Apfel risk score include: female sex, history of PONV, nonsmoking status, and the use of postoperative opioids

nonsmoking status, and use of postoperative opioids. The incidence of PONV was found to increase with each additional variable such that the risk of PONV with 0, 1, 2, 3, and 4 variables was 10%, 20%, 40%, 60%, and 80%, respectively. Patients can be categorized into low (0–1), medium (2–3), or high (4) risk based on the number of risk factors (Table 3.3b).

Treatment

The general principles of treatment for PONV include minimization of risk factors, prophylactic medication based on risk assessment, and rescue therapy for persistent symptoms (Fig. 3.2). Minimizing risk factors involves the choice of anesthetic, appropriate pain control, and adequate hydration. Using regional anesthesia, when appropriate, can significantly reduce the risk of developing PONV ninefold compared to the use of general anesthesia. Avoiding volatile anesthetics and nitrous oxide thus is key to reducing the risk for PONV. Total intravenous anesthesia (TIVA) with propofol also is associated with a lower incidence of PONV compared to volatile anesthetics [12]. Because opioids are associated with increased risk of PONV, managing postoperative pain with nonsteroidal anti-inflammatory medications such as NSAIDs or COX-2 inhibitors can lead to further reduction in PONV risk. Lastly, maintaining adequate hydration can lower the incidence of PONV. Studies have not demonstrated major differences in crystalloid vs. colloid solutions. However, studies have suggested that perioperative and postoperative use of dextrose-containing solutions can reduce the incidence of PONV and decrease the need for rescue antiemetics, when compared to normal saline [13].

Numerous classes of medication are available for prophylaxis and rescue therapy of PONV [9, 10]. For dosing guidelines, please refer to the supplementary table (Table 3.4). In general, each drug class is relatively similar in efficacy when used as a single agent, and combination

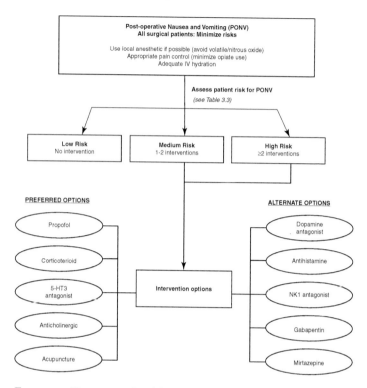

FIGURE 3.2 Treatment algorithm for postoperative nausea and vomiting. The initial treatment is aimed at assessing and minimizing the risk of developing symptoms. Multiple therapeutic options are available for treatment. The amount and type of therapy given should be guided by the level of risk for symptom development

therapy of multiple classes results in an additive effect and reduced incidence of PONV. The risk reduction of PONV for a single, two, and three agents is 20%, 40%, and 60%, respectively [10]. The major classes of medication used for treatment include histamine, dopamine, 5-HT_3, and NK1 receptor antagonists, as well as corticosteroids. Complementary techniques such as acupuncture stimulation (pericardium-6 point) also can be implemented as a prophylactic approach.

TABLE 3.4 Common medications, dose, and adverse effects for postoperative nausea and vomiting

Medication	Dose	Adverse effect
5-HT3 receptor antagonist		
Ondansetron	4 mg IV, 8 mg ODT	Headache, fatigue, malaise, constipation
Granisetron	0.35–3 mg IV	Headache, asthenia, constipation, fever, elevated LFTs
Palonosetron	0.075 mg IV	Headache, constipation, QT prolongation
Neurokinin-1 receptor antagonists		
Aprepitant	40 mg PO	Neutropenia, fatigue, headache, diarrhea, dyspepsia, abdominal pain
Rolapitant	70–200 mg PO	Anorexia, dizziness, hiccups, dyspepsia
Corticosteroids		
Dexamethasone	4–5 mg IV	Erythema, abdominal discomfort, rash, edema, diaphoresis, headache, elevated glucose
Methylprednisolone	40 mg IV	
Dopamine receptor antagonists		
Droperidol	0.625–1.25 mg IV	QT prolongation, drowsiness, tachycardia, hypotension, dizziness, rigors, dystonia, akathisia
Haloperidol	0.5–2 mg IM/IV	Extrapyramidal symptoms, tardive dyskinesia, akathisia, insomnia, anxiety, drowsiness
Metoclopramide	10 mg IM/IV	Drowsiness, restlessness, anxiety, insomnia, headache, dizziness

(continued)

TABLE 3.4 (continued)

Medication	Dose	Adverse effect
Antihistamine		
Dimenhydrinate	1 mg/kg IV	Drowsiness, dizziness, impaired coordination, headache, dry mucous membranes, urinary retention, hypotension
Meclizine	25–50 mg PO	
Anticholinergic		
Scopolamine	Transdermal patch	Xerostomia, dizziness, drowsiness, somnolence, urinary retention

It is recommended that adults at moderate risk for PONV receive one to two medications for prophylaxis and that two or more prophylactic approaches be used for adults at high risk [9]. When more than one prophylactic agent is implemented, it is recommended that medications from different classes be used to invoke the additive effects of modulating multiple receptor systems. An overview of preferred and alternative prophylactic strategies is provided in Fig. 3.2.

5-Hydroxytryptamine Receptor Antagonists

This class includes the medications ondansetron, granisetron, and palonosetron. Tropisetron and ramosetron have not been approved for use in the United States. This class of medication is a first-line option and is most effective when used as prophylactic medication. Ondansetron and granisetron are administered at the end of surgery. Palonosetron has a longer half-life and can be used prophylactically at the beginning of surgery. This class of medications is generally well tolerated with minimal side effects but may be associated with minor headache. At higher doses, they can also prolong the QTc interval.

Corticosteroids

Dexamethasone and methylprednisolone are used for prevention of PONV and are first-line options used prophylactically prior to surgery. Adverse effects may include elevated blood glucose and an increased risk of wound infection or poor wound healing, although recent studies have demonstrated it to be safe. Caution should be used in patients with poorly controlled type 2 diabetics.

Anticholinergics

Transdermal scopolamine commonly is used to reduce the risk of PONV. However, because of its slow onset of action, it is typically applied the night before or at least 2–3 h prior to surgery. Adverse events associated with this medication are mild but include visual disturbances, dry mouth, and dizziness.

Neurokinin-1 Receptor Antagonists

This class of medications includes aprepitant, casopitant, and rolapitant. Aprepitant is given orally, while casopitant and rolapitant are administered intravenously. The main limitation to the use of these medications is cost.

Dopamine Receptor Antagonists

This class includes droperidol, haloperidol, and metoclopramide. These medications carry a risk of QTc prolongation and arrhythmias and thus should be used with caution for patients with baseline prolonged QTc on EKG. Droperidol and haloperidol can also lead to extrapyramidal symptoms and are contraindicated in patients with Parkinson's disease or restless legs syndrome.

Antihistamines

Dimenhydrinate and meclizine are the drugs typically used from this class for PONV. They not only inhibit the H1 receptor but also possess anticholinergic properties. The major adverse effects include drowsiness, dry mouth, and urinary retention.

Other PONV Treatment Options

Additional medications that have been studied and found to reduce the incidence of PONV include mirtazapine [9], midazolam [11], and gabapentin [13]. Midazolam was associated with a significant reduction in PONV and decreased use of rescue antiemetics. Gabapentin effectively decreases the relative risk of PONV; the main adverse effect was its significantly increased rate of postoperative sedation.

Case Study: Follow-Up

Case 1   The patient was evaluated in the office, where her physical exam revealed some mild abdominal tenderness but was otherwise benign. Given her history of emesis, a urinalysis and basic metabolic panel were obtained, and both were unremarkable. She was diagnosed with nausea and vomiting of pregnancy. Instruction was given on lifestyle modifications including smaller, more frequent meals and avoiding greasy or fried food. She was started on the combination of doxylamine and pyridoxine, initially at bedtime, and then increased to the maximum of four tablets daily. On follow-up call 2 weeks later, her symptoms had significantly improved, and she was instructed to continue with this regimen through the remainder of the first trimester.

Case 2   This patient presented with multiple risk factors for postoperative nausea and vomiting prior to surgery including female sex, age, history of migraine headaches, and her planned surgical procedure (cholecystectomy). Given the multiple risk factors, the patient was treated with i.v. dexamethasone prior to surgery. Her persistent symptoms during postoperative recovery in the PACU led to a diagnosis of postoperative nausea and vomiting. No lab testing was performed. She was treated with IV fluids containing dextrose as well as sublingual ondansetron. With these interventions, her symptoms resolved within 2 h, and her postoperative course was otherwise uneventful.

Clinical Pearls

- Nausea and vomiting of pregnancy usually is diagnosed between 6 and 8 weeks' gestation. Symptoms arising past 9 weeks should prompt investigation of other causes.
- The diagnosis of nausea and vomiting of pregnancy is a clinical one. For mild symptoms without other clinical features of concern, laboratory testing is not necessary.
- Postoperative nausea and vomiting is a common disorder, with the incidence predicted by the number of risk factors manifested by the patient.
- Calculation of risk for postoperative nausea and vomiting allows the provider to appropriately treat with prophylactic medications based on this risk calculation.

Conflicts of Interest   None of the authors have any relevant conflicts of interest to report.

Self-Test Questions

Question 1. Which of the following is *NOT* a risk factor for the development of nausea and vomiting of pregnancy?

A. Symptoms in prior pregnancy
B. Family members who experienced symptoms
C. Tobacco use
D. Female sex of fetus
E. Increased placental mass

Question 2. Which of the following is *NOT* considered a first-line treatment for nausea and vomiting of pregnancy?

A. Prenatal vitamins
B. Ginger
C. Vitamin B6 (pyridoxine)
D. Ondansetron

Question 3. Which of the following increases the risk for post-operative nausea and vomiting?

A. Female sex
B. Tobacco use
C. Age > 50 years
D. Use of local anesthetic

Question 4. Aprepitant has been approved for use in postoperative nausea and vomiting. What is the mechanism of action of aprepitant?

A. 5-hydroxytryptamine receptor antagonists
B. Neurokinin-1 receptor antagonists
C. Dopamine receptor antagonist
D. Antihistamine
E. Anticholinergic

References

1. Committee on Obstetric Practice. ACOG practice bulletin no. 189: nausea and vomiting of pregnancy. Obstet Gynecol. 2018;131(1):e15–30.

2. O'Donnell A, McParlin C, Robson SC, Beyer F, Moloney E, Byant A, et al. Treatments for hyperemesis gravidarum and nausea and vomiting in pregnancy: a systematic review and economic assessment. Health Technol Assess. 2016;20(74):1366–5278.

3. McParlin C, O'Donnell A, Robson SC, et al. Treatments for hyperemesis Gravidarum and nausea and vomiting in pregnancy: a systematic review. JAMA. 2016;316(13):1392–401.

4. Festin M. Nausea and vomiting in early pregnancy. Clin Evid Handbook. 2015;92(6):516–7.

5. Vikanes A, Skjaerven R, Grjibovski AM, Gunnes N, Vangen S, Magnus P. Recurrence of hyperemesis gravidarum across generations: population based cohort study. BMJ. 2010;340:c2050.

6. Goodwin TM. Hyperemesis gravidarum. Obstet Gynecol Clin N Am. 2008;35(3):401–17.

7. Niemeijer MN, Grooten IJ, Vos N, Bais JM, van der Post JA, Mol BW, et al. Diagnostic markers for hyperemesis gravidarum: a systematic review and meta-analysis. Am J Obstet Gynecol. 2014;211(2):150.e1.

8. Quigley EM, Hasler WL, Parkman HP. AGA technical review on nausea and vomiting. Gastroenterology. 2001;120(1):263–86.

9. Gan TJ, Diemunsch P, Habib AS, Kovac A, Kranke P, Meyer TA, Watcha M, Chung F, Angus S, Apfel CC, Bergese SD, Candiotti KA, Chan MT, Davis PJ, Hooper VD, Lagoo-Deenadayalan S, Myles P, Nezat G, Philip BK, Tramer MR. Consensus guidelines for the management of postoperative nausea and vomiting. Anesth Analg. 2014;118:85–113.

10. Wiesmann T, Kranke P, Eberhart L. Postoperative nausea and vomiting – a narrative review of pathophysiology, pharmacotherapy and clinical management strategies. Expert Opin Pharmacother. 2015;16(7):1069–77.

11. Mishra A, Pandey RK, Sharma A, Darlong V, Punj J, Goswami D, Sinha R, Rewari V, Chandralekha C, Bansal VK. Is perioperative administration of 5% dextrose effective in reducing the incidence of PONV in laparoscopic cholecystectomy?: a randomized control trial. J Clin Anesth. 2017;40:7–10.

12. Grant MC, Kim J, Page AJ, Hobson D, Wick E, Wu CL. The effect of intravenous midazolam on postoperative nausea and vomiting: a meta-analysis. Anesth Analg. 2016;122(3):656–63.

13. Grant MC, Lee H, Page AJ, Hobson D, Wick E, Wu CL. The effect of preoperative gabapentin on postoperative nausea and vomiting: a meta-analysis. Anesth Analg. 2016;122(4):976–85.

Essential Reading List

Committee on Obstetric Practice. ACOG practice bulletin no. 189: nausea and vomiting of pregnancy. Obstet Gynecol. 2018;131(1):e15–30. An authoritative overview on diagnosis and treatment of nausea and vomiting of pregnancy

McParlin C, O'Donnell A, Robson SC, et al. Treatments for hyperemesis Gravidarum and nausea and vomiting in pregnancy: a systematic review. JAMA. 2016;316(13):1392–401. An excellent overview of the treatment for nausea and vomiting in pregnancy and hyperemesis gravidarum.

Gan TJ, Diemunsch P, Habib AS, Kovac A, Kranke P, Meyer TA, Watcha M, Chung F, Angus S, Apfel CC, Bergese SD, Candiotti KA, Chan MT, Davis PJ, Hooper VD, Lagoo-Deenadayalan S, Myles P, Nezat G, Philip BK, Tramer MR. Consensus guidelines for the management of postoperative nausea and vomiting. Anesth Analg. 2014;118:85–113. Comprehensive review of the diagnosis and treatment of post-operative nausea and vomiting.

Chapter 4
Cyclic Vomiting Syndrome and Cannabinoid Hyperemesis Syndrome

Michael J. Kingsley and David J. Levinthal

Case Study

A 28-year-old male is referred with a history of six episodes of sudden-onset, severe nausea and forceful vomiting over the last year. The episodes are accompanied by epigastric pain, and he vomits dozens of times per day during a typical 3–4 day episode. The episodes awaken him in the early AM hours with a sensation of warmth, and he experiences diaphoresis prior to the onset of abdominal pain, nausea, and

M. J. Kingsley
Department of Medicine, Division of Gastroenterology, Hepatology, and Nutrition, University of Pittsburgh Medical Center, Pittsburgh, PA, USA

Department of Medicine, VA Pittsburgh Healthcare System, Pittsburgh, PA, USA

D. J. Levinthal (✉)
Department of Medicine, Division of Gastroenterology, Hepatology, and Nutrition, University of Pittsburgh Medical Center, Pittsburgh, PA, USA
e-mail: levinthald@upmc.edu

© Springer Nature Switzerland AG 2019   75
B. E. Lacy et al. (eds.), *Essential Medical Disorders of the Stomach and Small Intestine*,
https://doi.org/10.1007/978-3-030-01117-8_4

vomiting. He is unable to do anything during an episode beyond spending time in bed or near a toilet. He subsequently feels extremely fatigued and depleted after his episodes subside.

The patient presented to the emergency department several times over the past year during an episode. He reports being informed "nothing was wrong" or that he had "a stomach bug," after negative evaluations including two unrevealing CT scans, urinalysis, and bloodwork that only confirmed mild dehydration and a normal EGD. He reported vomiting blood during his most recent episode and subsequently underwent another EGD with only a superficial Mallory-Weiss tear near the gastroesophageal junction; stomach biopsies were negative for *H. pylori*. In the ED, he has received IV fluids, ondansetron, and diphenhydramine with some mitigation of symptoms.

He reports feeling otherwise well between episodes, with a good appetite and no dyspepsia, nausea, or vomiting. Although his weight drops during an episode, he regains the lost weight easily, and his weight is stable overall. His past history is notable for moderate anxiety, allergic rhinitis, and a prior appendectomy. He does not use cannabis. His family history is significant for migraines in his mother. He is stressed about his job and is concerned about missing work on several occasions. He is particularly concerned about the unpredictable nature of these events and relates their negative impact on many aspects of his life.

Objectives

1. Recognize the clinical features of CVS and CHS and their common comorbid conditions.
2. Understand the role of limited evaluation in the diagnostic workup of likely CVS or CHS.
3. Review the treatment options for CVS and CHS, including prophylactic medications, and therapeutic strategies to abort attacks.

Epidemiology

Cyclic vomiting syndrome (CVS) was initially described in adults in 1988 [1] approximately 100 years after its initial description in children [2]. Perhaps due to the longer period of clinical recognition, more is now known about pediatric CVS than adult CVS. For example, the prevalence of CVS among children has been estimated between 0.04% and 3.8% [1, 3, 4], but the prevalence of the disorder among all adults remains unclear. A recent report of adult patients seen in a gastroenterology consultation clinic determined the prevalence of CVS to be as high as 10.8% [5], suggesting that CVS in adults is not as uncommon as previously believed.

An additional factor confounding assessments of the prevalence of CVS in adults is the general lack of recognition of the diagnosis. Indeed, in the work reporting a 10.8% prevalence of CVS in an outpatient gastroenterology clinic (based on recorded symptoms and using standardized criteria to identify cases), only 4% of those identified as CVS patients were ultimately diagnosed with CVS by their specialist [5]. Such a sobering finding is consistent with the fact that most adult CVS patients often suffer for several years before receiving a CVS diagnosis and appropriate treatment [2]. Unfortunately, these patients also commonly have extensive rounds of frequently negative diagnostic testing, in addition to surgeries that fail to relieve symptoms – about 25% of CVS patients may needlessly have undergone cholecystectomy [6].

Etiology/Pathophysiology

The pathophysiology of CVS remains incompletely understood, but a number of potential underlying pathways and predisposing factors have been described. Notably, CVS patients commonly report a number of comorbid conditions, such as a personal or family history of migraines; mood disorders such as anxiety, depression, and panic disorder; high rates of substance abuse; and an increased likelihood of exposure to past or current abuse [6, 7]. Such associations suggest that there could be a neural basis for CVS pathogenesis.

The most commonly recognized comorbidity of patients with CVS is migraine, with as many as 82% of pediatric CVS patients noted to have a personal or family history of migraines [8] and nearly half of adult patients reporting the same. Moreover, CVS shares a characteristic episodic pattern of distinct phases (Fig. 4.1) that is similarly observed in migraines, epilepsy, and panic disorder, further suggesting overlapping pathophysiologic mechanisms [9]. Indeed, each of these disorders shares similar triggers including physiologic and psychological stressors [9], and the risk of developing adult CVS, migraines, epilepsy, and panic disorder are all increased by exposure to prior traumatic or adverse life events. In further support of a potential neurologic basis for CVS, autonomic dysfunction has also been linked to CVS in between 43% and 90% of adult patients [10, 11].

Although strong data are lacking, several studies have supported a potential genetic contribution to CVS, notably in genes linked with mitochondria or mitochondrial function. This association is strongest in children [12, 13], and mitochondrial dysfunction is independently linked with autonomic dysregulation in CVS [2], as well as migraines in adults.

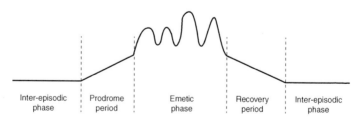

| Inter-episodic phase | Prodrome period | Emetic phase | Recovery period | Inter-episodic phase |

FIGURE 4.1 The four phases of cyclic vomiting syndrome (CVS) and cannabinoid hyperemesis syndrome (CHS)

Interestingly the polymorphisms associated with CVS in children and adult migraine are not strongly linked to adult-onset CVS [13], which suggests that despite a similar phenotype, there are divergent mechanisms for adult and pediatric-onset CVS. For example, polymorphisms in the RYR2 gene, which encodes a stress-induced calcium channel, may contribute to autonomic dysfunction associated with adult CVS [14].

Environmental factors also play an important role in CVS. Early adverse life events and chronic stress may be associated with the autonomic dysfunction in CVS and shape the severity of the disease course [15]. Importantly, marijuana use constitutes an additional environmental factor believed to elicit a CVS-like illness – cannabinoid hyperemesis syndrome (CHS). Whether CHS is a truly distinct disorder from CVS remains a topic of great debate. A significant proportion of patients with a cyclic pattern of vomiting have reported daily or frequent marijuana use [16, 17]. The recent Rome IV criteria for functional GI disorders created CHS as a separately defined entity with a cyclic pattern of vomiting seen in patients who use marijuana regularly. Paradoxically, however, marijuana is also known to acutely reduce nausea and vomiting [1], and many CVS patients use marijuana to abort an attack. Ultimately, there may be significant overlap between CHS and CVS, and the distinction may not be necessary if marijuana is viewed as a dose-dependent trigger for CVS. For example, it has been proposed that chronic, rather than intermittent, cannabinoid use may impact autonomic regulation [15] and secondarily lower the "CVS threshold" needed for a vomiting attack to occur [9] (Fig. 4.2).

Additionally, cannabinoid receptor polymorphisms have been recently described to be associated with CVS [18], and this may explain the differential sensitivity of individuals to cannabis exposures. Much of the underlying pathophysiology of CVS and CHS remains to be elucidated, but the growing body of evidence suggests that a number of distinct factors influence neurally mediated manifestations of nausea and vomiting.

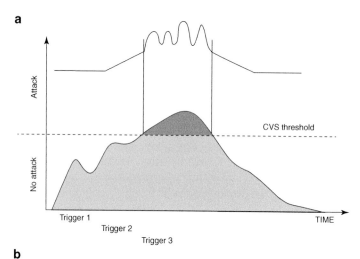

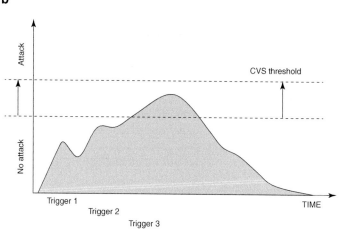

FIGURE 4.2 Graphical illustration of the "CVS threshold" concept. (**a**) Exposure to one or more triggers may elicit a CVS attack. (**b**) The use of prophylactic medications effectively raise the CVS threshold, such that exposure to the same triggers now fails to cross the threshold needed to elicit a CVS attack

Symptoms

CVS is defined by intermittent, repetitive episodes of debilitating nausea and vomiting separated by periods of relative symptom relief, according to Rome IV criteria [19] (Table 4.1). CHS is also defined by Rome IV criteria in those with significant prior cannabis use and subsequent relief from symptoms following a complete cessation of cannabis (Table 4.1). The Rome IV criteria now acknowledge that CVS patients may have milder symptoms between episodes. CVS is difficult to recognize in patients with a coalescent form of the disorder,

TABLE 4.1 The Rome IV criteria for cyclic vomiting syndrome (CVS) and cannabinoid hyperemesis syndrome (CHS)

Cyclic vomiting syndrome (CVS)

Stereotypical episodes of vomiting regarding onset (acute) and duration (less than 1 week)

A. At least three discrete episodes in the prior year and two episodes in the past 6 months, occurring at least 1 week apart

B. Absence of vomiting between episodes, but other milder symptoms can be present between cycles

Supportive remarks: PMH or FH of migraine headaches

Cannabinoid hyperemesis syndrome (CHS)

A. Stereotypical episodic vomiting resembling CVS in terms of onset duration and frequency[a]

B. Presentation after prolonged, excessive cannabis use

C. Relief of vomiting episodes by sustained cannabis cessation

Supportive remarks: May be associated with prolonged hot showers or baths

[a]Criteria must be filled for the last 3 months with symptom onset >6 months before diagnosis

typically associated with narcotic or heavy cannabis use, characterized by attacks of high frequency with essentially no symptom-free days. Yet, even these patients often describe an initial presentation more classic for CVS.

CVS can be divided into four distinct phases (Fig. 4.1). During the inter-episodic phase, patients are often relatively symptom-free. In the prodrome phase (minutes to hours), patients often experience symptoms in early AM hours that herald a CVS attack such as nausea and abdominal pain but also diaphoresis, diarrhea, fatigue, feelings of panic, or photophobia [8, 15]. The emetic phase begins with frequent, violent emesis and uncontrollable retching that may last hours to several days [1]. Some patients exhibit "guzzle-and-vomit" behavior (consuming large volumes of water despite ongoing frequent emesis) as a means of alleviating discomfort [6]. Although the use of hot showers or baths to relieve symptoms was thought to be pathognomonic for CHS, this behavior is also common in CVS patients [17]. In the final phase, the recovery period, vomiting ceases and patients begin to tolerate an oral diet but with dyspepsia that may resolve within a day or two.

Diagnostic Evaluation

As outlined in the Rome IV criteria, CVS and CHS remain clinical diagnoses based on symptoms. Classically, many patients may have undergone extensive diagnostic testing before the CVS/CHS diagnosis is considered. In a patient with uninvestigated nausea and vomiting, however, a limited clinical evaluation may be warranted to rule out additional etiologies which may present with similar symptoms. These tests could include a complete blood count, serum electrolytes and glucose, liver and pancreatic enzymes, pregnancy testing, and a urinalysis. Biochemical testing may reasonably investigate hypothyroidism or Addison's disease. An esophagogastroduodenoscopy (EGD) should also be considered. In performing an EGD, however, it is important not to overinterpret epiphenomena of recent vomiting as causal. For example, a Mallory-Weiss tear, defined as a laceration of the gastric cardia due to mechanical disruption from forceful vomiting, may reflect sequelae of a CVS attack rather than a cause of symptoms. A small bowel follow-through may also provide useful information to exclude obstructive structural lesions. In a patient with uncontrolled diabetes or other risk factors for gastroparesis, a gastric emptying study can be considered. Notably, patients with CVS typically have rapid or normal gastric emptying times, but a small subset of patients may have also exhibit delayed emptying [20]. Gastric emptying studies should not be performed during a CVS episode. In patients with any localizing neurological symptoms, brain imaging would be warranted. Ultimately, specialized testing should be targeted to particular symptoms or risk factors. In pursuing a diagnostic evaluation to rule out additional etiologies, the goal is to avoid an endless workup, as this may delay initiation of therapy and undermine a patient's confidence in the diagnosis and clinician.

Treatment

CVS severity should guide management decisions, particularly regarding prophylaxis using daily medications (Fig. 4.3). The primary factors of a severity assessment are CVS episode frequency (>4 episodes/year being more severe) and typical episode length (>3 days being more severe). CVS/CHS treatment both require a multifaceted approach to achieve optimal outcomes. Lifestyle modifications should be addressed in all patients and include avoidance of triggers such as particular foods (such as chocolate, cheese, monosodium glutamate, and red wine), emotional stressors, disrupted or reduced sleep, and energy-depleted states [1]. Those heavily using cannabis (thus having suspected CHS) should be counseled on marijuana cessation strategies. In addition, all patients should be provided with access to abortive therapies at home.

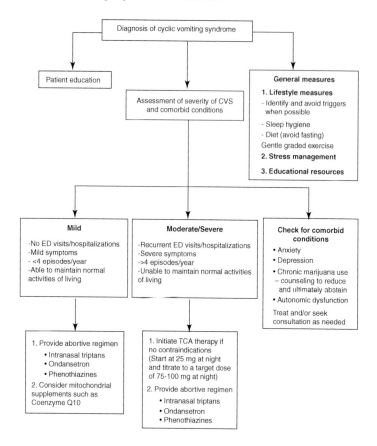

FIGURE 4.3 A treatment algorithm for patients diagnosed with CVS or CHS, from Bhandari and Venkatesan [21]

In patients who qualify for prophylactic therapy, first-line options include a tricyclic antidepressant (TCA) such as amitriptyline, nortriptyline, or doxepin or the anti-epileptic drug topiramate. TCAs should be initiated at low doses with titration to 75–100 mg/day (approximately 1 mg/kg/day) [22–24]. Topiramate (50–100 mg/day) is particularly attractive in patients with migraine headaches or obesity, and topiramate can be effective in those who failed to respond to TCAs [7] and is likely superior to propranolol prophylaxis [25]. Several alternative prophylactic medications can be considered in those non-responsive to TCAs or topiramate (Table 4.2). Theoretically, all of these agents effectively raise the CVS threshold (Fig. 4.2), therefore preventing an attack despite exposure to potential CVS triggers.

Treatment of comorbid conditions, particularly functional GI disorders and psychiatric illnesses, is an oftentimes overlooked aspect of optimal CVS management. For example, patients with treated anxiety may reduce healthcare utilization and experience reduced CVS attack frequency [36]. Additional mind-body focused modalities such as cognitive behavioral therapy, mindfulness meditation, biofeedback, and movement-based therapies (yoga, Pilates, tai chi) may also build resilience to stressors, secondarily reducing the impact of stress in driving CVS attacks [37]. Additional comorbid conditions such as GERD, IBS, migraines, and autonomic dysfunction should also be addressed.

Patients should attempt to abort a CVS attack at their first recognition of prodromal symptoms, as abortive interventions delivered earlier tend to be more effective. If available, orally dissolvable pills, nasal sprays, and subcutaneously injectable or suppository forms of medications should be offered to optimize systemic absorption. Abortive therapy should include an antiemetic such as ondansetron, promethazine, or prochlorperazine. Triptans, traditionally used for aborting migraines, have demonstrated promising efficacy in aborting CVS attacks [38, 39]. Although abdominal pain may be a feature of the prodrome, narcotic medications should be avoided as routine abortive therapy. Aprepitant may be effective in CVS, both as an abortive therapy as well as a prophylactic therapy [32]. Anxiolytics such as benzodiazepines, or other sedating medications such as diphenhydramine or hydroxyzine, are often useful abortive adjuncts [1]. Lastly, some patients can better abort an attack by resting quietly in a dark room, meditating, or taking hot showers or baths.

During the emetic phase of a CVS attack, further interventions are supportive and focus on prevention of secondary

TABLE 4.2 Prophylactic therapies for cyclic vomiting syndrome (CVS) and cannabinoid hyperemesis syndrome (CHS)

Agent	Goal dosage	Monitoring parameters/side effects	References
TCA (Amitriptyline, nortriptyline, doxepin)	75–100 mg (1 mg/kg/day)	Measure QTc; dry mouth, constipation, somnolence, mild hallucinations, blurred vision	[22–24]
Topiramate	50–100 mg daily (single or in divided doses)	Metabolic acidosis, kidney stones	[7, 25, 32]
Coenzyme Q10	300–400 mg daily	Elevated liver enzymes	[7, 27, 28]
L-carnitine	500–1500 mg BID		[27, 29, 30]
Levetiracetam	500 to 3000 mg/day	CBC; CNS depression, hypertension	[31]
Zonisamide	100 to 400 mg/day	Metabolic profile (including BUN, creatinine, and serum bicarbonate)	[31]
Aprepitant	125 mg twice weekly	Neutropenia, fatigue	[32]
Propranolol	1 mg/kg/day	Bradycardia, hypotension	[33]
Cyproheptadine	2–4 mg BID-TID	Somnolence	[34, 35]

complications such as those linked to dehydration. Patients with frequent CVS attacks and ED visits may also benefit from an individualized ED protocol, which often includes IV fluids, IV antiemetics, mildly sedating medications such as IV benzodiazepines or antihistamines, and IV pain medications such as ketorolac. Opioids are also often considered for pain control in the ED but should be avoided if possible. Frequent use of opioids may cloud a patient's clinical presentation, as opioid withdrawal symptoms may become indistinguishable from a CVS attack [15]. Moreover, chronic opioid use exposure itself may predict increased hospitalization rates among CVS patients [40].

Case Study: Follow-Up

The physical exam was normal, as was a small bowel follow-through ordered during the initial consultative visit. Based upon his consistent history and negative evaluations, the patient was diagnosed with cyclic vomiting syndrome (CVS). Given the frequency of attacks and their severity, the patient was offered prophylaxis using nortriptyline, titrated to 75 mg PO daily, and coenzyme Q10 300 mg PO daily. He was prescribed with ondansetron 4 mg orally dissolving tablets and a sumatriptan 20 mg intranasal spray to be used in combination to abort an impending CVS attack. He was encouraged to seek cognitive behavioral treatment for anxiety.

Over the following 6 months, the patient did not experience any severe CVS attacks and did not visit the ED. He notes only one minor CVS episode, during which he recognized the onset of diaphoresis and nausea as a prodrome similar to past CVS attacks. As a result, he administered intranasal sumatriptan and sublingual ondansetron and subsequently rested in a quiet, dark room. His nausea abated soon thereafter without progression to emesis or abdominal pain. His anxiety also improved on nortriptyline and with cognitive behavioral therapy. His clinical gains continued unabated over the following 12 months.

Clinical Pearls

- Patients with suspected CVS/CHS should undergo only limited diagnostic workup.
- TCAs and topiramate are first-line medications for CVS/CHS prophylaxis.
- Abortive therapies for CVS/CHS should ideally use orally dissolvable, nasal spray, or suppository forms of medications, administered as early as possible during the prodrome phase.
- Treating comorbid psychiatric and medical disorders may reduce CVS/CHS frequency.

Self-Test

Question 1. Which of the following clinical patterns of CVS attack frequency and duration would *not* warrant the use of daily prophylactic medications?

A. Six attacks per year, typically 5 days per episodes, all of which have led to ED visits and/or hospital admission

B. Eight attacks per year, typically 3 days per episode, with the ability to abort most attacks at home using sumatriptan

C. Three attacks per year, typically 12–18 h per episode, none of which have led to ED visits or hospital admission

D. Four attacks per year, typically 4 days per episode, with the ability to abort most attacks in the ED using IV ondansetron, alprazolam, and diphenhydramine

E. Five attacks per year, typically 2 days per episode, with the ability to generally avoid ED visits using home treatments that include alprazolam, ondansetron, hot showers, and rest

Question 2. Which of the following medications is *not* recognized as a useful prophylactic agent for CVS?

A. Topiramate
B. Nortriptyline
C. Levetiracetam
D. Alprazolam
E. Coenzyme Q10

Question 3. Which of the following medical disorders is the most closely associated comorbidity in those with CVS?

A. Epilepsy
B. Hypertension
C. GERD
D. Migraine
E. Type II diabetes

References

1. Abell TL, Adams KA, Boles RG, Bousvaros A, Chong SK, Fleisher DR, et al. Cyclic vomiting syndrome in adults. Neurogastroenterol Motil. 2008;20(4):269–84.
2. Hejazi RA, McCallum RW. Review article: cyclic vomiting syndrome in adultsDOUBLEHYPHENrediscovering and redefining an old entity. Aliment Pharmacol Ther. 2011;34(3):263–73.
3. Li BU, Misiewicz L. Cyclic vomiting syndrome: a brain-gut disorder. Gastroenterol Clin N Am. 2003;32(3):997–1019.
4. Chogle A, Velasco-Benitez CA, Koppen IJ, Moreno JE, Ramírez Hernández CR, Saps M, et al. A Population-Based Study on the Epidemiology of Functional Gastrointestinal Disorders in Young Children. J Pediatr. 2016;179:139–43.
5. Sagar RC, Sood R, Gracie DJ, Gold MJ, To N, Law GR, et al. Cyclic vomiting syndrome is a prevalent and under-recognized condition in the gastroenterology outpatient clinic. Neurogastroenterol Motil. 2018;30(1):e13174.
6. Fleisher DR, Gornowicz B, Adams K, Burch R, Feldman EJ. Cyclic vomiting syndrome in 41 adults: the illness, the patients, and problems of management. BMC Med. 2005;3:20.

7. Kumar N, Bashar Q, Reddy N, Sengupta J, Ananthakrishnan A, Schroeder A, et al. Cyclic Vomiting Syndrome (CVS): is there a difference based on onset of symptoms--pediatric versus adult? BMC Gastroenterol. 2012;12:52.

8. Li BU, Murray RD, Heitlinger LA, Robbins JL, Hayes JR. Is cyclic vomiting syndrome related to migraine? J Pediatr. 1999;134(5):567–72.

9. Levinthal DJ. The cyclic vomiting syndrome threshold: a framework for understanding pathogenesis and predicting successful treatments. Clin Transl Gastroenterol. 2016;7(10):e198.

10. Venkatesan T, Prieto T, Barboi A, Li B, Schroeder A, Hogan W, et al. Autonomic nerve function in adults with cyclic vomiting syndrome: a prospective study. Neurogastroenterol Motil. 2010;22(12):1303–7, e339.

11. Hejazi RA, Lavenbarg TH, Pasnoor M, Dimachkie M, Foran P, Herbelin L, et al. Autonomic nerve function in adult patients with cyclic vomiting syndrome. Neurogastroenterol Motil. 2011;23(5):439–43.

12. Boles RG, Chun N, Senadheera D, et al. Cyclic vomiting syndrome and mitochondrial DNA mutations. Lancet. 1997;350:1299–300.

13. Boles RG, Zaki EA, Lavenbarg T, et al. Are pediatric and adult-onset cyclic vomiting syndrome (CVS) biologically different conditions? Relationship of adult-onset CVS with the migraine and pediatric CVS-associated common mtDNA polymorphisms 16519 T and3010 A. Neurogastroenterol Motil. 2009;21:936–72.

14. Lee J, Wong SA, Li BU, Boles RG. NextGen nuclear DNA sequencing in cyclic vomiting syndrome reveals a significant association with the stress-induced calcium channel (RYR2). Neurogastroenterol Motil. 2015;27(7):990–6.

15. Levinthal DJ, Bielefeldt K. Adult cyclical vomiting syndrome: a disorder of allostatic regulation? Exp Brain Res. 2014;232(8):2541–7.

16. Namin F, Patel J, Lin Z, Sarosiek I, Foran P, Esmaeili P, et al. Clinical, psychiatric and manometric profile of cyclic vomiting syndrome in adults and response to tricyclic therapy. Neurogastroenterol Motil. 2007;19(3):196–202.

17. Venkatesan T, Sengupta J, Lodhi A, Schroeder A, Adams K, Hogan WJ, et al. An Internet survey of marijuana and hot shower use in adults with cyclic vomiting syndrome (CVS). Exp Brain Res. 2014;232(8):2563–70.

18. Wasilewski A, Lewandowska U, Mosinska P, Watala C, Storr M, Fichna J, et al. Cannabinoid receptor type 1 and mu-opioid receptor polymorphisms are associated with cyclic vomiting syndrome. Am J Gastroenterol. 2017;112(6):933–9.

19. Stanghellini V, Chan FKL, Hasler WL, Malagelada JR, Suzuki H, Tack J, et al. Gastroduodenal Disorders. Gastroenterology. 2016;150(6):1380–92.

20. Hejazi RA, Lavenbarg TH, McCallum RW. Spectrum of gastric emptying patterns in adult patients with cyclic vomiting syndrome. Neurogastroenterol Motil. 2010;22(12):1298–302, e338.

21. Bhandari S, Venkatesan T. Novel treatments for cyclic vomiting syndrome: beyond ondansetron and amitriptyline. Curr Treat Options Gastroenterol. 2016;14:495–506.

22. Prakash C, Clouse RE. Cyclic vomiting syndrome in adults: clinical features and response to tricyclic antidepressants. Am J Gastroenterol. 1999;94(10):2855–60.

23. Hejazi RA, Reddymasu SC, Namin F, Lavenbarg T, Foran P, McCallum RW. Efficacy of tricyclic antidepressant therapy in adults with cyclic vomiting syndrome: a two-year follow-up study. J Clin Gastroenterol. 2010;44(1):18–21.

24. Hejazi RA, Lavenbarg TH, Foran P, McCallum RW. Who are the nonresponders to standard treatment with tricyclic antidepressant agents for cyclic vomiting syndrome in adults? Aliment Pharmacol Ther. 2010;31(2):295–301.

25. Sezer OB, Sezer T. A new approach to the prophylaxis of cyclic vomiting: topiramate. J Neurogastroenterol Motil. 2016;22(4):656–60.

26. Hejazi RA, McCallum RW. Cyclic vomiting syndrome: treatment options. Exp Brain Res. 2014;232:2549–52.

27. Boles RG. High degree of efficacy in the treatment of cyclic vomiting syndrome with combined co-enzyme Q10, L-carnitine and amitriptyline, a case series. BMC Neurol. 2011;11:102.

28. Boles RG, Lovett-Barr MR, Preston A, Li BU, Adams K. Treatment of cyclic vomiting syndrome with co-enzyme Q10 and amitriptyline, a retrospective study. BMC Neurol. 2010;10:10.

29. McLoughlin LM, Trimble ER, Jackson P, Chong SK. L-carnitine in cyclical vomiting syndrome. Arch Dis Child. 2004 Dec;89(12):1180.

30. Van Calcar SC, Harding CO, Wolff JA. L-carnitine administration reduces number of episodes in cyclic vomiting syndrome. Clin Pediatr (Phila). 2002;41(3):171–4.

31. Clouse RE, Sayuk GS, Lustman PJ, Prakash C. Zonisamide or levetiracetam for adults with cyclic vomiting syndrome: a case series. Clin Gastroenterol Hepatol. 2007;5(1):44–8.

32. Cristofori F, Thapar N, Saliakellis E, Kumaraguru N, Elawad M, Kiparissi F, et al. Efficacy of the neurokinin-1 receptor antagonist aprepitant in children with cyclical vomiting syndrome. Aliment Pharmacol Ther. 2014;40(3):309–17.

33. Haghighat M, Rafie SM, Dehghani SM, Fallahi GH, Nejabat M. Cyclic vomiting syndrome in children: experience with 181 cases from southern Iran. World J Gastroenterol. 2007;13(12):1833–6.

34. Andersen JM, Sugerman KS, Lockhart JR, Weinberg WA. Effective prophylactic therapy for cyclic vomiting syndrome in children using amitriptyline or cyproheptadine. Pediatrics. 1997;100(6):977–81.

35. Badihian N, Saneian H, Badihian S, Yaghini O. Prophylactic therapy of cyclic vomiting syndrome in children: comparison of amitriptyline and Cyproheptadine: a randomized clinical trial. Am J Gastroenterol. 2018;113(1):135–40.

36. Bhandari S, Venkatesan T. Clinical characteristics, comorbidities and hospital outcomes in hospitalizations with cyclic vomiting syndrome: a Nationwide analysis. Dig Dis Sci. 2017;62(8):2035–44.

37. Slutsker B, Konichezky A, Gothelf D. Breaking the cycle: cognitive behavioral therapy and biofeedback training in a case of cyclic vomiting syndrome. Psychol Health Med. 2010;15(6):625–31.

38. Hikita T, Kodama H, Kaneko S, Amakata K, Ogita K, Mochizuki D, et al. Sumatriptan as a treatment for cyclic vomiting syndrome: a clinical trial. Cephalalgia. 2011;31(4):504–7.

39. Calhoun AH, Pruitt AP. Injectable sumatriptan for cyclic vomiting syndrome in adults: a case series. Headache. 2014;54(9):1526–30.

40. Saligram S, Bielefeldt K. The two sides of opioids in cyclical vomiting syndrome. N Am J Med Sci. 2014;6(3):114–8.

Essential Reading

Abell TL, Adams KA, Boles RG, Bousvaros A, Chong SK, Fleisher DR, et al. Cyclic vomiting syndrome in adults. Neurogastroenterol Motil. 2008 Apr;20(4):269–84.

Fleisher DR, Gornowicz B, Adams K, Burch R, Feldman EJ. Cyclic vomiting syndrome in 41 adults: the illness, the patients, and problems of management. BMC Med. 2005;3:20.

Hejazi RA, McCallum RW. Review article: cyclic vomiting syndrome in adults--rediscovering and redefining an old entity. Aliment Pharmacol Ther. 2011;34(3):263–73.

Stanghellini V, Chan FKL, Hasler WL, Malagelada JR, Suzuki H, Tack J, et al. Gastroduodenal Disorders. Gastroenterology. 2016;150(6):1380–92.

Chapter 5
Chronic Intestinal Pseudo-Obstruction

Sobia N. Laique and Scott L. Gabbard

Case Study

A 53-year-old female was referred by her local gastroenterologist for 4 years of progressive gastrointestinal (GI) symptoms. She initially presented to her internist with symptoms of constipation and abdominal bloating. Her internist began an evaluation by ordering a complete blood count (CBC), thyroid-stimulating hormone level (TSH), and colonoscopy – all of which were normal. Based on her symptoms, a normal physical examination, and her normal tests, she was diagnosed with IBS and treated with PEG-3350. She then noted

S. N. Laique
Internal Medicine, Cleveland Clinic, Cleveland, OH, USA
e-mail: laique.sobia@mayo.edu

S. L. Gabbard (✉)
Digestive Disease Institute, Cleveland Clinic, Cleveland, OH, USA
e-mail: gabbars@ccf.org

© Springer Nature Switzerland AG 2019
B. E. Lacy et al. (eds.), *Essential Medical Disorders of the Stomach and Small Intestine*,
https://doi.org/10.1007/978-3-030-01117-8_5

95

increasing episodes of upper abdominal bloating and early satiety. Upper endoscopy including biopsies of the duodenum and stomach was normal. Over the next year, she noted difficulty eating due to postprandial nausea; she lost approximately 15 pounds (10% of the total body weight). Abdominal x-ray revealed dilated loops of small intestine. CT enterography was negative for mechanical obstruction but did demonstrate diffusely dilated loops of small intestine. The patient was diagnosed with chronic intestinal pseudo-obstruction (CIPO).

Objectives

- Discuss the epidemiology, etiology, and pathogenesis of patients with CIPO.
- Outline a stepwise diagnostic approach for patients with suspected CIPO.
- Review treatment strategies for patients with CIPO with an emphasis on optimizing nutritional status (oral, enteral, and parenteral), therapies to improve intestinal motility, and endoscopic and surgical management options.

Epidemiology

Chronic intestinal pseudo-obstruction (CIPO) is a rare and debilitating condition. Patients show severe impairment of gastrointestinal (GI) propulsion leading to symptoms and/or signs suggestive of partial or complete intestinal obstruction in the absence of any mechanical obstruction. Most estimates of the incidence and prevalence of CIPO are from tertiary referral centers. One estimate from a pediatric tertiary care center is that approximately 100 infants are born with CIPO each year in the United States. This figure does not provide a good estimate on prevalence, however, as it does not include patients who develop CIPO later in life. In a national survey in Japan, the estimated prevalence of CIPO was 0.80 to 1.00 per 100,000, with an incidence of 0.21–0.24 per 100,000 [1]. The mean age at diagnosis was 63.1 years for males and 59.2 for females.

CIPO remains a challenge for most clinicians for several reasons. First, most physicians fail to recognize CIPO patients early due to their limited experience; second, symptoms of CIPO are non-specific. This may lead patients to be subjected to inadequate management including ineffective, and potentially dangerous, surgical procedures. Third, CIPO is an "umbrella term" covering a wide heterogeneous group of patients, i.e., congenital versus acquired/secondary to metabolic/endocrinological, neurological, and paraneoplastic disorders or idiopathic, with no apparent cause underlying the dysmotility. Finally, most CIPO patients show a variable outcome; some patients remain clinically stable over long periods of time, whereas others rapidly decline requiring parenteral nutrition to prevent severe malnutrition and death. These challenges and intrinsic difficulties hinder thorough phenotyping of patients, mechanistic studies, and disease management.

Classification

Several different classification schemes have been used to categorize CIPO patients. The authors prefer to categorize CIPO patients into three broad categories: congenital, acquired/secondary, and idiopathic (Table 5.1). Each of these groups can be further subdivided into three histological categories, neuropathies, myopathies, and mesenchymopathies, although some patients may have coexisting pathological abnormalities. A large proportion of patients are classified under the idiopathic category because no histological abnormality can be identified despite extensive testing.

TABLE 5.1 Classification of patients with chronic intestinal pseudo-obstruction

Onset	Variant	Typical related conditions
Congenital	CAID syndrome (SGOL 1 mutation)	Associated megacystis-microcolon-intestinal hypoperistalsis syndrome
	ACTG2 gene	Females. Periventricular nodular heterotopia, cardiac complications, thrombocytopenia, Ehlers-Danlos syndrome
	Mutations in *FLNA* and *L1CAM*	MNGIE, MELAS, MERRF
	Mitochondrial diseases (Mutations of TP or ECGF1)	Ehlers-Danlos syndrome
	Small bowel α-actin deficiency	
	Deficient interstitial cells of Cajal	
Acquired	Autoimmune	SLE, systemic sclerosis, dermatomyositis/polymyositis, autoimmune myositis, autoimmune ganglionitis
	Infectious/postinfectious	Chagas' disease, CMV, EBV, VZV, JC virus, Kawasaki disease, post-viral neuropathy
	Endocrine	Diabetes, hypothyroidism, hypoparathyroidism
	Oncology/hematology	Paraneoplastic (anti-Hu antibodies) syndrome small cell lung cancers/carcinoid tumors/malignant thymoma, chemotherapy and/or BM/stem cell transplant, radiation injury, pheochromocytoma
	Muscle disorders	Myotonic dystrophy, Duchenne muscular dystrophy
	Toxins	Fetal alcohol syndrome, alcohol abuse
	Drugs	Diltiazem and nifedipine, clonidine, cyclopentolate/phenylephrine eye drops (neonates), anti-Parkinsonians

Pathology	
Extrinsic autonomic nervous system	Stroke, encephalitis, calcification of basal ganglia, orthostatic hypotension, diabetes
Enteric nervous system	Hirschsprung's disease, Chagas disease, Von Recklinghausen disease
Mixed enteric neuromyopathy	Paraneoplastic (central nervous system neoplasms, bronchial carcinoid, leimyosarcoma, viral infections
Enteric smooth muscle layer	Systemic sclerosis, dermatomyositis, Ehlers-Danlos, jejunal diverticulosis, amyloidosis, diabetes
Idiopathic	Myotonic dystrophy, progressive systemic sclerosis, degenerative leiomyopathy, intestinal leiomyositis

CMV cytomegalovirus, *EBV* Epstein-Barr virus, *ECGF1* endothelial cell growth factor-1, *FLNA* filamin A gene, *JC virus* John Cunningham virus, *L1CAM* L1 cell adhesion molecule, *MELAS* mitochondrial encephalopathy with lactic acidosis and stroke-like episodes, *MERRF* myoclonus epilepsy associated with ragged-red fibers, *MNGIE* mitochondrial neurogastrointestinal encephalomyopathy, *SLE* systemic lupus erythematosus, *TP* thymidine phosphorylase gene, *VZV* varicella zoster virus

Etiology and Pathophysiology

Pathophysiologically, CIPO patients either have an impairment of the enteric nervous system, the intestinal smooth muscle, or the interstitial cells of Cajal (ICC), individually or in combination. Regardless of the cause, the end result is severe impairment of GI propulsion. These pathophysiologic abnormalities may arise due to another disease (secondary CIPO) or be idiopathic in nature. Approximately half of the cases of CIPO are secondary to neurologic, paraneoplastic, autoimmune, metabolic/endocrine, and infectious diseases [2].

Neuropathies

Neurologic disorders can affect the extrinsic autonomic nerve pathways supplying the gut (e.g., encephalitis, Parkinson's disease, or after a cerebrovascular accident) or the enteric nervous system (ENS) due to either an inflammatory (myenteric ganglionitis) or degenerative process. Degenerative neuropathies (paraneoplastic or immune-mediated) may result from several putative pathogenetic mechanisms, including altered calcium signaling, mitochondrial dysfunction, and production of free radicals, leading to degeneration and loss of gut intrinsic neurons. In paraneoplastic syndromes associated with small cell lung cancers, carcinoid tumors, or malignant thymoma, the circulating antineuronal (anti-Hu) antibodies are thought to target both the neurons in the submucosa and myenteric ganglia ENS damaging the enteric reflexes, thereby causing dysmotility. Immune-mediated pseudo-obstruction is seen in systemic sclerosis (SSc), dermatomyositis, and systemic lupus erythematosus. Neurotropic viruses (Herpes viridae, John Cunningham virus) may cause morphologic (i.e., inflammatory) or functional changes of the enteric nervous system and extrinsic neural pathways supplying the gut [3–5].

Congenital forms of neuropathies include genetic neuromuscular denervation or aganglionosis, Hirschsprung's disease, mitochondrial cytopathies such as mitochondrial encephalopathy with lactic acidosis and stroke-like episodes (MELAS), myoclonus epilepsy associated with ragged-red fibers (MERRF), and syndromes such as Waardenburg-Shah syndrome (deafness and pigmentary abnormalities in association with aganglionic megacolon) associated with mutations in neural crest-derived cells [6].

The interstitial cells of Cajal (ICC) are present within the submucosal, intramuscular, and intermuscular layers of the GI tract and serve as pacemaker cells, generating bioelectric slow-wave potentials leading to enteric smooth muscle contraction. Decreased number of ICCs, along with structural abnormalities, such as loss of processes and damaged intracellular cytoskeleton and organelles, has been reported in children (congenital) and adults (autoimmune diseases like SSc) with CIPO.

Intestinal Myopathies

The muscularis propria of the intestinal tract is normally composed of two layers, external (longitudinal) and internal (circular), oriented perpendicularly. These may be affected in some patients with CIPO. In degenerative leiomyopathy, there is a progressive loss of enteric smooth muscle and replacement with fibrous tissue. Symptoms of CIPO may not develop until adolescence. Patients with smooth muscle involvement may have impaired urinary bladder function. Intestinal leiomyositis, characterized by dense and diffuse lymphocytic infiltration of the muscularis propria, is another rare disease which predominantly affects children, and less than 12 patients have been reported in the world literature. In addition to the aforementioned diseases, secondary myopathies due to bowel ischemia, drug toxicity, radiation injury, and autoimmune disorders (myotonic dystrophy, progressive systemic sclerosis) are also seen [7].

Mesenchymopathies

More than one element of the neuromuscular apparatus of the gastrointestinal tract may be affected by various disease processes. For example, in SSc, immune-mediated destruction of the enteric nerves occurs before smooth muscle involvement. Similarly, mitochondrial cytopathy may result in neuropathy and subsequently myopathy. In diabetes mellitus, the extrinsic autonomic nerves and the ICCs are affected, whereas amyloidosis may cause an extrinsic neuropathy followed by myopathy.

Symptoms

Symptoms of CIPO vary from patient to patient based on the location and the extent of the GI tract involved. Symptoms may be acute, recurrent, or chronic. Abdominal pain and distension are reported by most (80%) patients. Nausea and vomiting occur in 75% and 40–50% of cases with documented gastroparesis (e.g., confirmed with a 4-h solid-phase gastric emptying scan). Esophageal dysmotility has been reported in approximately 70% of patients, while constipation occurs in 40%, and diarrhea (rarely steatorrhea) occurs in about 20–30% of cases (Table 5.2) [8, 9]. Diarrhea may be related to small intestinal bacterial overgrowth (SIBO) due to intestinal stasis and usually results in malabsorption and nutritional deficiencies in most patients. Although predominantly chronic in nature, these symptoms worsen during acute sub-occlusive episodes characterized by the abrupt onset of intense, cramping abdominal pain, distention, nausea, and vomiting. Intestinal volvulus must be excluded during an acute episode.

Patients may also have symptoms due to the underlying disorder (e.g., dysphagia due to esophageal involvement in CIPO related to SSc, proximal muscle weakness in patients with polymyositis/dermatomyositis, and bladder dysfunction in neuropathic and myopathic CIPO). Urinary bladder dys-

TABLE 5.2 Symptoms reported by patients with chronic intestinal pseudo-obstruction

Symptom	Reported frequency [8, 20]
Abdominal pain	58–80%
Abdominal distension	75–80%
Nausea	49–75%
Vomiting	40–50%
Heartburn/regurgitation	~50%
Dysphagia	70%
Early satiety	~40%
Constipation	40–50%
Diarrhea	20–30%

function (with or without megacystis and megaureter) often coexists with CIPO, more commonly detectable in children with an underlying myopathic derangement of the GI tract. Finally, CIPO patients may develop depression and/or other psychological disorders as a consequence of the disabling nature of this condition and the frustrating ineffectiveness of most prokinetic drugs.

Diagnosis

As yet, no single diagnostic test or pathognomonic finding indicative of CIPO has been identified. Thus, a stepwise diagnostic approach is recommended, aimed at ruling out mechanical obstruction, identifying underlying diseases, and understanding the pathophysiological features.

A thorough history and physical examination must be performed first. This should cover the patient's current medical conditions (autoimmune, connective tissue disorders), prior surgeries (the presence of adhesions, diverticula), family history (GI malignancies, similar constellation of symptoms), medication use, and any previous diagnostic tests performed in the evaluation of their symptoms. Warning signs, such as unintentional weight loss (more than 10% of the ideal body weight), hematemesis, and hematochezia, or signs of complete obstruction if present, warrant a more urgent workup and possible early surgical intervention.

To diagnose CIPO, patients should have symptoms for at least 6 months. The initial evaluation should aim at differentiating the patient with pseudo-obstruction from those with mechanical obstruction (Fig. 5.1). All patients should have a plain X-ray of the abdomen; air-fluid levels and dilated bowel loops with the patient in upright position are mandatory to suspect CIPO. In current clinical practice, dedicated enterography by computerized tomography (CT) or magnetic resonance imaging (MRI) is preferred as it more accurately demonstrates air-fluid levels, helps rule out mechanical causes as well as intestinal wall adhesions, and allows for transit time examination (Fig. 5.2). Cine MRI is an emerging, non-invasive, radiation-free technique to assess GI motility in CIPO patients. Fuyuki and colleagues studied 33 patients using cine MRI and demonstrated that the mean luminal diameter and contraction ratio in the CIPO group differed significantly from healthy volunteers [10]. Further validation of this method is necessary. Upper endoscopy and colonoscopy should be performed to help exclude mechanical occlusions and collect routine mucosal biopsies to exclude rare instances in which celiac disease or eosinophilic gastroenteropathy may be associated with dysmotility.

If imaging studies and endoscopy raise suspicion for CIPO and exclude mechanical (either intraluminal or extraluminal) obstruction, it is important to investigate potential underlying diseases and secondary causes of CIPO. Routine laboratory tests including a complete blood count, metabolic panel, hemoglobin A1C, and thyroid-stimulating hormone should be obtained. Appropriate laboratory tests and diagnostic studies should be considered to evaluate and then treat potential secondary causes of pseudo-obstruction including systemic autoimmune rheumatic diseases, autonomic neuropathies, endocrinopathies, viral etiologies, and malignancies/paraneoplastic processes.

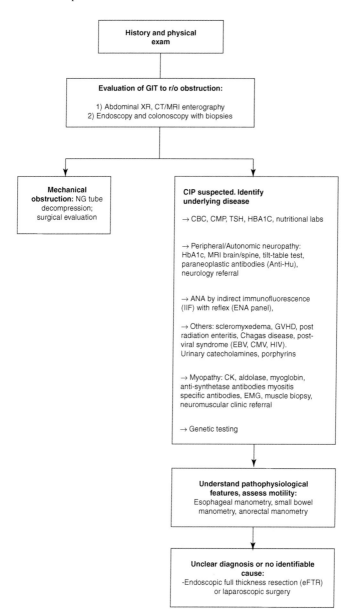

FIGURE 5.1 Diagnostic algorithm for evaluation of patients with suspected chronic intestinal pseudo-obstruction

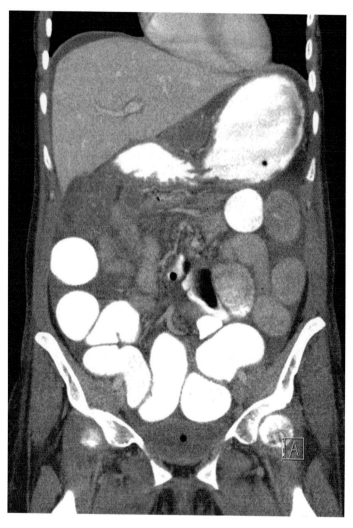

FIGURE 5.2 Computerized tomography (coronal view) image demonstrating air-fluid levels and dilated small bowel loops in patient with chronic intestinal pseudo-obstruction

Esophageal and/or small bowel manometry may provide pathophysiologic information on the mechanisms underlying dysmotility in CIPO patients (e.g., neuropathic vs myopathic patterns). Although this does not affect management, the evidence of a propulsive pattern (i.e., migrating motor complexes) predicts successful adaptation to jejunal feeding in children. Esophageal manometry may predict survival, inability to maintain adequate oral feeding, and parenteral nutrition requirement. Anorectal manometry is indicated in patients with intractable constipation and marked colonic distension to exclude Hirschsprung's disease. A manometric assessment of the entire GI tract is also essential prior to intestinal transplantation as it may provide clues about the outcome of isolated versus multivisceral transplantation in carefully selected patients.

The availability of minimally invasive procedures such as laparoscopic and endoscopic surgery have refueled interest in histopathological analysis of full-thickness intestinal biopsies [9]. These samples may demonstrate smooth muscle atrophy in the primary myopathic processes, neuropathic degeneration in the primary neuropathic disorders, and various findings for the secondary causes of CIP, including fibrosis in primary systemic sclerosis or evidence of amyloid or lymphoma. Recently, Valli and colleagues used endoscopic, full-thickness resection (eFTR) in four CIPO patients with suspected neuromuscular gut disorders. Large colonic full-thickness tissue samples obtained helped identify neuromuscular changes in all four patients with no adverse events suggesting that eFTR may be used as a safe and minimally invasive technique for obtaining biopsies [11].

Treatment

CIPO remains a challenge to treat. Once the diagnosis is made, therapy should focus on (1) avoidance of unnecessary surgery, (2) maintenance of adequate nutritional status including fluid and mineral balances, (3) improvement of intestinal propulsion, and (4) minimization of symptoms such as nausea, vomiting, bloating, and pain. Additionally, the underlying etiology (i.e., SSc) should be aggressively treated.

Nutrition Assessment

Nutritional evaluation should begin with anthropometric measures alongside a thorough dietary history, including oral intake and diet restrictions. Laboratory testing to evaluate the severity of the illness may include serum albumin, prealbumin, lymphocyte count, and C-reactive protein. Because of poor intake or absorption, it is also reasonable to measure calcium, iron, vitamin B12, folate, and fat-soluble vitamins. Thiamine and nicotinamide deficiencies have been reported in severe cases of SIBO; clinicians should be aware of these possible deficiencies and test as appropriate. Patients should undergo a formal nutrition evaluation by a registered dietician with experience in treating patients with CIPO [5].

Oral Diet

In patients with adequate intestinal absorption, maximization of oral intake is preferred as it has been found to be an independent predictor of survival [12]. Patients should be encouraged to take small, frequent meals (5–6 per day), with an emphasis on liquid calories and protein, while avoiding meals with high fat, high residue (delaying gastric emptying), and high lactose/fructose (evoking bloating/discomfort). Nutritional deficiencies also need to be corrected particularly fat-soluble vitamins (A, D, E, and K) as well as B12 and folate if bacterial overgrowth is present. Elemental feeding and dietary supplements with medium-chain fatty acids may also be used in combination when the aforementioned dietary changes are not successful [5, 13].

Enteral Nutrition Considerations

In cases of inadequate oral intake, enteral nutrition with a standard, non-elemental formula should be the next consideration [14]. Enteral nutrition starting with a slow infusion and continuous feeding or cyclical feeding (e.g., overnight) is preferred to large bolus feedings, especially if the feeding tube is distal to the pylorus. Before the placement of a permanent feeding tube, it is mandatory that a trial of nasogastric or nasojejunal feeding be performed using an enteral formula at the predetermined goal rate. If tolerated without significant discomfort, permanent enteral access may be placed.

Patients should be assessed for delayed gastric emptying, and if present, and there is objective evidence of malnutrition, a feeding tube should be placed distal to the pylorus. Antroduodenal manometry can help predict those who will tolerate enteral feeding; a study in children found that jejunal tube feeds were tolerated in all patients with an MMC on antroduodenal manometry compared to 33% of those without.

Parenteral Nutrition Considerations

In the most severe cases, total parenteral nutrition is required to maintain nutritional support and an adequate level of hydration once aforementioned therapies have failed. If patients are dependent on parenteral nutrition (PN) exclusively, they should receive approximately 25 kcal/kg/d, and lipids should supply approximately 30% of total parenteral calories with 1.0–1.5 g/kg/d protein and dextrose providing the remainder of required calories [5, 13].

Use of PN is not without risk, with a recent retrospective analysis of 51 patients receiving PN for an average of 8.3 years found 180 episodes of catheter-related sepsis, nine episodes of acute pancreatitis (two-thirds due to metabolic condition, one-third due to gallstones), five cases of D-lactic acidosis encephalopathy, and four patients with progression to cirrhosis; one death was directly related to a PN complication (catheter-related sepsis) in this population. Overall survival was 75% at 10 years compared with 48% at 5 years that had previously been reported [14]. As previously noted, oral intake is a major independent factor associated with better survival; thus, patients receiving PN should be encouraged to maximize oral intake as tolerated while receiving PN.

Medications and Other Therapies

Medications are often the first treatment attempted to try to ameliorate symptoms and improve nutritional intake. The various classes of medications used include (1) prokinetic agents to improve GI motility, (2) antiemetics, (3) pain medications, and (4) antibiotics to treat SIBO (Table 5.3). Regardless of the underlying process, all patients with CIPO have disordered GI tract motility, and so prokinetic agents remain one of the mainstays of treatment. Few investigational studies have been available to demonstrate their efficacy. In practice, the association of different prokinetic drugs and/or their rotation may be a strategy useful to increase therapeutic efficacy while minimizing tachyphylaxis and side effects. Similarly, antiemetics are used with variable efficacy and should be individualized based on the clinical presentation.

The most common symptom, however, is abdominal pain. Unfortunately, many patients with CIPO eventually require opiates for pain control. Few medications have demonstrated benefit for pain in CIPO. Non-opiate pain modulators such as tricyclic antidepressants, serotonin-norepinephrine reuptake inhibitors, and GABA analogues may be employed while monitoring for significant side effects such as constipation or drowsiness. Tramadol, a μ-opioid receptor agonist, can also be used and may be less constipating than opiates. If opiates are used, careful attention should be paid to antimotility effects, as well as the development of tolerance. Transdermal buprenorphine has been studied in children with idiopathic

TABLE 5.3 Medications that have been used for chronic intestinal pseudo-obstruction

Medication	Comments
Prokinetics	
Erythromycin	Off-label use, macrolide antibiotic with motilin agonist properties Efficacy at a dose of 1.5–2 g/day in adults, or 3–5 mg/kg/day in children. Accelerates gastric emptying and symptom relief. Tachyphylaxis is common
Metoclopramide	Available in the United States. Exerts prokinetic effects via type 2 dopamine receptor antagonism. Mainly used for acute episodes. Chronic use increases risk for severe extrapyramidal side effects
Cisapride	Taken off the US market in 1999 due to cardiac arrhythmia issues and drug interactions, available by FDA compassionate use
Domperidone	Available in the United States through FDA IND Dopamine agonist but does not pass the blood-brain barrier May be useful for gastroparesis, effective for nausea QTc prolongation or arrhythmia may occur
Tegaserod	Taken off the US market in 2007 for concerns of increased cardiac issues, not available in the United States except by FDA compassionate use

(continued)

TABLE 5.3 (continued)

Medication	Comments
Octreotide	Long-acting somatostatin analogue. Used at a dose of 50 mcg SQ every evening. Reported beneficial in scleroderma patients with CIPO and has also been studied with erythromycin May improve enteral nutrition tolerance, better studied in children
Leuprolide	Gonadotropin-releasing hormone analogue shown to decrease symptoms in patients with irritable bowel syndrome and CIPO – no large trials
Prucalopride	Highly selective 5-hydroxytryptamine 4 ($5\text{-}HT_4$) receptor agonist, not available in the United States Enhances motility through stomach, small bowel, and colon Studied in a small, randomized, placebo-controlled, single-center study
Lubiprostone, linaclotide	Stimulates ClCN-2 channels and intestinal guanylate cyclase receptors, respectively. Used to treat chronic constipation and irritable bowel syndrome with constipation Not systematically studied in CIPO

Antiemetics

Antihistamines (diphenhydramine, promethazine)	No single agent is particularly suited for the treatment of nausea and vomiting in CIPO. Rather, each patient needs to be assessed individually to determine current medication use, previous trials of antiemetics, adverse reactions, and financial status
Anticholinergics (scopolamine)	
Phenothiazines (prochlorperazine, promethezine)	
Butyrophenones (haloperidol, droperidol)	
Dopaminergic antagonists (metaclopramide, domperidone)	
Serotonin receptor antagonist (ondansetron, granistron)	
Miscellaneous (ginger, trimethobenzamide, lorazapem, dronabinol)	

(continued)

TABLE 5.3 (continued)

Medication	Comments
Antibiotics Rifaximin Amoxicillin and clavulanic acid Gentamicin Cephalosporin and metronidazole Tetracycline	Aimed at treating small intestinal bacterial overgrowth (see Chap. 20) Non-absorbable antibiotics, such as rifaximin, can be administered, although broad-spectrum antibiotics, such as amoxicillin and clavulanic acid, gentamicin, and metronidazole, often with antifungal compounds (e.g., nystatin or fluconazole), can be used for 1–2 week cycles alternated with antibiotic-free periods. Recently, amoxicillin-clavulanate has been demonstrated to accelerate intestinal transit in children, thus representing an interesting therapeutic option combining antibiotic and prokinetic effects
Pain control	Non-narcotic pain modulators, tricyclic antidepressants, selective serotonin reuptake inhibitors, and GABA analogues, used with caution because of their significant side effects – constipation and/or drowsiness Tramadol. In patients with chronic and unsustainable visceral pain, careful use of opiates paying attention to their known antimotility effects Transdermal buprenorphine
Fecal transplant	In the United States, an IND is required for use other than treatment of severe or recurrent *C. difficile* infection Small open-label study from China showed some reduction in symptoms and increased tolerance of enteral nutrition via nasojejunal tube

CIPO, with three of four children reporting adequate pain relief and none requiring further dose increases [11]. Other μ-opioid receptor antagonists (methylnaltrexone, naloxegol, naldemedine) have not been prospectively studied in CIPO.

Often patients will require rotating antibiotics to treat SIBO to help relieve symptoms of diarrhea and bloating and improve the nutritional status. No controlled trials have been performed to determine which antibiotics are best, but many clinicians recommend a rotating schedule of different antibiotics every month for 7–10 days over a 5- to 6-month cycle (please see Chap. 20 for specific information regarding treatment regimens).

Fecal Transplant

Fecal transplant is an intriguing potential treatment option for CIPO. A small open-label study from China prospectively studied nine adult patients for 8 weeks after receiving fecal transplant from volunteer donors via nasojejunal tube (NJT) daily for 6 days after 3 days of daily NJT administration of 500 mg of liquid vancomycin. This reportedly resulted in significant reduction in symptoms and increased tolerance of enteral nutrition via NJT [7]. However, based on this one study, there are many more questions that need to be answered.

GI Decompression

As bowel distension is commonly associated with pain and other symptoms in CIPO patients, intestinal segment decompression therapy represents one of the key aspects in CIPO management. No pharmacological therapies to date have been shown to achieve effective, non-invasive decompression in CIPO. Decompression may be attempted using conventional methods such as intermittent nasogastric suction, rectal tubes/colonoscopic decompression, or via surgical proce-

dures, such as feeding/venting gastrojejunostomies/jejunosto-
mies (or other intestinal "ostomies"). Ohkuba and colleagues
assessed the efficacy and safety of percutaneous endoscopic
gastrojejunostomy (PEG-J) decompression therapy in seven
CIPO patients. A significant decrease in the number of days
without abdominal symptoms was observed in six out of the
seven patients, along with the improvement in malnutrition
and wasting [15]. Surgically placed gastrostomy tubes have
been shown to decrease hospital admissions (0.2 admissions
per patient year) from baseline before tube placement (1.2
admissions per patient year) [16].

If the use of venting procedures does not provide adequate relief, then subtotal enterectomy has been performed
for palliation. This may be in addition to long-term PN and/
or in preparation to an intestinal transplant. In general,
attempts should be made to avoid surgery when possible
given the high postoperative morbidity (58.2%) and mortality rates (7.9%) and frequent CIPO-related reoperations
(44% at 1 year, 66% at 5 years) as demonstrated by Sabbagh
et al. in their analysis of 63 patients who underwent surgery
for CIPO [17]. Surgery also has a high rate of stoma prolapse
along with considerable risk of dehydration due to enteric
fluid losses [17, 18].

Small Intestinal Transplantation

Intestinal transplantation has been increasingly used for the
management of intestinal failure and irreversible TPN complications secondary to CIPO, accounting for about 9% of the
transplants performed and can be a life-saving procedure with
good long-term survival for selected patients. The severity of
bowel disease and liver status dictates the type of the transplant, isolated small bowel, or multivisceral transplantation.
Recent United Network for Organ Sharing data in children
demonstrated 1- and 5-year survival rates for patients trans-
planted for functional disorders of 75% and 57%, respectively; these rates are comparable to the overall survival rates
for intestinal transplant [19]. Infectious and opportunistic
complications are seen at similar rates between patients with

CIPO and those with other indications for transplant. Early referral to specialized tertiary centers is critical, allowing for timely intervention and ultimately a better outcome.

Case Study Follow-Up

A 4-h solid-phase gastric emptying scan revealed 95% gastric emptying at 4 h (normal). Esophageal manometry revealed ineffective esophageal motility but no evidence of a myopathic process affecting the smooth muscle of the esophagus; it was presumed that her CIPO was secondary to a neuropathic etiology. A nonabsorbable antibiotic was used to empirically treat for presumed small intestine bacterial overgrowth, which improved bloating by approximately 50%. Because of continued symptoms, octreotide 50 mcg was administered subcutaneously each night, which further helped symptoms. The patient was seen by a dietician and started on liquid nutrition supplementation, which allowed her to regain 5 pounds. While the patient has continued episodes of bloating/distention, her quality of life has improved significantly with the above therapies.

Clinical Pearls
- CIPO is a rare and debilitating GI motility disorder, characterized by clinical symptoms of either continuous or intermittent of bowel obstruction (abdominal pain, abdominal distension, nausea, and vomiting) in the absence of mechanical obstruction.
- The diagnostic workup should include imaging, manometry studies, and, occasionally, full-thickness bowel biopsies alongside workup to determine secondary causes.
- Treatment goals should include optimizing the nutritional status, avoiding surgery, and preventing or delaying the development of intestinal failure.

Self-Test

Question 1. A patient with chronic abdominal bloating and distention is found to have severely dilated loops of small bowel visualized on enterography. She has undergone exploratory laparotomy, without evidence of mechanical obstruction. Which of the following tests is not indicated in identifying the cause of the patient's presentation?

A. TSH
B. Fasting glucose
C. Fasting gastrin level
D. ANA

Question 2. A patient with known chronic intestinal pseudo-obstruction (CIPO) presents with chronic abdominal bloating and weight loss of 10 pounds (7.5% of total body weight). Which of the following therapies has been shown to improve bloating in patients with CIP?

A. Simethicone 80 mg PO TID
B. Octreotide 50 mcg subcutaneous QHS
C. Omeprazole 40 mg PO BID
D. Polyethylene glycol 3350 1 capful PO BID

Question 3. A 45-year-old female with known chronic intestinal pseudo-obstruction (CIPO) presents with recurrent episodes of vomiting, leading to hospitalization. Which of the following therapies has been shown to reduce hospitalization in patients with CIPO?

A. Venting gastrostomy tube
B. Cisapride 20 mg PO TID
C. Metoclopramide 10 mg PO ACHS
D. Pyloroplasty

References

1. Iida H, Ohkubo H, Inamori M, Nakajima A, Sato H. Epidemiology and clinical experience of chronic intestinal pseudo-obstruction in Japan: a nationwide epidemiologic survey. J Epidemiol. 2013;23(4):288–94.
2. De Giorgio R, Sarnelli G, Corinaldesi R, Stanghellini V. Advances in our understanding of the pathology of chronic intestinal pseudo-obstruction. Gut. 2004;53(11):1549–52.
3. El-Chammas K, Sood MR. Chronic intestinal pseudo-obstruction. Clin Colon Rectal Surg. 2018;31(2):99–107.
4. Di Nardo G, Blandizzi C, Volta U, Colucci R, Stanghellini V, Barbara G, et al. Review article: molecular, pathological and therapeutic features of human enteric neuropathies. Aliment Pharmacol Ther. 2008;28(1):25–42.
5. Gabbard SL, Lacy BE. Chronic intestinal pseudo-obstruction. Nutr Clin Pract. 2013;28(3):307–16.
6. Sekino Y, Inamori M, Yamada E, Ohkubo H, Sakai E, Higurashi T, et al. Characteristics of intestinal pseudo-obstruction in patients with mitochondrial diseases. World J Gastroenterol. 2012;18(33):4557–62.
7. Gu L, Ding C, Tian H, Yang B, Zhang X, Hua Y, et al. Serial frozen fecal microbiota transplantation in the treatment of chronic intestinal pseudo-obstruction: a preliminary study. J Neurogastroenterol Motil. 2017;23(2):289–97.
8. Stanghellini V, Cogliandro RF, De Giorgio R, Barbara G, Morselli-Labate AM, Cogliandro L, et al. Natural history of chronic idiopathic intestinal pseudo-obstruction in adults: a single center study. Clin Gastroenterol Hepatol. 2005;3(5):449–58.
9. Di Nardo G, Di Lorenzo C, Lauro A, Stanghellini V, Thapar N, Karunaratne TB, et al. Chronic intestinal pseudo-obstruction in children and adults: diagnosis and therapeutic options. Neurogastroenterol Motil. 2017;29(1).
10. Fuyuki A, Ohkubo H, Higurashi T, Iida H, Inoh Y, Inamori M, et al. Clinical importance of cine-MRI assessment of small bowel motility in patients with chronic intestinal pseudo-obstruction: a retrospective study of 33 patients. J Gastroenterol. 2017;52(5):577–84.

11. Prapaitrakool S, Hollmann MW, Wartenberg HC, Preckel B, Brugger S. Use of buprenorphine in children with chronic pseu-doobstruction syndrome: case series and review of literature. Clin J Pain. 2012;28(8):722–5.

12. Amiot A, Joly F, Cazals-Hatem D, Merrouche M, Jouet P, Coffin B, et al. Prognostic yield of esophageal manometry in chronic intestinal pseudo-obstruction: a retrospective cohort of 116 adult patients. Neurogastroenterol Motil. 2012;24(11):1008–e542.

13. Kirby DF, Raheem SA, Corrigan ML. Nutritional interventions in chronic intestinal Pseudoobstruction. Gastroenterol Clin N Am. 2018;47(1):209–18.

14. Scolapio JS, Ukleja A, Bouras EP, Romano M. Nutritional management of chronic intestinal pseudo-obstruction. J Clin Gastroenterol. 1999;28(4):306–12.

15. Ohkubo H, Fuyuki A, Arimoto J, Higurashi T, Nonaka T, Inoh Y, et al. Efficacy of percutaneous endoscopic gastro-jejunostomy (PEG-J) decompression therapy for patients with chronic intestinal pseudo-obstruction (CIPO). Neurogastroenterol Motil. 2017;29(12).

16. Pitt HA, Mann LL, Berquist WE, Ament ME, Fonkalsrud EW, Den Besten L. Chronic intestinal pseudo-obstruction. Management with total parenteral nutrition and a venting enterostomy. Arch Surg Chic. 1985;120(5):614–8.

17. Sabbagh C, Amiot A, Maggiori L, Corcos O, Joly F, Panis Y. Non-transplantation surgical approach for chronic intestinal pseudo-obstruction: analysis of 63 adult consecutive cases. Neurogastroenterol Motil. 2013;25(10):e680–6.

18. Pakarinen MP, Kurvinen A, Koivusalo AI, Ruuska T, Mäkisalo H, Jalanko H, et al. Surgical treatment and outcomes of severe pediatric intestinal motility disorders requiring parenteral nutrition. J Pediatr Surg. 2013;48(2):333–8.

19. Lao OB, Healey PJ, Perkins JD, Horslen S, Reyes JD, Goldin AB. Outcomes in children after intestinal transplant. Pediatrics. 2010;125(3):e550–8.

20. Di Nardo G, Karunaratne TB, Frediani S, De Giorgio R. Chronic intestinal pseudo-obstruction: progress in management? Neurogastroenterol Motil. 2017;29(12).

Essential Reading

El-Chammas K, Sood MR. Chronic intestinal pseudo-obstruction. Clin Colon Rectal Surg. 2018;31(2):99–107. This article provides a detailed overview of the classification and pathophysiology of CIPO

Di Nardo G, Karunaratne TB, Frediani S, De Giorgio R. Chronic intestinal pseudo-obstruction: Progress in management? Neurogastroenterol Motil. 2017;29 This article provides a comprehensive overview on the advances in management for CIPO

Kirby DF, Raheem SA, Corrigan ML. Nutritional interventions in chronic intestinal Pseudoobstruction. Gastroenterol Clin N Am. 2018;47:209–18. This article provides an authoritative overview on the treatment, particularly nutritional interventions for CIPO patients

Part II

Dyspepsia and Other Disorders of Neuromuscular Function

Chapter 6
A Diagnostic Approach to Dyspepsia

Kimberly Harer and William L. Hasler

Case Study

A 66-year-old man with known hypertension presents to the gastroenterology clinic with a 6-month history of increasing epigastric burning, belching, and bloating. His symptoms began insidiously without any obvious triggering event. Prior to this, he was asymptomatic. He also reports feeling full after meals and has noticed he stops eating earlier than normal due to this sense of fullness. He denies vomiting but has experienced mild nausea on a few occasions. He denies weight loss, heartburn, regurgitation, dysphagia, melena, hematochezia, diarrhea, or constipation. His medications include verapamil for hypertension and occasional sildenafil for erectile dysfunction. He does not use nonsteroidal anti-inflammatory drugs (NSAIDs). He reports a 25-pack-year history of smoking, but has not used tobacco products for

K. Harer · W. L. Hasler (✉)
Division of Gastroenterology, University of Michigan Health System, Ann Arbor, MI, USA
e-mail: kharer@umich.edu; whasler@umich.edu

© Springer Nature Switzerland AG 2019
B. E. Lacy et al. (eds.), *Essential Medical Disorders of the Stomach and Small Intestine*,
https://doi.org/10.1007/978-3-030-01117-8_6

more than a decade. His family history is negative for gastrointestinal malignancy. On review of systems, he notes no other associated new extraintestinal symptoms. On physical examination, he exhibits mild epigastric tenderness with a negative Carnett's sign. His stool is hemoccult negative. Laboratory studies obtained at his most recent clinic visit with his primary physician included a normal hemoglobin, renal function, liver chemistries, and serum amylase. He has never undergone *Helicobacter pylori* testing or treatment, nor has he ever undergone esophagogastroduodenoscopy (EGD) for any indication. His last colonoscopy at age 61 was normal.

Objectives

- Review the symptom components of dyspepsia.
- Discuss the differential diagnosis for dyspepsia.
- Understand the diagnostic approach to uninvestigated dyspepsia.

Epidemiology

The prevalence of dyspepsia is typically quoted in the range from 20% to 40% [1–5]. However, estimating the prevalence has proven to be a difficult undertaking, due to the use of varying diagnostic criteria and the fact that symptoms overlap with those of other gastrointestinal conditions, such as gastroparesis and functional gastrointestinal disorders. Additionally, many studies investigate the prevalence of "uninvestigated dyspepsia," which encompasses both patients with dyspepsia secondary to organic causes and those with functional dyspepsia. The true prevalence is also likely underestimated due to the fact that many patients with dyspepsia do not seek medical care.

Identified risk factors for dyspepsia include female gender, smoking, NSAID use, and *Helicobacter pylori* (*H.*

pylori) infection [2]. Studies have also demonstrated an association with other gastrointestinal disorders, most notably irritable bowel syndrome (IBS) and gastroesophageal reflux disease (GERD). A systematic review and meta-analysis reported a pooled prevalence of IBS in patients with dyspepsia of 37% [6]. Similarly, a European study demonstrated 34% of patients with dyspeptic symptoms had concomitant reflux [7]. This symptom overlap has led to the hypothesis that these disorders are part of a spectrum that share common underlying pathophysiologic disruptions [5].

Patients with dyspeptic symptoms are subdivided into two groups based on whether an underlying organic etiology of their symptoms is identified during evaluation. If an etiology is identified, the patient is classified as having secondary dyspepsia. If no organic cause is identified, the patient is classified as having functional dyspepsia. For the purpose of this chapter, our focus will be on the diagnostic approach to excluding secondary causes of dyspepsia. Functional dyspepsia is discussed in detail in Chap. 8.

Etiology and Pathophysiology

The diagnostic approach to dyspepsia is often a challenge, due to the wide-ranging list of potential organic etiologies that can induce dyspeptic symptoms, as well as the high prevalence of functional gastroduodenal disorders that can be clinically indistinguishable from dyspepsia caused by an organic condition. The most common organic etiologies of dyspepsia include peptic ulcer disease (PUD), NSAID use, GERD, and malignancy. Less prevalent organic causes include gastrointestinal dysmotility, hepatopancreaticobiliary disorders, inflammation, ischemia, and musculoskeletal disorders. A more comprehensive list of specific disorders is outlined in Table 6.1.

EGD is often performed during the evaluation of dyspepsia. The endoscopic findings in pooled data from nine

TABLE 6.1   Etiologies of dyspepsia

Gastritis/Peptic Ulcer Disease

Helicobacter pylori infection

Chemical gastritis (NSAID[a], bile acid, etc.)

Autoimmune gastritis

Gastroesophageal Reflux Disease (GERD)

Gastrointestinal Dysmotility

Gastroparesis

Infiltrative disorders (amyloid, sarcoid)

Esophageal dysmotility

Malignancy

Esophageal

Gastric

Small bowel

Hepatobiliary

Pancreatic

Lymphoma

Ischemia

Mesenteric or celiac artery compromise

Inflammatory

Inflammatory bowel disease (IBD)

Eosinophilic gastroenteritis

Celiac disease

Hepatopancreaticobiliary Disorders

Cholelithiasis

Chronic pancreatitis

Hepatitis

TABLE 6.1 (continued)

Musculoskeletal Pain
Chronic abdominal wall pain
Costochondritis
Diabetic thoracic radiculopathy
Functional Gastroduodenal Disorders
Functional dyspepsia
Chronic nausea and vomiting syndrome
Visceral hypersensitivity
Irritable bowel syndrome

[a]Nonsteroidal Anti-inflammatory Drugs

studies that evaluated patients with dyspepsia demonstrated PUD in 11%, erosive esophagitis in 6%, Barrett's esophagus in 0.8%, gastroesophageal malignancy in 0.2%, and normal results in 82% [5]. This report highlights the most common causes of organic dyspepsia, as well as the high percentage of normal endoscopic studies performed for uninvestigated dyspepsia.

In concert with the broad differential, the underlying pathophysiology of dyspepsia also includes a wide variety of proposed mechanisms. Direct gastric mucosal injury, such as with NSAIDs or *H. pylori* infection, is one of the straight forward mechanisms. Vagal injury and other causes of gastric neuromuscular dysfunction can impair gastric motility or fundal accommodation, which can subsequently induce symptoms of early satiety and/or postprandial fullness. Impaired mucosal integrity may contribute to symptoms in inflammatory causes of dyspepsia. Celiac or superior mesenteric artery stenosis can lead to impaired intestinal perfusion and subsequent chronic, episodic ischemia. Several factors may contribute to symptom generation in functional dyspepsia including abnormal gastric emptying, blunted fundal relaxation after eating (e.g., abnormal accommodation), heightened sensitivity to gastric distention or duodenal acid exposure, and duodenal eosinophilia. These mechanisms are described in more detail in Chap. 8.

Symptoms

Patients with dyspepsia may report epigastric pain/burning, early satiety, postprandial fullness, and nausea. Epigastric pain or burning may be postprandial with some organic causes, as well as the postprandial distress syndrome, variant of functional dyspepsia. Alternatively, epigastric pain may be unaffected by meals in some conditions and in a proportion of patients with the epigastric pain syndrome functional dyspepsia subset. Some individuals with PUD even report symptom improvements with meal ingestion. Patients often use the term bloating to describe the sensation of fullness during or after a meal, and they may use the term heartburn to describe epigastric burning. Thus, it is imperative to delve deeper into the patient's symptoms and clarify what is truly meant when ill-defined symptoms such as heartburn or bloating are reported. Figure 6.1 highlights the component symptoms of dyspepsia and their characteristics. Prominent chest pain and vomiting are not commonly included in the description of dyspepsia.

Taking a detailed symptom history is critical to aid in identifying the most likely etiology of dyspepsia, all of which can present with similar dyspeptic symptoms of epigastric pain, early satiety, and postprandial fullness. Understanding the patient's predominant symptoms, as well as the associated symptoms, helps provide a guide to identifying the most likely underlying diagnosis. Predominant heartburn or regurgitation symptoms point toward GERD. Significant nausea or vomiting is often seen in gastroparesis. Colicky and episodic pain that may radiate to the right side is often an indication of a pancreaticobiliary pathology, such as cholelithiasis or chronic pancreatitis.

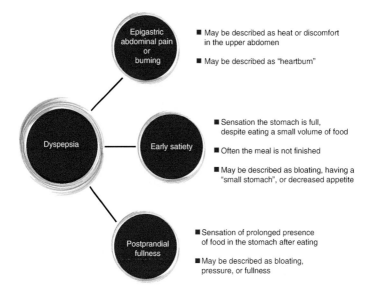

FIGURE 6.1 Dyspepsia symptoms and descriptions

Unintentional weight loss and progressive symptoms raise concern for malignancy.

Diagnostic Evaluation

The goal of the diagnostic approach to dyspepsia is to identify any causative factors and rule out more sinister etiologies in at-risk populations. Diagnostic evaluation is based on a detailed patient history and examination, patient age, and the presence or absence of alarm features. Alarm features include unintentional weight loss, progressive or new dysphagia, odynophagia, persistent vomiting, unexplained iron deficiency anemia, a palpable mass or lymphadenopathy, a family history of upper gastrointestinal malignancy, or spending childhood in a country with high risk for gastrointestinal malignancy (e.g., Southeast Asia or parts of South America) (Table 6.2).

TABLE 6.2 Alarm features worrisome for malignancy in dyspepsia

Alarm Features
Unintentional weight loss (5% of body weight)
Progressive or new dysphagia or odynophagia
Persistent vomiting
Unexplained iron deficiency anemia
Palpable mass or lymphadenopathy
Family history of upper gastrointestinal malignancy
Childhood in country with high risk for gastrointestinal malignancy[a]

[a]Southeast Asia, parts of South America

Patients presenting with dyspepsia who are younger than 60 years should undergo *H. pylori* testing via stool antigen testing or urea breath test, with subsequent treatment if testing indicates active infection [5]. Prior recommendations to exclude *H. pylori* infection only in geographic regions with high prevalence rates were eliminated in the most recent guidelines, given the uncertainties relating to exposure to the infection for any given patient [8]. Following therapy, it is important to ensure patients undergo eradication testing via stool antigen or urea breath test 4 weeks after therapy concludes. The patient should not take a proton pump inhibitor (PPI) in the 4 weeks prior to eradication testing, as this may result in a false-negative test result [9]. Caveats to the *H. pylori* "test and treat" diagnostic recommendation in patients under 60 years old include the presence of more than one alarm feature, clinically significant weight loss (typically >5% of baseline body weight), overt gastrointestinal bleeding, or a rapidly progressive alarm feature. If any of these clinical criteria are met, initial evaluation with EGD is recommended despite a younger age. Patients age 60 years or older should undergo initial evaluation via EGD with gastric biopsies, regardless of the presence of alarm features, due to

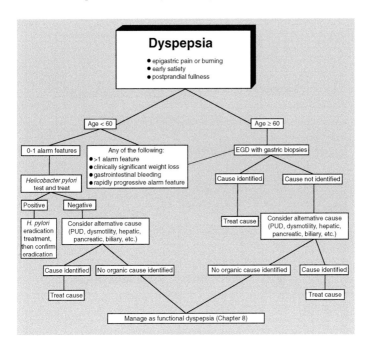

FIGURE 6.2 Diagnostic algorithm for dyspepsia

elevated malignancy risk in this age group [5]. Figure 6.2 outlines a suggested approach to evaluation.

If an EGD is performed, gastric biopsies should be obtained from the lesser and greater curvature of the antrum, lesser and greater curvature of the body, and incisura angularis to ensure detection of *H. pylori*, if present [10]. Additionally, patients who are immunocompromised or have undergone a bone marrow transplant should have duodenal biopsies obtained to evaluate for opportunistic infections or graft-versus-host disease [11]. Duodenal biopsies should also be obtained if there is clinical suspicion for inflammatory conditions such as celiac disease or eosinophilic gastroenteritis.

The algorithm for dyspepsia evaluation seems relatively straight forward, but there is significant overlap in symptoms

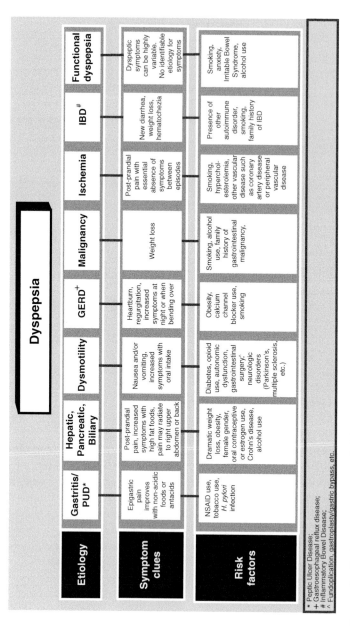

FIGURE 6.3 Patient symptoms and risk factors for various causes of dyspepsia

* Peptic Ulcer Disease;
+ Gastroesophageal reflux disease;
# Inflammatory Bowel Disease;
^ Fundoplication, gastroplasty/gastric bypass, etc.

with other organic and functional disorders, such as gastroparesis. If initial evaluation with *H. pylori* testing or EGD is unrevealing, consideration of alternative etiologies should be entertained, based on the patient's symptoms and risk factors. Not all patients will require additional testing; however, it is imperative to consider the diagnoses outlined in Table 6.1. For example, gastroparesis presents with symptoms of dyspepsia; however, patients commonly report more prominent nausea and vomiting. If a patient is at risk for gastroparesis and presents with predominant symptoms of nausea and vomiting, further evaluation with a gastric emptying study may be warranted. If a patient has a history of vascular disease and complains of pain only with meals, evaluation for ischemia should be considered. Laboratory testing can also be used to exclude metabolic, hepatopancreaticobiliary, and inflammatory conditions. If evaluation for an organic cause is negative, a diagnosis of functional dyspepsia should be made and treatment commenced. Figure 6.3 describes some of the common causes of dyspepsia, along with their clinical clues and patient risk factors.

Treatment

Treatment of dyspepsia is based on the presence or absence of an identified organic etiology. If *H. pylori* is detected in the setting of dyspeptic symptoms, eradication treatment should be pursued. As discussed above, successful eradication should be confirmed via stool antigen or urea breath test 4 weeks after therapy is completed. PPI therapy should not be used in the interim since it can lead to false-negative test results. Specific therapies of other identified organic causes of dyspepsia should be offered. PUD unrelated to *H. pylori* infection can be managed with acid suppression regimens and withholding of NSAID intake, if appropriate. GERD is managed with aggressive PPI programs, with additional medication or surgery options advocated for patients who do not respond to PPI. Specific treatments of hepatopancreaticobiliary, ischemic, or inflammatory etiologies should be recommended. If gastroparesis is identified, treatment with antiemetics or prokinetics should be considered.

If the evaluation for an organic cause is unrevealing, a diagnosis of functional dyspepsia should be made. An initial course of PPI is offered, to be followed by sequential trials of therapy with a tricyclic antidepressant and then a prokinetic for PPI treatment failures, as recommended in a recent guideline document [8]. A more detailed discussion of functional dyspepsia treatment is provided in Chap. 8.

Case Study: Follow-Up

The 66-year-old man discussed at the beginning of the chapter presented with unexplained dyspepsia. Given his age greater than 60 years, clinical guidelines dictated that an EGD with gastric biopsies should be performed. The EGD was normal and gastric biopsies were also unremarkable. The patient's clinical presentation and history did not warrant further evaluation at this time. Given the unremarkable evaluation for an organic cause of dyspepsia, the patient was diagnosed with functional dyspepsia and empirically started on a PPI for 4 weeks. On outpatient follow-up, he reported complete symptom resolution on twice daily PPI therapy. He was maintained on a regimen of once daily PPI dosing with good symptom control.

Clinical Pearls

- Patients with dyspepsia report epigastric pain/burning, early satiety, postprandial fullness, and/or nausea.
- Patients with dyspepsia younger than 60 years of age should undergo *H. pylori* testing, and eradication treatment should be given if testing is positive.

- EGD evaluation should be performed for patients aged 60 years and over and for patients under age 60 years with (1) more than 1 alarm feature, (2) clinically significant weight loss, (3) gastrointestinal bleeding, or (4) rapidly progressive alarm features.
- If no etiology for dyspepsia is identified, management of functional dyspepsia should be pursued as described in Chap. 8.

Self-Test

Question 1. A 34-year-old woman presents to your clinic with complaints of epigastric burning, bloating and fullness after meals, and intermittent nausea for the past 5 months. She denies dysphagia, heartburn, melena, hematochezia, vomiting, or weight loss. Recent laboratory evaluation demonstrates normal hemoglobin, white blood cell count, and iron levels. Ranitidine 150 mg was tried without significant benefit. Her mother was recently diagnosed with gastric cancer at age 61. What is the next best step?

A. Prescribe PPI BID.
B. Perform EGD with gastric biopsies.
C. Perform gastric emptying testing.
D. Order *H. pylori* stool antigen testing.

Question 2. A 75-year-old man with uncontrolled diabetes presents for evaluation of epigastric burning, bloating and fullness after meals, and intermittent nausea for the past 4 months. He denies dysphagia, heartburn, melena, hematochezia, vomiting, or weight loss. His colonoscopy within the past year was normal. He has not tried any medications for his symptoms. What is the next best step?

A. Prescribe PPI BID.
B. Perform EGD with gastric biopsies.

C.   Perform gastric emptying testing.
D.   Order *H. pylori* stool antigen testing.

Question 3. A 62-year-old woman with a past medical history of hypertension presents to your clinic complaining of epigastric burning, which is associated with mild nausea. She also reports that she has been unable to eat the entire turkey and cheese sandwich she previously would enjoy for lunch. She denies dysphagia, heartburn, melena, hematochezia, vomiting, or weight loss. Her only medication is aspirin 81 mg daily. EGD with gastric biopsies was normal including rapid urease testing of the gastric biopsy tissue. Laboratory evaluation including complete blood count, metabolic panel, and liver panel were unremarkable. A 4-week trial of PPI therapy was not helpful. What is the most likely diagnosis at the present time?

A.   Gastroparesis
B.   Functional dyspepsia
C.   NSAID-induced chemical gastritis
D.   GERD

References

1. El-Serag HB, Talley NJ. Systemic review: the prevalence and clinical course of functional dyspepsia. Aliment Pharmacol Ther. 2004;19:643–54.
2. Ford AC, Marwaha A, Sood R, Moayyedi P. Global prevalence of, and risk factors for, uninvestigated dyspepsia: a meta-analysis. Gut. 2015;64:1049–57.
3. Mahadeva S, Goh KL. Epidemiology of functional dyspepsia: a global perspective. World J Gastroenterol. 2006;12:2661–6.
4. Castillo EJ, Camilleri M, Locke GR, Burton DD, Stephens DA, Geno DM, Zinsmeister AR. A community-based, controlled study of the epidemiology and pathophysiology of dyspepsia. Clin Gastroenterol Hepatol. 2004;2:985–96.
5. Stanghellini V, Chan FK, Hasler WL, Malagelada JR, Suzuki H, Tack J, Talley NJ. Gastroduodenal disorders. Gastroenterology. 2016;150:1380–92.

6. Ford AC, Marwaha A, Lim A, Moayyedi P. Systematic review and meta-analysis of the prevalence of irritable bowel syndrome in individuals with dyspepsia. Clin Gastroenterol Hepatol. 2010;8:401–9.

7. Piessevaux H, De Winter B, Louis E, Muls V, De Looze D, Pelckmans P, Deltenre M, Urbain D, Tack J. Dyspeptic symptoms in the general population: a factor and cluster analysis of symptom groupings. Neurogastroenterol Motil. 2009;21:378–88.

8. Moayyedi PM, Lacy BE, Andrews CN, Enns RA, Howden CW, Vakil N. ACG and CAG clinical guideline: management of dyspepsia. Am J Gastroenterol. 2017;112:988–1013.

9. Courillon-Mallet A. Confirmation of helicobacter pylori eradication following first line treatment. How and when? Gastroenterol Clin Biol. 2003;27:473–7.

10. Dixon MF, Genta RM, Yardley JH, Correa P. Classification and grading of gastritis. The updated Sydney system. International workshop on the histopathology of gastritis, Houston 1994. Am J Surg Pathol. 1996;20:1161–81.

11. Yang Y, Brill J, Krishnan P, Leontiadis G, Clinical Guidelines Committee. American Gastroenterological Association Institute guideline on the role of upper gastrointestinal biopsy to evaluate dyspepsia in the adult patient in the absence of visible mucosal lesions. Gastroenterology. 2015;149:1082–7.

Essential Reading

Ford AC, Marwaha A, Sood R, Moayyedi P. Global prevalence of, and risk factors for, uninvestigated dyspepsia: a meta-analysis. Gut. 2015;64:1049–57. This article presents a rigorous description of the epidemiology and clinical features of patients presenting with uninvestigated dyspepsia.

Moayyedi PM, Lacy BE, Andrews CN, Enns RA, Howden CW, Vakil N. ACG and CAG clinical guideline: management of dyspepsia. Am J Gastroenterol. 2017;112:988–1013. This article presents the most updated guidelines by the American College of Gastroenterology and Canadian Association of Gastroenterology describing the diagnostic and treatment approaches to uninvestigated dyspepsia.

Stanghellini V, Chan FK, Hasler WL, Malagelada JR, Suzuki H, Tack J, Talley NJ. Gastroduodenal disorders. Gastroenterology.

2016;150:1380–92. This article presents the Rome IV criteria for functional gastroduodenal disorders including functional dyspepsia in relation to organic disorders presenting with similar symptoms.

Yang Y, Brill J, Krishnan P, Leontiadis G, Clinical Guidelines Committee. American Gastroenterological Association Institute Guideline on the role of upper gastrointestinal biopsy to evaluate dyspepsia in the adult patient in the absence of visible mucosal lesions. Gastroenterology. 2015;149:1082–7. This article presents the updated recommendations of the American Gastroenterological Association on indications and methods of endoscopic biopsy performance in patients with unexplained dyspepsia.

Chapter 7
Helicobacter pylori and Related Diseases

Muhammad Ali Khan and Colin W. Howden

Case

A 45-year-old man, who recently emigrated to the USA from Eastern Europe, complains of intermittent pain in the epigastrium that has bothered him for years. The pain is described as "gnawing" in character and is often worse before eating, slightly improved after eating, and sometimes wakes him from sleep. He has no other gastrointestinal symptoms. His weight has been steady. About 10 years ago, he had a minor episode of hematemesis. Endoscopy at that time revealed a small duodenal ulcer; gastric mucosal biopsies were positive for *Helicobacter pylori* (*H. pylori*) infection. However, he did not follow-up at that time and was never treated for the infection. He has recently been self-medicating with an over-the-counter H_2-receptor antagonist (H_2RA) for intermittent epigastric pain. He has had no

M. A. Khan · C. W. Howden (✉)
Division of Gastroenterology, University of Tennessee Health Science Center, Memphis, TN, USA
e-mail: mkhan24@uthsc.edu; chowden@uthsc.edu

© Springer Nature Switzerland AG 2019   141
B. E. Lacy et al. (eds.), *Essential Medical Disorders of the Stomach and Small Intestine*,
https://doi.org/10.1007/978-3-030-01117-8_7

further episodes of gastrointestinal bleeding. His general health is otherwise good. He is on no prescription medicines. Family history is unremarkable. He smokes up to a pack of cigarettes daily and has one or two alcoholic drinks on most evenings. He does not use aspirin or nonsteroidal anti-inflammatory drugs (NSAIDs). He has no known drug allergies and does not recall being treated with antibiotics in the past. He has read on the Internet that *H. pylori* infection is associated with ulcers and with stomach cancer, and he now wishes to be retested and, if appropriate, treated for the infection. A urea breath test (UBT) was positive, confirming *H. pylori* infection. He was advised to undergo treatment with a combination of omeprazole, clarithromycin, amoxicillin, and metronidazole for 14 days. He was also advised to stop smoking.

Objectives

- Understand the association between *H. pylori* infection and peptic ulcer.
- Identify appropriate patients who should be tested for *H. pylori* infection.
- Recognize the strengths and limitations of different diagnostic tests for *H. pylori* infection.
- Review appropriate treatment options for *H. pylori* infection.

Epidemiology

H. pylori infection is extremely common worldwide, especially in less developed countries. A systematic review and meta-analysis of studies from 73 countries reported an overall prevalence of 44.3% [1] but with marked variation between, and within, continents. In developing countries, the overall prevalence was 50.8%, as compared with 34.7% in the developed world. Men may be slightly more likely than women to have *H. pylori* infection; overall prevalence rates were, respectively, 46.3% and 42.7%. *H. pylori* infection is usually acquired in childhood, although the precise mode of infection is unclear. Low socioeconomic status and large family size during childhood are risk factors for infection. Children born to *H. pylori*-infected mothers are at particularly high risk of infection in early childhood [2]. Although men may have a slightly higher prevalence of infection than women, male and female children have similar rates of infection [3]. People born in the earlier decades of the twentieth century are more likely to be infected than those born in later decades; there is, therefore, evidence of a birth cohort effect regarding *H. pylori* prevalence. Among veterans in the USA, prevalence among those born before 1920 was 73%, compared with 22% in those born after 1980 [4]. Ethnic and racial groups in the USA with the highest rates of infection include African Americans, Hispanic Americans, Native Americans, and Alaskan natives [4, 5].

Etiology and Pathophysiology

H. pylori is a spiral, microaerophilic, Gram-negative bacterium that is highly adapted to the human stomach. It resides beneath the mucous layer, tightly attached to the gastric epithelium, and damages the gastric mucosa by disrupting the mucous protection barrier through the release of toxins. Damage is exacerbated by the host inflammatory response. *H. pylori* can only survive on gastric-type mucosa.

H. pylori induces chronic inflammation in the gastric mucosa and alters the physiology of gastric acid secretion. In most individuals, this is asymptomatic. However, in a subset, this altered gastric secretory activity, when coupled with a host inflammatory response, can lead to peptic ulcer disease. Furthermore, chronic gastritis in certain patients can progress to atrophy, intestinal metaplasia, and, ultimately, gastric adenocarcinoma. In rare circumstances, persistent lymphoid stimulation by *H. pylori* antigens can lead to gastric mucosa-associated lymphoid tissue (MALT) lymphoma [6].

People who acquire *H. pylori* in developed countries generally have inflammation that is most marked in the gastric antrum. Inflammation from *H. pylori* infection leads to increased release of gastrin, which increases parietal cell mass in the stomach and – therefore – gastric acid secretion. Over many years, this excess secretion of acid by the stomach may produce areas of gastric metaplasia in the duodenum. *H. pylori* can colonize these areas; the resulting inflammation impairs mucosal defense allowing acid and pepsin from the stomach to produce ulceration [6].

In less developed countries, *H. pylori* infection is likely to cause inflammation of the entire stomach including the acid-producing corpus. Chronic inflammation from *H. pylori* infection leads to progressive loss of parietal cells with a reduction in acid secretion. Some infected individuals will develop chronic atrophic gastritis and are at increased risk of gastric cancer [6, 7].

Symptoms

H. pylori infection may be asymptomatic or may cause dyspeptic symptoms. Only a relatively small proportion of infected individuals go on to develop a duodenal or gastric ulcer. Typical ulcer symptoms include pain in the epigastrium that may be described as "burning" or "gnawing" in character. Severity of the pain typically fluctuates over weeks or months, and patients may be pain-free for periods. Classically, pain is worse at night and may wake patients from sleep. Pain is often helped by eating small quantities of food or by taking antacids or acid-suppressing medicines. Vomiting is an unusual symptom (unless chronic ulceration has led to gastric outflow obstruction) but, if present, may be associated with an improvement in pain. Weight loss in peptic ulcer is also unusual. The main complications of peptic ulcer disease are bleeding, perforation, and gastric outlet obstruction. Bleeding may present with hematemesis and/or melena or – if particularly brisk – hematochezia. Perforation is characterized by the abrupt onset of intense upper abdominal pain, followed by the development of more generalized abdominal pain from peritonitis. Gastric outlet obstruction typically presents with persistent vomiting that may be accompanied by upper abdominal discomfort and weight loss.

Some infected individuals will ultimately develop gastric cancer; typical symptoms include upper abdominal pain, vomiting, gastrointestinal bleeding, poor appetite, and weight loss.

Patients with gastric MALT lymphoma generally have non-specific dyspeptic symptoms.

Diagnostic Evaluation

The 2017 American College of Gastroenterology (ACG) treatment guideline on *H. pylori* infection [8] included recommendations for testing particular groups of patients for the infection; these are summarized in Table 7.1.

Diagnostic tests for *H. pylori* can be divided into endoscopic and non-endoscopic. Endoscopy should not be performed solely for the diagnosis of *H. pylori* infection. Endoscopic tests, which require the collection of gastric mucosal biopsies, include histology, biopsy-based urease tests, and, rarely, culture and sensitivity testing. Non-endoscopic tests include serology, urea breath test (UBT), and fecal antigen tests. Apart from serology, all are considered tests of active infection. Serological testing cannot distinguish between current and past infection. In low-prevalence areas, including much of the USA, the positive predictive value of serology is unacceptably low; positive serological tests should be confirmed by a test of active infection. In general, tests of active infection are preferred over serological testing [8–10].

Patients who do not require endoscopy can be tested for *H. pylori* infection with the UBT or fecal antigen test. In

TABLE 7.1 Indications for testing for *H. pylori* infection along with strength of recommendation and quality of evidence

Indication	Strength of recommendation	Quality of evidence
Peptic ulcer disease	Strong	High
History of peptic ulcer disease[a]	Strong	High
Low-grade gastric MALT lymphoma	Strong	Low
Endoscopic resection of early gastric cancer	Strong	Low
Uninvestigated dyspepsia under age 60 without alarm features	Conditional	High for efficacy Low for age threshold
Dyspepsia patients having endoscopy	Strong	High
Long-term, low-dose aspirin therapy	Conditional	Moderate
Initiating chronic NSAID treatment	Strong	Moderate
On NSAID treatment	Conditional	Low
Unexplained iron deficiency anemia	Conditional	Low
Idiopathic thrombocytopenic purpura	Conditional	Very low

Adapted with permission from American College of Gastroenterology practice guideline on *H. pylori* infection (Chey et al. [8])

Abbreviations used: *MALT* mucosa-associated lymphoid tissue, *NSAID* nonsteroidal anti-inflammatory drug

[a]unless previous cure of *H. pylori* infection has been documented

those who do require endoscopy, *H. pylori* status can be determined by a biopsy-based test and/or histology. Importantly, proton pump inhibitors (PPIs), bismuth compounds, and antibiotics decrease the sensitivity of all tests for active infection. Therefore, PPIs should be held for 2 weeks prior to testing, and antibiotics and bismuth should be avoided for 4 weeks. If necessary, patients who are taking a PPI can be switched to standard dose H_2RA treatment for 2 weeks before testing.

The UBT and biopsy-based urease tests are based upon the bacterium's urease activity. Normally, the human stomach is devoid of urease. If urease activity is detected, this therefore confirms the presence of *H. pylori*. In the UBT, labeled urea (with either nonradioactive ^{13}C or radioactive ^{14}C) is given by mouth; through its urease activity, *H. pylori* metabolizes urea with the release of labeled CO_2 that can be detected in breath samples. The sensitivity and specificity of the UBT are both around 95% [11]. *H. pylori* antigens can be detected in fecal samples. Sensitivity and specificity of fecal antigen testing is around 93% [11]. Both the UBT and fecal antigen test can be used after treatment to determine whether *H. pylori* infection has been cured. Posttreatment testing should be delayed for at least 4 weeks after completing treatment, and patients should not take a PPI for the 2 weeks before testing.

Treatment

Treatment of *H. pylori* infection generally requires a combination of at least three – and preferably four – medicines taken together for 10–14 days. National and regional treatment guidelines have been established for many countries and are likely to continue to evolve [8–10]. Treatment regimens for *H. pylori* infection are not uniformly effective in eradicating the infection. Failure of eradication is most often due to antimicrobial resistance, inadequate patient compliance, or some combination of the two.

The 2017 ACG treatment guideline for *H. pylori* infection recommended a variety of regimens [8], although not all had been evaluated in trials conducted within North America. Some general principles of treatment should be followed. For example, clarithromycin should not be used in patients who have previously been treated with it, or another macrolide antibiotic, for any reason. Patients who self-report as being "penicillin allergic" should be tested by an allergy specialist for this. Many such patients are not truly allergic and may safely be treated with a regimen containing amoxicillin. This is important, as resistance to amoxicillin by *H. pylori* is very rare; consequently, amoxicillin remains a very useful and important agent for *H. pylori* infection. The two most reliable four-drug combinations endorsed in the ACG guideline [8] are bismuth quadruple therapy and concomitant therapy; details of these are given in Table 7. 2.

Ideally, the choice of antimicrobials for treatment of *H. pylori* infection would be based on the results of sensitivity testing. However, this is not generally available. Therefore, treatment is largely empiric but can be guided by the answers to two questions: "Has the patient used macrolides before for any reason?" and "Is the patient truly penicillin allergic?" Fig. 7. 1, taken from the 2017 ACG practice guideline [8], illustrates how these two key questions can guide treatment selection.

Since eradication is not always achieved after a single course of treatment, routine posttreatment testing is now recommended [8, 10]. This should be with a test of active infection – such as the UBT or fecal antigen test – and not with serology. Patients with persistent infection after an initial course of treatment should be retreated with a different regimen. Importantly, clarithromycin and levofloxacin should not be included in the second treatment, if they have been used as part of the first. Medicines that can be included in both first and subsequent treatments include bismuth, amoxicillin, and tetracycline, since resistance to these is very rare. Bismuth-based quadruple therapy (i.e., a PPI, a bismuth salt, tetracycline, and metronidazole) is an appropriate regimen both first line and second line, especially for patients who

TABLE 7.2 Four-drug combinations recommended for the treatment of *H. pylori* infection

Regimen	Drugs and doses	Dosing frequency	Duration
Bismuth quadruple	PPI (standard dose)	*b.i.d.*	10–14 days
	Bismuth subcitrate (120–300 mg) or subsalicylate (300 mg)	*q.i.d.*	
	Tetracycline (500 mg)	*q.i.d.*	
	Metronidazole (250–500 mg)	*q.i.d.* (for 250 mg) *t.i.d.* or *q.i.d.* (for 500 mg)	
Concomitant	PPI (standard dose)	*b.i.d.*	10–14 days
	Clarithromycin (500 mg)		
	Amoxicillin (1000 mg)		
	Nitroimidazole[a] (500 mg)		

Adapted with permission from American College of Gastroenterology practice guideline on *H. pylori* infection (Chey et al. [8])
Abbreviations used: *b.i.d.* twice daily, *t.i.d.* three times daily, *q.i.d.* four times daily
[a]either metronidazole or tinidazole

have failed treatment with a clarithromycin-containing regimen or who are truly penicillin allergic.

Patients who fail two or more treatment regimens should be referred to a specialist. Antimicrobial sensitivity testing, if available, should be considered for such patients. However, since this is not widely available, rescue treatment is often on an empiric basis and should be guided by which antimicrobial agents the patient has already received. Figure 7.2, taken from the 2017 ACG treatment guideline [8], illustrates the process of selection of a rescue regimen.

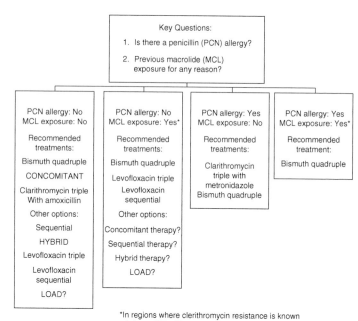

FIGURE 7.1 Selection of a first-line treatment regimen for *H. pylori* infection. (Reproduced with permission from American College of Gastroenterology practice guideline on *H. pylori* infection (Chey et al. [8]))

Case Study: Follow-Up

The patient successfully completed the 14-day course of omeprazole, clarithromycin, amoxicillin, and metronidazole and reported that he had been fully compliant. He noticed a marked improvement in his abdominal pain while on treatment. He had mild diarrhea and taste disturbance during treatment but had been advised in advance that those side effects might occur. These resolved after completing the

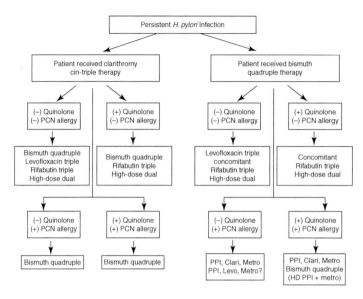

FIGURE 7.2 Selection of a salvage treatment regimen for persistent *H. pylori* infection. (Adapted with permission from American College of Gastroenterology practice guideline on *H. pylori* infection (Chey et al. [8]))

course of therapy. He had also been advised to avoid alcohol while on the treatment, because of concerns about an interaction with metronidazole. He sought advice from his primary care physician about smoking cessation programs. He stopped all medicines after the 14-day course and took only occasional doses of his over-the-counter H_2RA. Six weeks after completing treatment for *H. pylori* infection, a repeat UBT was negative, indicating cure of the infection. He was advised that the chances of reinfection with *H. pylori* were very small and that he should not experience further problems with peptic ulcer, unless he started aspirin or a NSAID. Therefore, he was also advised that he should not need to continue to use H_2RAs or other acid-suppressing medicines.

Clinical Pearls

- *H. pylori* infection is usually asymptomatic but can lead to peptic ulcer or gastric cancer.
- Testing for *H. pylori* infection should be with a test of active infection, such as the UBT or fecal antigen test, rather than serology.
- Treatment for *H. pylori* infection should be with a four-drug combination for 10–14 days.
- All patients treated for *H. pylori* infection should be appropriately retested to see if the infection has been cured.

Self-Test

Question 1. A patient was treated for *H. pylori* infection with a 14-day course of a PPI, clarithromycin, and amoxicillin. Four weeks after completing treatment, and with the patient off the PPI for 4 weeks, a UBT was positive. What is the appropriate course of action?

A. Treat with a PPI, clarithromycin, and metronidazole for 14 days
B. Treat with a PPI, clarithromycin, and amoxicillin for 28 days
C. Treat with a PPI, amoxicillin, and metronidazole for 14 days
D. Treat with a PPI, bismuth, tetracycline, and metronidazole for 14 days

Question 2. To which of the following antibiotics is *H. pylori* least likely to become resistant?

A. Amoxicillin
B. Clarithromycin
C. Levofloxacin
D. Metronidazole

Question 3. A 45-year-old man has completed a 14-day course of a four-drug combination for *H. pylori* infection. He continues to take omeprazole 20 mg daily for mild, intermittent heartburn. How should he be retested to determine cure of *H. pylori* infection?

A. Continue omeprazole and perform a UBT
B. Continue omeprazole and perform a fecal antigen test
C. Discontinue omeprazole for 5 days and perform a UBT
D. Discontinue omeprazole for 14 days and perform a UBT

References

1. Zamani M, Ebrahimtabar F, Zamani V, Miller WH, Alizadeh-Naevaeu R, Shokri-Shirvani J, Derakshan MH. Systematic review with meta-analysis: the worldwide prevalence of *Helicobacter pylori* infection. Aliment Pharmacol Ther. 2018;47(7):868–76.

2. Weyermann M, Rothenbacher D, Brenner H. Acquisition of *Helicobacter pylori* infection in early childhood: independent contributions of infected mothers, fathers and siblings. Am J Gastroenterol. 2009;104(1):182–9.

3. de Martel C, Parsonnet J. *Helicobacter pylori* infection and gender: a meta-analysis of population-based prevalence surveys. Dig Dis Sci. 2006;51(12):2292–301.

4. Nguyen T, Ramsey D, Graham D, Shaib Y, Shiota S, Velez M, et al. The prevalence of *Helicobacter pylori* remains high in African American and Hispanic veterans. Helicobacter. 2015;20(4):305–15.

5. Goodman KJ, Jacobson K, Veldhuyzen van Zanten S. *Helicobacter pylori* infection in Canadian and related Arctic aboriginal populations. Can J Gastroenterol. 2008;22(3):289–95.

6. Suerbaum S, Michetti P. *Helicobacter pylori* infection. N Engl J Med. 2002;347:1175–86.

7. Bornschein J, Malfertheiner P. *Helicobacter pylori* and gastric cancer. Dig Dis. 2014;32(3):249–64.

8. Chey WD, Leontiadis GI, Howden CW, Moss SF. ACG clinical guideline: treatment of *Helicobacter pylori* infection. Am J Gastroenterol. 2017;112(2):212–39.

9. Fallone CA, Chiba N, van Zanten SV, Fischbach L, Gisbert JP, Hunt RH, et al. The Toronto consensus for the treatment

of *Helicobacter pylori* infection in adults. Gastroenterology. 2016;151(1):51–69.

10. Malfertheiner P, Megraud F, O'Morain CA, Gisbert JP, Kuipers EJ, Axon AT, et al. Management of *Helicobacter pylori* infection-the Maastricht V/Florence consensus report. Gut. 2017;66(1):6–30.

11. Vaira D, Vakil N. Blood, urine, stool, breath, money and *Helicobacter pylori*. Gut. 2001;48(3):287–9.

Essential Reading

Chey WD, Leontiadis GI, Howden CW, Moss SF. ACG clinical guideline: treatment of *Helicobacter pylori* infection. Am J Gastroenterol. 2017;112(2):212–39.

Fallone CA, Chiba N, van Zanten SV, Fischbach L, Gisbert JP, Hunt RH, et al. The Toronto consensus for the treatment of *Helicobacter pylori* infection in adults. Gastroenterology. 2016;151(1):51–69.

Suerbaum S, Michetti P. *Helicobacter pylori* infection. N Engl J Med. 2002;347:1175–86.

Vaira D, Vakil N. Blood, urine, stool, breath, money and *Helicobacter pylori*. Gut. 2001;48(3):287–9.

Chapter 8
Functional Dyspepsia

Nicholas J. Talley and Dane R. Cook

Case

A 57-year-old woman with a background history of mild
asthma and allergic rhinitis presents with a 30-year history
of unexplained gnawing, or sometimes burning, epigastric
pain after eating. She also reports feeling bloated and
uncomfortable after most meals and an inability to finish a
meal as large as her sister or husband (early satiety). When
asked about food triggers, ingestion of wheat was identified, but reduced ingestion of gluten gave limited relief.
She also described what had been labelled as heartburn a
few days per week (lower retrosternal and epigastric burning), but no acid regurgitation or dysphagia. Her bowel
habits were normal, and there was no history of weight
loss, vomiting, or dysphagia. There was no history of an
infection preceding the onset of symptoms. She had a

N. J. Talley (✉) · D. R. Cook
Global Research, The University of Newcastle,
New Lambton, NSW, Australia
e-mail: nicholas.talley@newcastle.edu.au

© Springer Nature Switzerland AG 2019
B. E. Lacy et al. (eds.), *Essential Medical Disorders
of the Stomach and Small Intestine*,
https://doi.org/10.1007/978-3-030-01117-8_8

155

history of anxiety, but not depression. Ten years ago, an esophagogastroduodenoscopy (EGD) was normal, including testing for *H. pylori*, and she was treated with a standard-dose proton pump inhibitor (PPI) with only slight improvement. The dominant symptoms remained postprandial fullness and early satiety and were at times bad enough to result in time off work. Her sleep was affected. Physical examination revealed a normal weight female, with a soft and non-tender abdomen. The working diagnosis was PPI-resistant non-erosive gastroesophageal reflux disease (GERD), and she was referred for a second opinion and further workup.

A repeat EGD was normal with no evidence of peptic ulceration or esophagitis. Duodenal biopsies from the second portion were obtained, with confirmation that the patient was eating gluten at the time of biopsy. There was no evidence of celiac disease, but the duodenal eosinophil count in 5 high-power fields (5 HPF) was increased to 39/5 HPF (normal <22/5 HPF). Gastric biopsies were normal. An oesophageal impedance-pH study off PPI therapy was normal. A diagnosis of functional dyspepsia (FD) (postprandial distress (PDS) subtype) was made.

Objectives

- Recognise patients presenting with symptoms of FD in clinical practice.
- Differentiate FD from other causes of dyspepsia, especially GERD.
- Understand current treatment options for FD.

Epidemiology

Unexplained fullness after eating, early satiety, and/or epigastric pain or burning are common complaints in the community and in clinical practice. Although there is a broad list of differential diagnoses for these symptoms, including peptic ulcer disease, GERD, medication side effects (e.g. non-steroidal anti-inflammatory drugs (NSAIDs)), and rarely gastroesophageal malignancy or gastroparesis, the majority of those who consult have no explanation identified by EGD or other routine tests and are labelled as having FD [1].

In the USA, about 10% of the population report typical FD symptoms, although many are mislabelled as having GERD. Heartburn and FD symptoms overlap more than expected by chance, suggesting a common underlying pathophysiology, and therefore in some cases, it can be difficult to differentiate the two conditions. One clue is early satiety; this symptom is a good discriminator and points to FD rather than GERD [1, 2]. Frequent dominant heartburn on the other hand points to GERD.

Expert consensus subdivides FD into those with PDS, characterised by postprandial fullness and/or early satiety at least 3 days per week (in fact usually patients have symptoms after most meals), and epigastric pain syndrome (EPS), characterised by intermittent episodes of pain or burning at least 1 day per week. PDS and EPS often overlap, but in the general population, PDS is more prevalent, accounting for about two-thirds of FD cases [2]. FD is important because the symptoms impact on quality of life, including work and relationships. Anxiety and depression, as well as sleep disturbances, are highly prevalent in patients with FD.

Etiology and Pathophysiology

The pathogenesis of FD is not completely understood and is likely multifactorial in nature. Traditionally FD has been considered a disorder arising from the stomach, and most attention has focussed on this organ. Fullness after eating points to a gastric motility problem, and although one in five patients with FD have slower than normal gastric emptying, this abnormality correlates poorly, if at all, with symptoms. Vomiting is not a feature of FD but is frequent in gastroparesis and may help distinguish these two overlapping conditions [3]. Further, there is good evidence that a subset with FD have gastric fundus relaxation failure, and this is associated with the inability to finish a normal-sized meal [4]. Normally, the gastric fundus relaxes after eating creating a pleasant feeling of satiety, but if there is a failure of this normal vagal mechanism, then early satiety often occurs. Certain drugs that relax the gastric fundus can reduce PDS symptoms, including early satiety [5]. In addition to disordered motility, hypersensitivity to mechanical or chemical stimuli is frequently observed in FD, although as with gastric emptying the relationship between this and symptoms of dyspepsia is not completely understood [2].

There is increasing evidence that abnormalities in the duodenum may lead to FD, particularly PDS. Increased duodenal inflammation has been identified in a subset with PDS, most notably increased duodenal eosinophils [6] (defined as >22 eosinophils after counting 5 HPFs) (Fig. 8.1). Further, duodenal eosinophils in FD are associated with increased small intestinal permeability and changes in neuronal structure and function, which may explain intestinal hypersensitivity [7]. In some cases, mast cells can also be seen to be increased along with eosinophils, if special stains are applied [8]. Immune activation has been documented in FD (cytokines and circulating homing small intestinal T cells), and immune activation is associated with (and might explain) slow gastric emptying [1].

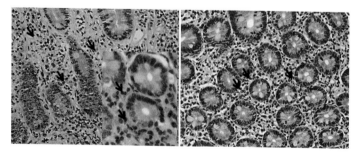

FIGURE 8.1 Duodenal mucosa, showing eosinophils in clusters in the lamina propria around glands (arrowed)

Although epigastric pain or burning can be a feature of FD, and some patients respond to acid suppression [9], gastric acid secretion is normal. Eradication therapy for *H. pylori* leads to complete symptom resolution in only a minority of FD patients. The FD subgroup most likely to respond reports EPS. This suggests epigastric pain may arise from gastric pathology in some FD cases.

Infections other than *H. pylori* may be associated with FD. As in irritable bowel syndrome (IBS), there is good evidence that FD can arise after an acute intestinal infection, such as *Salmonella* (post-infectious FD) [10]. It is therefore important to ask for a history of infective symptoms prior to the onset of dyspepsia, although this may be difficult to ascertain in most due to a delay in presentation.

Other putative mechanisms have been suggested and are current areas of investigation. For example, many patients with FD report that certain foods may induce symptoms, such as gluten. It is conceivable that, just as in celiac disease, there is an abnormal immune response to gliadin in FD [11, 12]. The gastroduodenal microbiome has been shown to be perturbed in patients with FD, when compared with non-FD patients. 'Normalisation' of gut flora through the use of probiotics may represent a potential therapeutic option, although a Japanese study that investigated this did not report on clinical outcomes [13]. An underlying genetic predisposition is possible but remains to be firmly established. For example, a subgroup with FD have clinical evidence of Ehlers-Danlos type III, but the genetics are unknown [14].

A summary of proposed disease mechanisms based on current understanding is presented in Table 8.1.

Symptoms

The key symptoms are early satiety, postprandial fullness (often described as bloating by patients, unless specific questioning is conducted), epigastric pain, and epigastric burning; these are now considered to constitute dyspepsia [15, 16]. Early satiety is common but is often missed unless specifically

TABLE 8.1 Proposed mechanisms for functional dyspepsia

Mechanism	Clinical significance
Duodenal inflammation (characterised by eosinophilia)	Present in up to 40% of patients and may be associated with early satiety and pain. May be improved with acid suppression
Infection	Certain infections may cause acute or post-infectious symptoms. Eradication of *H. pylori* alleviates symptoms in a minority of patients
Impaired gastric emptying	Present in one in five patients, but correlation with symptoms is unclear. Consider a trial of a prokinetic
Impaired gastric accommodation	Present in up to one-third of patients, particularly PDS, although correlation with symptoms is unclear
Gastric and duodenal hypersensitivity	Hypersensitivity to mechanical distension or chemical stimuli has been observed, but the relationship to symptoms is unclear
Food allergens	Food triggers should be sought. Gluten restriction may be helpful in a minority of patients
Psychosocial factors – brain-gut axis	A relationship between psychiatric disorders, particularly depression and anxiety, is common and should be sought in patients with FD
Genetic factors	An underlying genetic predisposition is possible
Gut microbiome	The small intestinal microbiome may be abnormal, but the role of small intestinal bacterial overgrowth is unclear

asked for whilst eliciting the patient's history. Patients often describe this as a vague discomfort or excess gas after eating, although what they really mean is that they cannot finish a normal-sized meal because they feel full or uncomfortable. Other symptoms may co-occur, including nausea and heartburn, but these are not considered primary dyspeptic symptoms any longer and may arise through separate mechanisms. Certain symptoms, such as vomiting, require evaluation for alternative or coexistent disease such as gastroparesis. The Rome IV criteria (Table 8.2) provides a symptom-based framework for diagnosing FD [2].

Diagnostic Evaluation

A careful history and examination should be performed in patients presenting with epigastric symptoms. Epigastric pain can arise from many other causes, including biliary and pancreatic pathology. If the pattern of the pain is suggestive (severe, episodic, lasting for hours, radiating to the back) or if there are risk factors for biliary tract disease, appropriate testing is indicated, but beware of false-positive results (e.g. abdominal ultrasound finding incidental gallstones). Peptic ulcers may cause EPS, or less often PDS, so a history of NSAID use and testing for *H. pylori* is a routine part of the evaluation as, in the absence of these risk factors, peptic ulcer disease is highly unlikely.

Current expert consensus recommends an EGD for any patient aged ≥60 years with dyspeptic symptoms, primarily to exclude gastroesophageal malignancy [17]. On the other hand, performing an EGD in younger patients with dyspepsia generally has a low yield, but should be considered on a case-by-case basis if certain 'alarm features' or 'red flags' are present. These include vomiting, dysphagia and/or odynophagia, evidence or suspicion of gastrointestinal bleeding, unexplained weight loss, a palpable mass or lymphadenopathy, or a family history of upper gastrointestinal malignancy [2, 17]. However, even in the presence of a red flag, few

TABLE 8.2 Rome IV criteria for functional dyspepsia

Functional dyspepsia (FD)
Diagnostic criteria

1. One or more of the following:
    a. Bothersome postprandial fullness
    b. Bothersome early satiety
    c. Bothersome epigastric pain
    d. Bothersome epigastric burning
and
2. No evidence of structural disease to explain symptoms

Postprandial distress syndrome (PDS)

Diagnostic criteria	Supportive remarks

1. Must include one or both of the following at least 3 days a week:
    a. Bothersome postprandial fullness
    b. Bothersome early satiety
and
2. No evidence of organic, systemic, or metabolic disease to explain symptoms
	Postprandial epigastric discomfort, epigastric bloating, excessive belching, and nausea may be present
	Vomiting should prompt consideration for alternative diagnoses
	Heartburn may coexist, but is not considered a dyspeptic symptom
	Symptoms that are relieved by evacuation of faeces or gas are not considered part of dyspepsia
	Other gastrointestinal disorders such as gastro-oesophageal reflux and irritable bowel may coexist with PDS

TABLE 8.2 (continued)

Functional dyspepsia (FD)

Epigastric pain syndrome (EPS)	
Diagnostic criteria	Supportive remarks

1. Must include at least one of the following symptoms at least 1 day a week
  a. Bothersome epigastric pain
and/or
  b. Bothersome epigastric burning
and
2. No evidence of organic, systemic, or metabolic disease to explain symptoms
	Pain has no clear relationship to meals and may be induced or alleviated after ingestion of a meal
	Postprandial epigastric bloating, belching and nausea may be present
	Vomiting should prompt consideration for alternative diagnoses
	Heartburn may coexist, but is not considered a dyspeptic symptom
	The pain does not fulfil biliary pain criteria
	Symptoms that are relieved by evacuation of faeces or gas are not considered part of dyspepsia
	Other gastrointestinal disorders such as gastro-oesophageal reflux and irritable bowel may coexist with EPS

Modified from Stanghellini et al. [2]

Notes: [a]The diagnosis of FD requires fulfilment of the criteria for PDS and/or EPS

[b]Criteria must be filled for at least 3 months with symptom onset at least 6 months before diagnosis

patients with typical FD symptoms will have malignancy identified at EGD [17].

Gastroparesis is rare, unlike FD [3]. If the patient is vomiting or losing weight, a gastric emptying study should be considered if the EGD and other tests are normal. However, it should be remembered that a mild degree of delayed gastric emptying is common in FD (20%) and is unlikely to adequately explain the symptoms [2].

GERD is common and overlaps with FD. This can make differentiating the two conditions troublesome. A rule of thumb is that the presence of early satiety most likely indicates true FD, not GERD. Some cases of PPI failure in patients thought to have non-erosive GERD are explained by misdiagnosis of FD as GERD [18]. IBS also overlaps with FD more than expected by chance, but altered bowel habits in association with bloating or pain characterise IBS, not FD. As with IBS, anxiety and less often depression are common in those with FD, and depression should be screened for, as its presence alters treatment. There is some evidence that these central nervous system disturbances may arise primarily from the gut in some cases, rather than the brain, indicating the communication is bidirectional [19].

Celiac disease is a great mimic and can present with dyspepsia. It is our practice to ask about wheat intolerance, check a complete blood count, and consider tissue transglutaminase testing for celiac disease. A diagnostic algorithm to workup suspected FD is shown in Fig. 8.2.

Treatment

A firm diagnosis, followed by reassurance, explanation, and a treatment plan work best in clinical practice. The prognosis is excellent, and FD is not linked to any increase in mortality [20]. A treatment algorithm is shown in Fig. 8.3.

Helicobacter Pylori

If *H. pylori* is detected, either by non-invasive means (e.g. breath test, stool antigen) or on biopsies during EGD, eradication therapy should be offered [21]. Patients should be counselled regarding potential side effects, and it is important to remember that the majority of patients with FD will not respond symptomatically to eradication (suggesting the *H. pylori* infection is often incidental and asymptomatic).

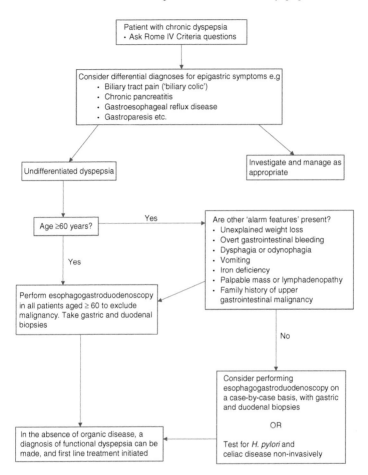

FIGURE 8.2 Diagnostic algorithm for functional dyspepsia

Acid Suppression

Acid suppression is otherwise first-line therapy [17]. A standard dose of a PPI before breakfast is superior to placebo. A double-dose PPI adds no established benefit. The mechanism by which a PPI works is unknown but may increase the duodenal pH, positively alter the microbiome, or possibly sup-

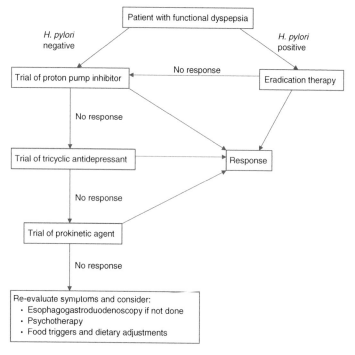

FIGURE 8.3 Treatment algorithm for functional dyspepsia

press duodenal eosinophils [22]. An alternative is a histamine type-2 receptor antagonist (H_2RA), although current evidence indicates that PPIs are slightly more effective, and the therapeutic effect of H_2RAs may wear off over time (tachyphylaxis).

Acid suppression appears to be more effective in PDS than in EPS, but given the significant overlap of these in real-world settings, and the potential for coexistent GERD, a trial of acid suppression is generally warranted in all patients with FD, regardless of subtype [9, 17].

Antidepressants

Tricyclic antidepressants (TCAs) are considered second-line therapy [17]. A systematic review found that the beneficial effect of antidepressants for treating FD was limited to TCAs, and highlighted the need to monitor for side effects [23].

Prokinetics

Trials that have compared prokinetic agents with PPI therapy in FD showed a trend towards PPIs being more effective. As such, prokinetic therapy is a potential second-line option [17]. In the USA, prokinetic options are limited, as most of the drugs that were evaluated in randomised trials (e.g. cisapride and mosapride) are not currently available. Prokinetic agents used to treat gastroparesis (e.g. metoclopramide, domperidone) have limited data regarding their efficacy in FD. Acotiamide, which acts by enhancing the release and duration of enteric acetylcholine, has been shown to be superior to placebo in reducing PDS symptoms and is currently available in Japan and India [5, 24].

Further Options

The non-absorbable antibiotic rifaximin provided relief of FD symptoms in one clinical trial, but the duration of benefit is unknown [25]. The benefit of probiotics has not been established. Herbal products such as peppermint oil and STW-5 (Iberogast) may also be of benefit in some patients.

Dietary therapy may be helpful. Just as in IBS, a diet low in fermentable oligo-, di-, and monosaccharides and polyols appears to help some cases, but randomised controlled trial evidence in FD is lacking. Food triggers should be considered, as some patients may respond to gluten restriction (those with early satiety in particular) [12]. Psychological therapies can help some patients, particularly if there is comorbid psychological distress, and we refer for cognitive behavioural therapy if patients are responding poorly. Depression should be treated if present.

Case Study: Follow-Up

As the patient was concerned about the potential side effects of PPI long term, she was switched to a H_2RA and reported substantial benefit initially, although this waned over months. A low dose of amitriptyline (starting at 10 mg at night for 1 month, then 25 mg for 1 month, then increasing to 50 mg at night for 6 months) was well-tolerated, improved sleep, and reduced all dyspeptic symptoms.

Clinical Pearls

- If a patient reports early satiety (remembering you need to ask specifically about this complaint), think about underlying FD high up on your differential diagnosis list.
- Increased duodenal eosinophils are linked to FD, particularly PDS – but you must ask your pathologist to count 5 high-power fields in order to detect the abnormality, otherwise this will be missed.
- A young patient (<60 years) with dyspeptic symptoms and no alarm features, no relevant drug history (e.g. NSAIDs), and no evidence of *H. pylori* on non-invasive testing has FD until proven otherwise; EGD then has a low yield. EGD should be performed in patients ≥60 years of age, and on a case-by-case basis in younger patients with alarm features.
- First-line therapeutic options for FD are acid suppression or, if *H. pylori* infected, eradication therapy.
- Low-dose tricyclic antidepressants and prokinetics are second-line options.

Self-Test

Question 1. A 45-year-old man consults regarding a 5-year history of epigastric discomfort, described as burning in nature. Early in its course, the pain was intermittent and tended to occur after meals, although he feels that it is occurring more frequently in recent times. He had a poor response to a PPI. In addition, he has noticed his stools have become increasingly loose and offensive and at times are difficult to flush. EGD with gastric and duodenal biopsies 2 years ago on a normal diet were unremarkable.

Which of the following investigations is most likely to help establish a diagnosis?

A. Repeat EGD and duodenal biopsies.
B. Urease breath test for *H. pylori*
C. Abdominal CT scan
D. Glucose hydrogen breath test
E. Celiac serology

Question 2. You are reviewing a 35-year-old female who has returned for follow-up after a normal EGD for symptoms of moderately severe persistent dyspepsia, with normal bowel habits. Gastric biopsies were normal, without evidence of *H. pylori*. Duodenal biopsies demonstrated an eosinophil count of 30/hpf, on at least 5 high-power fields. There were no typical changes of coeliac disease.
You make a diagnosis of FD, likely PDS, and discuss management options. Which of the following would you recommend as first-line based on randomised controlled trials?

A. Trial of PPI
B. Low FODMAP diet and psychotherapy
C. Trial of a TCA
D. No treatment indicated – reassurance and discharge to primary care physician
E. H_2RA

Question 3. The Rome IV criteria provide a symptom-based framework for the diagnosis of functional dyspepsia (FD) and its subtypes. Which of the following symptoms is *least* likely to occur in functional dyspepsia, and should alert clinicians to an alternative diagnosis?

A. Excessive belching
B. Heartburn less than once a week
C. Frequent postprandial vomiting
D. Nausea
E. Early satiety

References

1. Talley NJ, Ford AC. Functional dyspepsia. N Engl J Med. 2015;373(19):1853–63.
2. Stanghellini V, Chan FKL, Hasler WL, Malagelada JR, Suzuki H, Tack J, et al. Gastroduodenal disorders. Gastroenterology. 2016;150(6):1380–92.
3. Tack J, Carbone F. Functional dyspepsia and gastroparesis. Curr Opin Gastroenterol. 2017;33(6):446–54.
4. Carbone F, Tack J. Gastroduodenal mechanisms underlying functional gastric disorders. Dig Dis. 2014;32(3):222–9.
5. Ueda M, Iwasaki E, Suzuki H. Profile of acotiamide in the treatment of functional dyspepsia. Clin Exp Gastroenterol. 2016;9:83–8.
6. Walker MM, Aggarwal KR, Shim LSE, Bassan M, Kalantar JS, Weltman MD, et al. Duodenal eosinophilia and early satiety in functional dyspepsia: confirmation of a positive association in an Australian cohort. J Gastroenterol Hepatol. 2014;29(3):474–9.
7. Cirillo C, Bessissow T, Desmet A-S, Vanheel H, Tack J, Vanden Berghe P. Evidence for neuronal and structural changes in submucous ganglia of patients with functional dyspepsia. Am J Gastroenterol. 2015;110:1205.
8. Walker MM, Talley NJ, Prabhakar M, Pennaneac'H CJ, Aro P, Ronkainen J, et al. Duodenal mastocytosis, eosinophilia and intraepithelial lymphocytosis as possible disease markers in the irritable bowel syndrome and functional dyspepsia. Aliment Pharmacol Ther. 2009;29(7):765–73.

9. Pinto-Sanchez MI, Yuan Y, Hassan A, Bercik P, Moayyedi P. Proton pump inhibitors for functional dyspepsia. Cochrane Database Syst Rev. 2017;11:CD011194.

10. Mearin F, Pérez-Oliveras M, Perelló A, Vinyet J, Ibañez A, Coderch J, Perona M. Dyspepsia and irritable bowel syndrome after a Salmonella gastroenteritis outbreak: one-year follow-up cohort study. Gastroenterology. 2005;129(1):98–104.

11. Potter M, Walker MM, Talley NJ. Non-coeliac gluten or wheat sensitivity: emerging disease or misdiagnosis? Med J Aust. 2017;207(5):211–5.

12. Du L, Shen J, Kim JJ, He H, Chen B, Dai N. Impact of gluten consumption in patients with functional dyspepsia: a case–control study. J Gastroenterol Hepatol. 2018;33(1):128–33.

13. Igarashi M, Nakae H, Matsuoka T, Takahashi S, Hisada T, Tomita J, et al. Alteration in the gastric microbiota and its restoration by probiotics in patients with functional dyspepsia. BMJ Open Gastroenterol. 2017;4(1):e000144.

14. Fikree A, Chelimsky G, Collins H, Kovacic K, Aziz Q. Gastrointestinal involvement in the Ehlers–Danlos syndromes. Am J Med Genet C: Semin Med Genet. 2017;175(1):181–7.

15. Vakil NB, Howden CW, Moayyedi P, Tack J. White paper AGA: functional dyspepsia. Clinical Gastroenterol Hepatol. 2017;15(8):1191–4.

16. Enck P, Azpiroz F, Boeckxstaens G, Elsenbruch S, Feinle-Bisset C, Holtmann G, et al. Functional dyspepsia. Nat Rev Dis Primers. 2017;3:17081.

17. Moayyedi PM, Lacy BE, Andrews CN, Enns RA, Howden CW, Vakil N. ACG and CAG clinical guideline: management of dyspepsia. Am J Gastroenterol. 2017;112:988.

18. D'Alessandro A, Zito F, Pesce M, Andreozzi P, Efficie E, Cargiolli M, et al. Specific dyspeptic symptoms are associated with poor response to therapy in patients with gastroesophageal reflux disease. United European Gastroenterol J. 2017;5(1):54–9.

19. Koloski NA, Jones M, Talley NJ. Evidence that independent gut-to-brain and brain-to-gut pathways operate in the irritable bowel syndrome and functional dyspepsia: a 1-year population-based prospective study. Aliment Pharmacol Ther. 2016;44(6):592–600.

20. Ford AC, Forman D, Bailey AG, Axon ATR, Moayyedi P. Effect of dyspepsia on survival: a longitudinal 10-year follow-up study. Am J Gastroenterol. 2012;107:912.

21. Chey WD, Leontiadis GI, Howden CW, Moss SF. ACG clinical guideline: treatment of helicobacter pylori infection. Am J Gastroenterol. 2017;112:212.

22. Jackson MA, Goodrich JK, Maxan M-E, Freedberg DE, Abrams JA, Poole AC, et al. Proton pump inhibitors alter the composition of the gut microbiota. Gut. 2016;65(5):749–56.

23. Ford AC, Luthra P, Tack J, Boeckxstaens GE, Moayyedi P, Talley NJ. Efficacy of psychotropic drugs in functional dyspepsia: systematic review and meta-analysis. Gut. 2017;66(3):411–20.

24. Kusunoki H, Haruma K, Manabe N, Imamura H, Kamada T, Shiotani A, et al. Therapeutic efficacy of acotiamide in patients with functional dyspepsia based on enhanced postprandial gastric accommodation and emptying: randomized controlled study evaluation by real-time ultrasonography. Neurogastroenterol Motil. 2012;24(6):540–e251.

25. Tan VPY, Liu KSH, Lam FYF, Hung IFN, Yuen MF, Leung WK. Randomised clinical trial: rifaximin versus placebo for the treatment of functional dyspepsia. Aliment Pharmacol Ther. 2017;45(6):767–76.

Essential Reading

Moayyedi PM, Lacy BE, Andrews CN, Enns RA, Howden CW, Vakil N. ACG and CAG clinical guideline: management of dyspepsia. Am J Gastroenterol. 2017;112:988. Evidence-based guidelines for the diagnosis and management of patients with dyspepsia.

Stanghellini V, Chan FKL, Hasler WL, Malagelada JR, Suzuki H, Tack J, et al. Gastroduodenal disorders. Gastroenterol. 2016;150(6):1380–92. Provides a detailed overview of FD and other functional disorders, with reference to the Rome IV Criteria.

Talley NJ, Ford AC. Functional dyspepsia. N Engl J Med. 2015;373(19):1853–63. Expert overview of FD with explanation of disease mechanisms and discussion of relevant clinical trials.

Chapter 9
Rumination Syndrome

Neelima Bonthi, Magnus Halland, and David A. Katzka

Case Study

A 25-year-old man is referred for evaluation of refractory gastroesophageal reflux symptoms. His history started 1 year ago when he noted the onset of regurgitation of his meal immediately and for up to 30 min, following eating. This started intermittently, but within months started to occur with every meal. He does not describe the regurgitant as sour or acidic, and he does not experience heartburn. The food would commonly come up into his mouth, at which point he will either expectorate it or re-swallow it. The regurgitation does not appear related to the size of the meal and may occur with as little as a glass of water. There are no nocturnal symptoms, and he has not lost weight. He has become fearful of eating in social situations because of these symptoms. He saw his primary care physician, who prescribed omeprazole 40 mg

N. Bonthi · M. Halland · D. A. Katzka (✉)
Division of Gastroenterology and Hepatology, Mayo Clinic,
Rochester, MN, USA
e-mail: Katzka.david@mayo.edu

© Springer Nature Switzerland AG 2019
B. E. Lacy et al. (eds.), *Essential Medical Disorders of the Stomach and Small Intestine*,
https://doi.org/10.1007/978-3-030-01117-8_9

before breakfast, but his symptoms have not abated. A subsequent endoscopy was normal. He was referred to a thoracic surgeon for fundoplication but is coming to you for a second opinion. His past medical history is unremarkable. He denies cigarette use and drinks one beer per week. He is an attorney for the city government and exercises regularly. Physical examination was unremarkable.

Objectives

- Understand the clinical criteria by which rumination syndrome is diagnosed.
- Be able to differentiate rumination syndrome from unresponsive gastroesophageal reflux disease (GERD).
- Understand the pathophysiology of rumination syndrome.
- Understand the use of testing in rumination syndrome, particularly esophageal manometry as an objective means of diagnosis, and administering biofeedback therapy.

Epidemiology

The prevalence of rumination syndrome is unclear, given how few epidemiologic studies have been performed. It is more common in children, young adults, patients with fibromyalgia or eating disorders, and patients with pelvic floor dysfunction and constipation [1–5]. This last group has been termed REDRUM syndrome, representing a combination of rectal evacuation disorder and rumination [6]. Rumination is also more common in patients with learning or developmental delay disorders [7]. The incidence of rumination may also vary geographically. For example, studies from Colombia reported a prevalence of 5% [8], in contrast to Mexico [9] and Australia [1], where prevalence is <1%. Whether this truly represents different racial or geographic predispositions or more careful or different diagnostic criteria is unclear. Nevertheless, many, if not most, patients with rumination syndrome do not have evident medical or psychologic predisposing factors [10]. Finally, it is also likely that under-recognition of rumination leads to underestimation of its true prevalence.

Etiology and Pathophysiology

The etiology of rumination syndrome is unknown [11]. It appears to be a subconscious learned response, but a clear initiating event is not typically identified. The subconscious nature of this behavior is reinforced by an inability of normal subjects to induce rumination. The abnormal physiology is defined by an augmentation in gastric pressure, and a reduction in both the lower esophageal sphincter (LES) and upper esophageal sphincter (UES) pressures (Fig. 9.1) [12, 13]. With a gastric pressure that is higher than these sphincter pressures, there is a gradient that forces retrograde flow of the

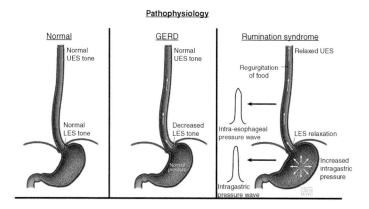

FIGURE 9.1 Pathophysiology of GERD and rumination syndrome. During or after a meal in: (**a**) normal person, (**b**) GERD (after 1 h) (**c**) Rumination syndrome (within 10–30 mins or during a meal). (Used with permission of Mayo Foundation for Medical Education and Research, all rights reserved)

stomach content proximally into the mouth [12, 13]. Whether this increase in gastric pressure is primary or passively transmitted through a rise in intra-abdominal pressure is unclear. The correlation of increased electromyographic (EMG) changes in the abdominal wall, concordant with rumination episodes, and the favorable response of rumination to diaphragmatic breathing supports the latter [14, 15]. A rumination event will only occur when all three of these pressure changes occur simultaneously. An isolated increase in gastric pressure is unlikely to be of sufficient magnitude to overcome a normal LES pressure. Further study of rumination has proposed three subtypes. Specifically, rumination may follow reflux events, supragastric belches, and classic rumination episodes in isolation. Each of these three types is associated with gastric strain. However, there is no clear data that demonstrates abnormalities of gastric motility, such as poor accommodation or delayed emptying, associated with increased pressure events.

Symptoms

The Rome diagnostic criteria to define rumination are persistent or recurrent regurgitation of recently ingested food into the mouth, with subsequent spitting, or remastication and swallowing. The regurgitation is not preceded by retching [16]. Supportive criteria include the fact that regurgitation events are usually not preceded by nausea, there is cessation of the process when the regurgitated material becomes acidic, and the regurgitant contains recognizable food with a pleasant taste. Using this as a starting template, patients with rumination may present with numerous variations including regurgitation of both liquids and solids, small- or large-volume regurgitation, symptoms that are independent of meal size, a sense of substernal reflux of gastric content, and usually maintenance of weight, although weight loss may be seen in up to 40% of patients. Another striking feature is the consistency of the symptoms occurring with virtually every meal in these patients. This consistency in symptoms often leads patients to a sense of complacency about their symptoms. Patients with rumination syndrome do not respond to therapy with proton pump inhibitors (PPIs); in fact PPI therapy may worsen symptoms in some patients, as the regurgitant remains non-acid for a longer period after meals. Indeed, rumination syndrome should be considered in the differential diagnosis of PPI refractory GERD. One of the most notable findings lacking in rumination syndrome is the absence of nocturnal symptoms, which is consistent with the need for a daytime unperceived increase in abdominal pressure in order to facilitate regurgitation. In addition to the postprandial regurgitation symptoms, dyspeptic symptoms such as early satiety, bloating, and epigastric discomfort are common among patients with rumination syndrome, and these also appear to lessen with treatment [13].

Diagnostic Evaluation

The diagnosis of rumination syndrome is most commonly made by a history that fulfills the Rome criteria, without concerning warning signs such as weight loss, nocturnal symptoms, chest pain, or severe heartburn (Fig. 9.2). One of the most helpful means of confirming the diagnosis is to observe the patient in your clinic during and after a meal. The clinical appearance of rumination episodes is different than reflux or regurgitation. One may also witness visible air swallowing preceding the regurgitation. Nevertheless, at times it can be difficult to distinguish rumination syndrome from regurgitation secondary to achalasia or GERD (Table 9.1). As a result, a well-performed esophagogram, or high-resolution esophageal manometry, can help exclude achalasia. In addition, adding a postprandial component to a high-resolution esophageal manometry can be used to objectively diagnose rumination. The most common feature is gastric strain >30 mmHg, manifest by a rapid-onset high-amplitude contraction originating from the stomach and migrating proximally with a pan-esophageal distribution [17]. This is typically accompanied by

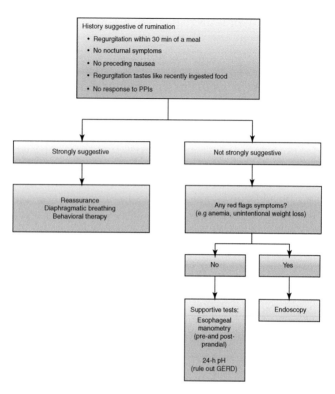

FIGURE 9.2 Diagnostic algorithm for rumination syndrome. (Used with permission of Mayo Foundation for Medical Education and Research, all rights reserved)

TABLE 9.1 Comparison of symptoms of rumination syndrome and disorders that may be confused with rumination

Etiology	Symptoms
Rumination syndrome	Regurgitation of normal tasting food during a meal or within 30 min of eating a meal, no nocturnal symptoms, halitosis
GERD	Regurgitation of sour/bitter tasting food after 1 h of eating a meal, nausea, nocturnal symptoms
Gastroparesis	Nausea, vomiting, and abdominal pain
Achalasia	Postprandial regurgitation, dysphagia, usually without re-swallowing

a retrograde flow of gastric contents into the esophagus, which can be detected by impedance [18, 19]. In addition to rapid increases in gastric pressure, other findings typically noted during this type of study during rumination events include a marked reduction in both LES and UES pressure [12], allowing regurgitation of content into the mouth. Although esophageal manometry is uncomfortable, and adding a meal challenge with the catheter in situ even more so, this provides the best opportunity to correlate symptoms with abnormal gastroesophageal physiology [12].

Treatment

Several treatments are used for rumination syndrome (Table 9.2). The most common is behavioral therapy with diaphragmatic breathing. The conversation starts with an explanation of the mechanism of rumination as an abnormal postprandial reflex of increased gastric pressure occurring with an increase in abdominal muscle tone, simultaneous with relaxation of the esophageal sphincters, allowing retrograde flow of gastric content. The main goal of diaphragmatic therapy is to reduce abdominal wall tone and increase the crural component of the LES during and after eating [12, 15]. Diaphragmatic breathing may be taught formally through biofeedback with EMG monitoring of the abdominal musculature [15], for the patient to see when they are successfully relaxing the abdominal wall, but as this technique is confined

TABLE 9.2 Rumination syndrome treatment options

Treatment of rumination syndrome
Behavioral therapy: diaphragmatic breathing is very effective, with good results noted within hours to weeks
Refractory symptoms: baclofen 10 mg thrice daily increases LES tone. Dose adjustment may be needed, based on central nervous system side effects, including drowsiness and dizziness
Treatment with uncertain benefit: surgery, with Nissen fundoplication

to a few expert centers, most patients are given simple instructions. The technique can be taught by the physician or any member of the physician care team [20]. Reinforcement of the technique is available through multiple Internet and multidisciplinary sources (e.g., yoga instructors, psychologists, voice therapists). The basic maneuver is teaching the patient to breathe with their diaphragm, rather than their chest. This is done by asking them to sit in a relaxed position, placing one hand on their abdomen and the other on their chest. The patient breathes by allowing the hand on the abdomen to move out with inspiration, while the hand on the chest remains still. Inspirations should be steady and deep, aiming for six to eight per minute. Sometimes it is helpful to ask patients to use a similar breathing pattern to when they are trying to go to sleep. Ideally the patient should learn to do this breathing while eating, and in the postprandial period, for as long as they feel rumination might occur. Alternatively, some patients can use the breathing when they sense the onset of regurgitation of food. At the beginning of therapy, patients are also instructed to practice diaphragmatic breathing as much as they can, whether eating or not. For some patients, where either confirmation of the diagnosis or proof of proper performance of the technique is needed, esophageal manometry may be performed during, and after, the postprandial period for therapy [12]. The patient is asked to alternate periods of regular and diaphragmatic breathing with observation of gastric pressure. The decrease in gastric pressurizations with proper diaphragmatic breathing can be easily seen by the patient and physician and appreciated when the favorable effects of the breathing are accompanied by a reduction in rumination episodes during monitoring.

There has been little experimentation with medications. One randomized trial demonstrated that preprandial baclofen may reduce rumination episodes [21]. Agents that enhance gastric accommodation, such as buspirone [22], may be tried, but there are no specific data determining their efficacy. Fundoplication has been tried in patients who are refractory to all other therapies [23].

Case Study: Follow-Up

This patient was diagnosed with rumination syndrome by the history and by observing the patient ruminate and re-swallow food in front of the physician multiple times. As a result, it was determined that no further diagnostic evaluation was needed. The patient was scheduled for a return appointment and asked to bring a meal. At this time, more detail was given on the pathophysiology of rumination syndrome and the principals by which diaphragmatic breathing can be effective. He was then taught over a 10-min period how to breathe with his diaphragm. After he learned this technique successfully, he was instructed to eat his meal and continue the breathing technique for 15 min. It was immediately noticeable to the patient that the episodes of regurgitation ceased. The patient was sent home and asked to continue to assiduously practice diaphragmatic breathing both while fasting and with meals, for the next 2 months. At follow-up, the patient noted a 90% reduction in the number of rumination episodes and was satisfied.

Clinical Pearls

- Rumination syndrome is likely a subconscious learned reflex of the patient during, and after, a meal in which there is an increase in gastric pressure transmitted through the abdominal wall, which is of sufficient magnitude to push gastric content against gravity through a hypotonic LES and UES.
- Rumination syndrome is best diagnosed by a careful history, but occasionally objective testing is needed to rule out other disorders and/or to confirm the diagnosis.
- Rumination differs from other disorders of regurgitation, such as achalasia or GERD, in that it is not dependent on the size of the meal, does not worsen in the supine position, is consistent at most meals, and is often not bothersome to the patient.

- The best treatment for rumination syndrome is diaphragmatic breathing to reverse the gastroesophageal pressure gradient. It is easily taught, and is highly effective, but requires practice.

Self-Test

Question 1. In order for an episode of rumination to occur, which of the following events must occur?

A. Decrease in UES pressure
B. Decrease in LES pressure
C. Increase in gastric pressure
D. All of the above

Question 2. The diagnosis of rumination is best made by which of the following?

A. A careful history
B. Barium esophagography
C. Ambulatory pH/impedance monitoring
D. Endoscopy

Question 3. Which of the following medications have been demonstrated to be effective in rumination syndrome?

A. Omeprazole
B. Hyoscyamine
C. Baclofen
D. Buspirone

References

1. Koloski NA, Talley NJ, Boyce PM. Epidemiology and health care seeking in the functional GI disorders: a population-based study. Am J Gastroenterol. 2002;97(9):2290–9.
2. Wang X, Luscombe GM, Boyd C, Kellow J, Abraham S. Functional gastrointestinal disorders in eating disorder patients: altered dis-

tribution and predictors using ROME III compared to ROME II criteria. World J Gastroenterol. 2014;20(43):16293–9.

3. Almansa C, Rey E, Sanchez RG, Sanchez AA, Diaz-Rubio M. Prevalence of functional gastrointestinal disorders in patients with fibromyalgia and the role of psychologic distress. Clin Gastroenterol Hepatol. 2009;7(4):438–45.

4. Rosen R, Rodriguez L, Nurko S. Pediatric rumination subtypes: A study using high-resolution esophageal manometry with impedance. Neurogastroenterol Motil. 2017;29(5):1–9.

5. Khan S, Hyman PE, Cocjin J, Di Lorenzo C. Rumination syndrome in adolescents. J Pediatr. 2000;136(4):528–31.

6. Vijayvargiya P, Iturrino J, Camilleri M, Shin A, Vazquez-Roque M, Katzka DA, et al. Novel association of rectal evacuation disorder and rumination syndrome: diagnosis, co-morbidities and treatment. United European Gastroenterol J. 2014;2(1):38–46.

7. Rogers B, Stratton P, Victor J, Kennedy B, Andres M. Chronic regurgitation among persons with mental retardation: a need for combined medical and interdisciplinary strategies. Am J Ment Retard. 1992;96(5):522–7.

8. Chogle A, Velasco-Benitez CA, Koppen IJ, Moreno JE, Ramirez Hernandez CR, Saps M. A population-based study on the epidemiology of functional gastrointestinal disorders in young children. J Pediatr. 2016;179:139–43. e1.

9. Lopez-Colombo A, Morgan D, Bravo-Gonzalez D, Montiel-Jarquin A, Mendez-Martinez S, Schmulson M. The epidemiology of functional gastrointestinal disorders in Mexico: a population-based study. Gastroenterol Res Pract. 2012;2012:606174.

10. Lee H, Rhee PL, Park EH, Kim JH, Son HJ, Kim JJ, et al. Clinical outcome of rumination syndrome in adults without psychiatric illness: a prospective study. J Gastroenterol Hepatol. 2007;22(11):1741–7.

11. O'Brien MD, Bruce BK, Camilleri M. The rumination syndrome: clinical features rather than manometric diagnosis. Gastroenterology. 1995;108(4):1024–9.

12. Halland M, Parthasarathy G, Bharucha AE, Katzka DA. Diaphragmatic breathing for rumination syndrome: efficacy and mechanisms of action. Neurogastroenterol Motil. 2016;28(3):384–91.

13. Absah I, Rishi A, Talley NJ, Katzka D, Halland M. Rumination syndrome: pathophysiology, diagnosis, and treatment. Neurogastroenterol Motil. 2017;29(4):1–8.

14. Barba E, Accarino A, Soldevilla A, Malagelada JR, Azpiroz F. Randomized, placebo-controlled trial of biofeed-

back for the treatment of rumination. Am J Gastroenterol. 2016;111(7):1007–13.

15. Barba E, Burri E, Accarino A, Malagelada C, Rodriguez-Urrutia A, Soldevilla A, et al. Biofeedback-guided control of abdominothoracic muscular activity reduces regurgitation episodes in patients with rumination. Clin Gastroenterol Hepatol. 2015;13(1):100–6. e1.

16. Schmulson MJ, Drossman DA. What is new in Rome IV. J Neurogastroenterol Motil. 2017;23(2):151–63.

17. Amarnath RP, Abell TL, Malagelada JR. The rumination syndrome in adults. A characteristic manometric pattern. Ann Intern Med. 1986;105(4):513–8.

18. Kessing BF, Bredenoord AJ, Smout AJ. Objective manometric criteria for the rumination syndrome. Am J Gastroenterol. 2014;109(1):52–9.

19. Kessing BF, Govaert F, Masclee AA, Conchillo JM. Impedance measurements and high-resolution manometry help to better define rumination episodes. Scand J Gastroenterol. 2011;46(11):1310–5.

20. Chitkara DK, Van Tilburg M, Whitehead WE, Talley NJ. Teaching diaphragmatic breathing for rumination syndrome. Am J Gastroenterol. 2006;101(11):2449–52.

21. Pauwels A, Broers C, Van Houtte B, Rommel N, Vanuytsel T, Tack J. A randomized double-blind, placebo-controlled, crossover study using baclofen in the treatment of rumination syndrome. Am J Gastroenterol. 2018;113(1):97–104.

22. Tack J, Janssen P, Masaoka T, Farre R, Van Oudenhove L. Efficacy of buspirone, a fundus-relaxing drug, in patients with functional dyspepsia. Clin Gastroenterol Hepatol. 2012;10(11):1239–45.

23. Oelschlager BK, Chan MM, Eubanks TR, Pope CE 2nd, Pellegrini CA. Effective treatment of rumination with Nissen fundoplication. J Gastrointest Surg. 2002;6(4):638–44.

Essential Reading

Barba E, Accarino A, Soldevilla A, Malagelada J-RR, Azpiroz F. Randomized, placebo-controlled trial of biofeedback for the treatment of rumination. Am J Gastroenterol. 2016;111(7):1007–13. This study demonstrates the efficacy of biofeedback for rumination syndrome.

Chitkara DK, Tilburg M, Whitehead WE, Talley NJ. Teaching diaphragmatic breathing for rumination syndrome. Am J Gastroenterol. 2006;101(11):2449–52. This article instructs clinicians how to teach diaphragmatic breathing in the office.

Halland M, Parthasarathy G, Bharucha AE, Katzka DA. Diaphragmatic breathing for rumination syndrome: efficacy and mechanisms of action. Neurogastroenterol Motil. 2016;28(3):384–91. This study demonstrates the pathophysiology of rumination syndrome and how diaphragmatic breathing works.

Chapter 10
Gas-Bloat Syndrome

Carolina Malagelada and Juan R. Malagelada

Case Study

A 42-year-old female patient presents for consultation at the gastroenterology outpatient clinic with the main symptom of painful upper abdominal distension. Relevant past medical history included atopic features in childhood (eczematous type rash and asthma) which remitted after age 10. When she was approximately 34 years old, following her first pregnancy, she developed frequent postprandial heartburn and subsequent diagnostic evaluation showed abnormal gastro-esophageal reflux, associated with a small hiatal hernia and grade B esophagitis on endoscopy. She was advised to control her symptomatic reflux condition with omeprazole 20 mg, initially on demand, and later on a daily basis. Although her heartburn was reasonably well controlled by the proton pump inhibitor, she experienced nightly episodes

C. Malagelada · J. R. Malagelada (✉)
Digestive System Research Unit, University Hospital Vall d'Hebron, Barcelona, Spain

Centro de Investigación Biomédica en Red de Enfermedades Hepáticas y Digestivas (Ciberehd), Barcelona, Spain

© Springer Nature Switzerland AG 2019
B. E. Lacy et al. (eds.), *Essential Medical Disorders of the Stomach and Small Intestine*,
https://doi.org/10.1007/978-3-030-01117-8_10

187

of heartburn and regurgitation that frightened and distressed her. Thus, at age 38 she underwent a surgical Nissen fundoplication that ameliorated her reflux symptoms considerably. After a brief period of post-fundoplication dysphagia, which subsided spontaneously, she began experiencing very uncomfortable postprandial bloating, initially restricted to the upper abdomen but gradually becoming more diffuse and accompanied by a remarkable abdominal distension that "made her look as though she was pregnant." At the same time, she began perceiving air-fluid sounds inside the abdomen, postprandial fullness with a feeling of "slow digestion," and flatulence that did not seem to decrease the bloating sensation or modify the accompanying abdominal distension.

Objectives

- Recognize key manifestations of the gas-bloat syndrome.
- Learn the relevant background features of the medical history.
- Understand the mechanisms of bloating and abdominal distension.
- Review treatment options for affected individuals.

Epidemiology

Many healthy people occasionally feel bloated, particularly after indulging in heavy meals. This type of bloating, although annoying, rarely elicits concern because it is regarded by most individuals as "normal." Even so, some individuals will request medical consultation on the grounds that it curtails their freedom to overindulge and binge without discomfort. However, medically significant gas-bloat syndrome refers to patients, as in the case study above, who experience chronic recurrent symptoms, which may reach a disabling level, and occur on a persistent basis, and not exclusively following heavy meals [1]. This type of clearly pathologic gas-bloat syndrome is much less common and deserves focused clinical management. However, precise figures about its prevalence are unavailable.

Etiology and Pathophysiology

The gas-bloat syndrome is usually caused by several interacting disease mechanisms (Table 10.1) although the relative weight of participating pathophysiological components varies considerably among affected individuals (Fig. 10.1). The most relevant are described below:

(a) *Excess accumulation of exogenous air and/or fluid inside the gastrointestinal tract*

Aerophagia is a term that refers to excess swallowing of air, potentially inducing bloating and distension. However, most aerophagics rapidly expel the swallowed air through their mouth or through the anus since air advancing from the stomach into the upper small bowel is rapidly cleared forward. Thus, aerophagia most often manifests clinically as chronic belching and/or excess flatulence rather than as bloating. However, there is a subset of individuals who show impaired disposal of intestinally infused gas loads [2]. When there is an imbalance between gas entering the gastrointestinal tract and gas clearance, there is a potential for developing bloating (which reflects both increased bowel wall tension and/or heightened perception) and abdominal distension intra-luminal gas (which determines expansion of the bowel) (Fig. 10.2).

Other intra-luminal components, besides gas, may distend the bowel and produce or accentuate the same phenomenon. Slowly absorbed carbohydrates such as fructose and mannitol may increase intestinal water content [3]. The presence of intra-luminal lipids, especially after heavy fatty meals, greatly increases gas retention and the sensation of bloating [2].

TABLE 10.1 Mechanisms of bloating and abdominal distension

Stretching gut walls

Stomach: swallowed air and CO_2

Intestine: expansion by intra-luminal fluid retained by osmotically active molecules

Colon: constipation with retained stool, gas accumulation

Increased perception of gut wall tension

Inflamed tissues

Neurosensitization

Gut wall

Autonomic nervous system, spinal pathways

Brain: stress emotion, anxiety, hypervigilance, somatization

Extraintestinal tissues and influences

Circadian pattern

Perimenstrual

Intra-abdominal adipose tissue increase

Abdominal reshaping by aberrant viscera-somatic responses

Intercostal muscle contraction with thoracic expansion

Diaphragmatic muscle contraction and descent

Anterior abdominal muscle relaxation

Another key factor is the accumulation of retained stool in the large bowel of constipated individuals. Fecal intra-colonic impaction may even slow down small bowel transit and further increase bloating, as evidenced by human experimental data on bloating induced by an oral load of psyllium which is a bulky, yet not fermentable, form of fiber [4].

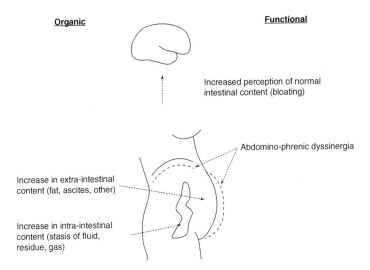

Organic

Functional

Increased perception of normal intestinal content (bloating)

Abdomino-phrenic dyssinergia

Increase in extra-intestinal content (fat, ascites, other)

Increase in intra-intestinal content (stasis of fluid, residue, gas)

FIGURE 10.1 Schematic representation of organic and functional causes of abdominal distension

(b) *Other sources of excess intra-luminal gas*

Endogenous generation of gas inside the bowel is another important factor potentially expanding the bowel with increased bowel wall tension, heightened perception, and abdominal distension. Excess intra-luminal gas production may be caused by bacteria in the small intestine (i.e., small intestine bowel overgrowth (SIBO)), by increased fermentation of intra-luminal substrates via an increased load of unabsorbed fermentable components of the diet or via modifications of the colonic microbiome with relative increases in gas-producing or reductions in gas-consuming bacterial species [5].

Impaired bowel gas-diffusion, particularly in the large bowel, may be another important factor resulting in increased intra-luminal gas. Both impaired blood flow, as in chronic ischemia, and mucosal low-grade inflammation may be responsible for diminished gas permeability.

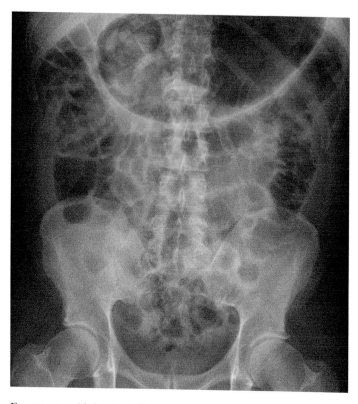

FIGURE 10.2 Abdominal distension caused by a marked increase in gastrointestinal gas content. This abdominal X-ray was performed during an acute episode of painful abdominal distension in a patient with a previous Nissen fundoplication. A CT scan was also performed and ruled out mechanical obstruction

(c) *Distorted perception of intestinal wall tension*

Differences in gas volume between symptomatic and asymptomatic individuals, and during symptomatic and asymptomatic periods in affected individuals, are minimal, but visceral hypersensitivity intervenes to induce a heightened conscious perception (bloating) [6] and to activate, as we will describe later, aberrant viscero-somatic reflexes that induce abdominal expansion (distension) [7].

The relevance of visceral hypersensitivity to the development of bloating and distension is highlighted by observations in patients with advanced intestinal neuropathy and enteric dysmotility, who may greatly distend their abdomens by a substantially different mechanism. In their case, symptomatic abdominal distension is directly produced by intraluminal accumulation of gas and other content due to ineffective peristalsis.

Visceral perception is modulated by a number of central mechanisms that influence the magnitude and character of bloating. In this regard, emotion and cognitive pain modulation are interlinked, helping to explain the relevance of stress, anxiety, and other psychological mood changes on central reception and representation of nociceptive inputs arising from the gut [8]. Bloating and its perceived intensity may, therefore, depend on a complex interaction between local gut conditions and multiple modulatory influences arranged along the gut-brain axis.

(d) *Other intra-abdominal organs and tissues*

Extraintestinal tissues inside the abdominal cavity may potentially influence the perception of bloating and abdominal distension. In particular, intra-abdominal fat is a highly relevant factor (Fig. 10.3). Certainly, rapid weight gain has been long identified as a precipitant factor for symptomatic bloating and abdominal distension. Extraintestinal fat may constrain bowel expansion during digestion, amplifying the stimulus of visceral and peritoneal sensory receptors. Furthermore, intra-abdominal fat appears to exert a pro-inflammatory action, due to its potential to release inflammatory cytokines. In addition, accumulation of fat inside the abdomen may produce mass distension increasing individual attention on this part of the anatomy. In turn, excessively focused attention (hypervigilance) may greatly enhance perception of abdominal nociceptive stimuli.

The menstrual female cycle also has substantial influence on the development of symptomatic bloating. In fact, bloating may be present in otherwise asymptomatic women during the

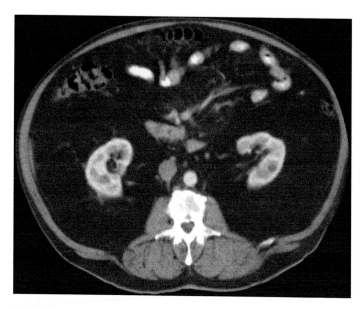

FIGURE 10.3 Abdominal distension caused by a marked increase in visceral fat. Note the modest amount of subcutaneous fat

premenstrual and ovulation phases. This appears to be due to enhanced visceral sensitivity via summation of intra-abdominal stimuli or hormonal influences [9].

Finally, meals and evacuation may influence bloating and distension, due to mass effects, and pooling of food, chyme, and fecal contents at various levels of the gastrointestinal tract via summation phenomena and also via stimulation by specific meal components [2]. Thus, heavy fatty meals and constipation are two relevant events that may substantially aggravate bloating and abdominal distension.

(e) *The relevance of viscero-somatic reflexes and induced changes in abdominal shape*

Unperceived reflexes are the physiological core of gut function. In healthy individuals, the digestive system tolerates customary loads of food, liquid, and gas without significant conscious perception of motor events. Hence, postprandial gut accommodation and propulsion are regulated by reflex neural activity that is unperceived. Unperceived reflex activity may, however, be modulated and upgraded by the central nervous system in an analogous fashion to consciously perceived nociceptive peripheral stimuli. Hence, viscero-somatic reflexes acting on diaphragmatic and abdominal wall muscle activity may be altered by central neural circuits, responding to either external or endogenous inputs. Abdominal distension may thus develop with or without concurrent bloating.

Normal individuals react to intestinal distension produced by infused gas by a reflex response consisting of contraction of the anterior abdominal muscles and relaxation of the diaphragm. Consequently, they accommodate the expanded intestinal volume without protrusion of the anterior abdominal wall. By contrast, patients with bloating and abdominal distension activate different viscero-somatic responses expressed as thoracic expansion, diaphragmatic contraction, and inferior oblique muscle relaxation. This abnormal set of responses reshapes the abdominal cavity without altering total intraperitoneal volume. The result is anterior abdominal wall protrusion and visible distension [7, 10].

This abnormal viscero-somatic response to intra-luminal bowel stimuli constitutes a highly prevalent mechanism for development of abdominal distension [11]. The bloating sensation, which represents the sensory counterpart of this abnormal response often, but not invariably, accompanies abdominal distension. Thus patients may complain of bloating, distension, or both in combination, or separately, on different occasions, or under different circumstances.

Symptoms

Bloating is a feeling of increased intra-abdominal pressure that may range in intensity from mildly uncomfortable to painful. Patients tend to describe it as a "gas bloat" because they perceive the symptom as if gas had been blown into their abdomen and as though relief could be obtained by quickly expelling it. This subjective impression is contrary to the actual pathophysiology data, which shows that intra-luminal gas is only marginally increased during symptomatic episodes. Abdominal distension often, but not invariably, accompanies the sensation. Abdominal distension is described as an enlargement of the waist and in severe cases as if it were "a pregnant abdomen." Both abdominal bloating and distension may present in isolation or, quite often, as part of another functional gastrointestinal disorder such as functional dyspepsia or irritable bowel syndrome (IBS) [12].

Bloating in functional dyspepsia tends to be described as centered in the upper abdomen, predominantly during the postprandial period. It may be clinically indistinguishable from the typical epigastric fullness that constitutes a key symptom of the postprandial distress subgroup of functional dyspepsia. Patients may even describe it as "indigestion" or "slow digestion." Sometimes it is accompanied by repeated belching. The latter encourages patients to attempt to obtain relief by forcefully belching, without realizing that air is simultaneously sucked into the stomach (aerophagia), defeating their intentions.

Bloating may elicit a broad range of personal attitudes and reactions. Some individuals accept postprandial bloating as a minor nuisance, whereas others consider it unbearable and actively seek medical attention, diagnostic evaluation, and subsequently demand effective treatment for relief. Bloating may coexist with flatulence, but these two clinical manifestations are not inextricably linked. When meal fermentable substrates reach the colon, gas production surges, and both flatulence and bloating may develop simultaneously [5]. However, gastrointestinal loads of non-fermentable fiber may cause a similar bloating sensation, without an increase in flatulence [13]. This dissociation is often acknowledged by patients who experience an increase in bloating when consuming large amounts of raw fiber, without necessarily developing flatulence or an increase in stool frequency.

Diagnostic Evaluation

Diagnosis depends primarily on symptom description by the patient. Physical examination is usually unhelpful, unless significant abdominal distension is an accompanying feature. Clinicians should be sensitive to patient suffering and at the same time must exercise judgment, to decide whether symptoms justify embarking on an in-depth evaluation, as this can be time-consuming, expensive, often invasive and occasionally risky. Patients complaining of bloating in the context of a functional gastrointestinal disorder, such as functional dyspepsia or IBS, may not require specific investigations. In this regard, consideration of extraintestinal manifestations, such as migraine headaches, urinary symptoms (e.g., interstitial cystitis), and joint pains, is helpful, because it reinforces a functional origin. Likewise, unconcerned patients with bloating may not require special testing, provided that "organic" forms of bloating and abdominal distension (infectious etiologies, celiac disease, ischemia, or portal hypertension) have been considered and excluded.

Functional bloating and abdominal distension have been defined by specific criteria that were developed by the Rome IV consensus process [12]. When complaints fulfill such criteria and are severe, protracted, and impinge substantially on the patient's quality of live, a set of ancillary diagnostic tests may be requested, always beginning with the simplest and least invasive (Fig. 10.4).

Tests to investigate the mechanism of bloating in individual patients can be divided into three categories:

1. *Tests directed to ascertain whether fermenting carbohydrate malabsorption is involved.*

These tests include breath tests for lactose and fructose malabsorption, tests to establish whether SIBO is a factor, and tests to assess the individual's microbiome looking for imbalances in microbial metabolism (gas-producing vs. gas-consuming bacteria) [14]. Unfortunately, these indirect tests are fraught with potential technical problems and

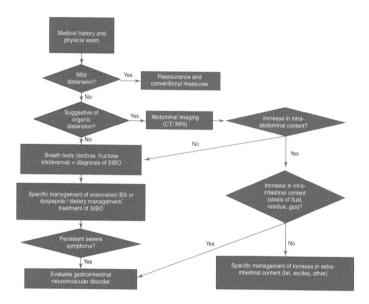

FIGURE 10.4 Diagnostic algorithm for abdominal distension

uncertainties. Most important there may be no correlation between test results and clinical relevance (i.e., a patient may show test evidence of lactose intolerance and fail to improve by removing lactose from their diet). Nevertheless, breath tests are relatively simple, and many patients expect, or even demand, this type of "food intolerance" evaluation. On the other hand, blood tests based on IgG reaction to food components have not been validated and should not be used.

2. *Tests to assess possible viscero-somatic dyssynergia in patients with bloating and abdominal distension.*

Two classes of tests are available, imaging tests and electromyographic tests. Imaging tests (CT or MRI) are most useful when comparing the same individual at baseline (not distended) and during a prominent episode of bloating with distension. Viscero-somatic dyssynergia is supported by finding lower diaphragm and anterior abdominal protrusion (reshaping of the abdominal cavity) during distension episodes [15]. Excess intra-luminal gas in the gut is often present, but in small amounts, and this feature is, therefore, an unreliable variable.

3. *Tests to evaluate concomitant neuromuscular disease*

Some patients develop bloating and abdominal distension as a manifestation of gut neuromuscular disease. In such instances, bloating and distension result from bowel expansion due to the accumulation of intra-luminal endogenous gas and secretions and exogenous food debris [16]. In severe cases, the diagnosis may be established by imaging tests showing stasis in parts of the gastrointestinal tract. However, there are more subtle clinical presentations that may require more sophisticated diagnostic tests, especially motility tests, such as esophageal manometry, gastric emptying tests, and small bowel manometry or endoluminal capsule motility tests to examine contractility patterns in the small bowel.

When severe pain accompanies the gas-bloat syndrome, a barostat study may be helpful to look for visceral hypersensitivity. This test, unfortunately, is only available at specialized centers and measures gastric tone, gastric accommodation, and gastric conscious sensitivity to distension all in one procedure. If appropriate, at the end of the test, the response to intravenous erythromycin (smooth muscle responsiveness) or glucagon (gastric relaxation) can be measured to obtain complete evaluation of gastric sensory and motor function.

Treatment

A reasonable treatment approach must take into account the severity and impact on quality of life perceived by the patient. It should be structured as a step-by-step series of increasingly complex and potent treatments that fit the magnitude of the problem to avoid undue medicalization and overmedication.

Mild forms of the gas-bloat syndrome may be successfully managed by explanation and reassurance, accompanied by simple time-honored measures such as eating slowly, chewing well, avoiding excess carbonated drinks and alcohol, exercising, etc. Somewhat more severe symptoms, but still not eliciting significant concern, warrant consideration of common pathogenetic factors that may play a contributory role. First, a detailed dietary history should be obtained to ascertain whether the patient is ingesting excessive fermentable products that unduly increase intestinal gas production, and addressed if present. Second, bowel movement pattern and effectiveness of defecation should be ascertained, with measures to correct constipation and pelvic floor dyssynergia if relevant. Third, recent excess weight gain must be evaluated and reversed by diet and exercise.

Patients with more severe and protracted symptoms warrant consideration of radical dietary modification and other approaches. First, a drastic reduction of fermentable dietary substrates, via a low FODMAP (fermentable oligo-, di-, monosaccharides, and polyols) diet, which has proven its effectiveness, may be implemented [17]. However, this imposes a significant burden on the patient, and long-term compliance may become an issue. Some investigators have proposed that simpler forms of dietary modification may produce comparable amelioration.

Microbiome modulation via antibiotics, probiotics, and prebiotics may also be considered. Broad-spectrum and non-absorbable antibiotics, such as rifaximin, are an option. They may act on SIBO, modify the colonic microbiota, or both. Rifaximin has shown efficacy in reducing IBS-associated bloating [18]. Probiotics are an alternative, with some trial data supporting their use but, overall, clinical efficacy remains to be conclusively proven. Finally, prebiotics constitute an interesting option, given their capacity to induce the proliferation of beneficial bacterial species. Although initially they may be associated with an increase in gas production and flatulence, after a 1- to 2-week adaptation period, gas production decreases and bloating appears to improve [19].

Pharmacological measures may be needed to improve symptoms in more severe cases. Promoting gas evacuation, via cholinomimetic agents, such as parenteral neostigmine or

oral pyridostigmine may help bloating and abdominal distension, although these agents perform better in acute distension, since tachyphylaxis reduces their effectiveness.
Prucalopride, linaclotide, and lubiprostone are laxative agents
but may also reduce bloating and distension via complementary effects on visceral sensitivity and gas clearance. In this
regard, anorectal biofeedback may also be useful to facilitate
stool evacuation in constipated patients with dyssynergia.

Attenuating, visceral hypersensitivity is also a key therapeutic objective. Visceral hypersensitivity represents a sen-
sorial amplification of the afferent stimulus generated by
gut wall tension. Such altered perception appears to be
present in a substantial number of patients with abdominal
pain. Furthermore, even at an unperceived level, signal
amplification and distortion may be responsible for the
abnormal viscero-somatic reflex activity that produces
abdominal distension without bowel expansion. Various
pharmacologic agents may reduce conscious perception of
increased wall tension. Traditionally, antispasmodic drugs
that purportedly relax bowel wall have been prescribed,
mostly to alleviate pain. Their efficacy in controlling bloating is uncertain.

Since visceral hyperalgesia probably involves multiple dis-
turbed mechanisms along the gut-brain axis, the use of centrally acting agents has been proposed. Antidepressants may
alleviate visceral pain, although their efficacy on bloating and
abdominal distension remains unproven [20]. Older tricyclic
antidepressants with multiple receptor affinity show anti-
hypersensitivity properties, even at relatively low doses, but
side effects may limit their use.

Among newer antidepressants, those inhibiting reuptake
of both norepinephrine, as well as serotonin, appear to be
more effective than those inhibiting only serotonin reuptake.
Since patients with severe symptoms are often anxious or
depressed, the primary action of antidepressants on mood
and anxiety is of added value. Purely anxiolytic agents such as
benzodiazepines may alleviate bloating on account of their
relaxing effect and inhibition of stress-induced symptoms, but
somnolence and the risk of addiction must be considered.

Psychotherapeutic approaches such as hypnotherapy and behavioral modification may also be effective, but the paucity of trained therapists is a limiting factor, as well as the time-intensive nature of these approaches [21]. Correction of abdominal distension via abdominal biofeedback treatment is emerging as a valid and useful therapy, particularly for patients with prominent abdominal distension accompanying bloating. Biofeedback therapy is facilitated by an abdominal electromyography recording technique, permitting visual control of abdominal muscle activity by the patient under the guidance of an experienced trainer [11]. The goal is to teach the patient to block distension by voluntarily inhibiting inter-costal and diaphragmatic activity, while increasing contraction of the anterior abdominal muscles.

Case Study: Follow-Up

The patient underwent upper gastrointestinal endoscopy that showed a well-constructed Nissen fundoplication with absent esophagitis and mild *Helicobacter pylori*-negative antral gas-tritis. A CT scan of her abdomen showed some gas inside her stomach and bowels, as well as moderate intra-abdominal lipomatosis. However, the magnitude of these features was judged insufficient to explain her complaints. A scintigraphic gastric emptying test showed a mild delay in meal evacuation. A barostat study was next performed to evaluate gastric con-tractility/relaxation. This test evidenced decreased gastric relaxation in response to duodenal nutrient infusion (impaired gastric accommodation) and a disproportionate painful response to graded gastric distension (visceral hypersensitiv-ity). An abdominal electromyographic study, performed dur-ing a significant distension episode, showed inappropriate relaxation of the anterior abdominal wall muscles. The patient was treated with 25 mg amitriptyline to alleviate her visceral hypersensitivity and several sessions of biofeedback treatment to correct the viscero-somatic dyssynergia that was considered largely responsible for her striking abdominal distension. At a 3-month follow-up visit, she felt pleased with the symptomatic improvement she had achieved and the return to normal life activities.

Clinical Pearls

- Potential organic causes for bloating and distension should be considered first, and discarded if not applicable.
- Discriminating between a functional abdominal disorder, such as the gas-bloat syndrome, and a neuromuscular gut disorder may be difficult on clinical grounds alone and may require special tests.
- Positivity of specific carbohydrate malabsorption breath tests such as lactose, fructose, and others does not necessarily prove this is the main etiology of the symptoms.
- A step-by-step application of therapeutic measures, beginning with simpler approaches such as reassurance and advice, is the most reasonable approach for gas-bloat syndrome.

Self-Test

Question 1. Abdominal biofeedback treatment of abdominal distension achieves its therapeutic goal by:

A. Promoting belching and expelling intragastric air
B. Promoting flatulence and expelling intra-colonic gases
C. Relaxing the patient and hence diminishing abdominal pain perception
D. Helping the patient inhibit intercostal and diaphragmatic muscular activity while contracting the anterior abdominal muscles to reduce distension
E. Reducing intra-luminal pressure via colon and omentum repositioning within the abdominal cavity

Question 2. Clinical factors that should be assessed because of their pathogenetic relevance to bloating and abdominal distension include:

A. Presence or absence of *Helicobacter pylori* infection
B. High dietary protein intake
C. Prior surgery such as anti-reflux Nissen-type fundoplication
D. Presence or absence of gallstones
E. Carcinoid syndrome due to multiple metastatic liver lesions

Question 3. Which of the following statements is correct?

A. Passing flatus frequently prevents bloating.
B. Ingestion of large amounts of psyllium fiber prevents both bloating and flatulence.
C. Frequent ingestion of carbonated beverages increases both bloating and flatulence.
D. Bloating may occur without flatulence and may resolve without apparent expelling of gas by mouth or anus.
E. Activated charcoal, which absorbs intestinal gas, relieves both flatulence and bloating.

References

1. Malagelada JR, Accarino A, Azpiroz F. Bloating and abdominal distension: old misconceptions and current knowledge. Am J Gastroenterol. 2017;112(8):1221–31.
2. Serra J, Salvioli B, Azpiroz F, Malagelada JR. Lipid-induced intestinal gas retention in irritable bowel syndrome. Gastroenterology. 2002;123(3):700–6.
3. Murray K, Wilkinson-Smith V, Hoad C, Costigan C, Cox E, Lam C, et al. Differential effects of FODMAPs (fermentable oligo-, di-, mono-saccharides and polyols) on small and large intestinal contents in healthy subjects shown by MRI. Am J Gastroenterol. 2014;109(1):110–9.
4. McRorie J. Clinical data support that psyllium is not fermented in the gut. Am J Gastroenterol. 2013;108(9):1541.

5. Mego M, Accarino A, Malagelada JR, Guarner F, Azpiroz F. Accumulative effect of food residues on intestinal gas production. Neurogastroenterol Motil. 2015;27(11):1621–8.

6. Agrawal A, Houghton LA, Lea R, Morris J, Reilly B, Whorwell PJ. Bloating and distention in irritable bowel syndrome: the role of visceral sensation. Gastroenterology. 2008;134(7):1882–9.

7. Villoria A, Azpiroz F, Burri E, Cisternas D, Soldevilla A, Malagelada JR. Abdomino-phrenic dyssynergia in patients with abdominal bloating and distension. Am J Gastroenterol. 2011;106(5):815–9.

8. Koloski NA, Jones M, Talley NJ. Evidence that independent gut-to-brain and brain-to-gut pathways operate in the irritable bowel syndrome and functional dyspepsia: a 1-year population-based prospective study. Aliment Pharmacol Ther. 2016;44(6):592–600.

9. Houghton LA, Lea R, Jackson N, Whorwell PJ. The menstrual cycle affects rectal sensitivity in patients with irritable bowel syndrome but not healthy volunteers. Gut. 2002;50(4):471–4.

10. Burri E, Barba E, Huaman JW, Cisternas D, Accarino A, Soldevilla A, et al. Mechanisms of postprandial abdominal bloating and distension in functional dyspepsia. Gut. 2014;63(3):395–400.

11. Barba E, Burri E, Accarino A, Cisternas D, Quiroga S, Monclus E, et al. Abdominothoracic mechanisms of functional abdominal distension and correction by biofeedback. Gastroenterology. 2015;148(4):732–9.

12. Drossman DA. Functional gastrointestinal disorders: history, pathophysiology, clinical features and Rome IV. Gastroenterology. 2016. pii: S0016-5085(16)00223-7. https://doi.org/10.1053/j.gastro.2016.02.032. [Epub ahead of print].

13. Furne JK, Levitt MD. Factors influencing frequency of flatus emission by healthy subjects. Dig Dis Sci. 1996;41(8):1631–5.

14. Mego M, Bendezú A, Accarino A, Malagelada JR, Azpiroz F. Intestinal gas homeostasis: disposal pathways. Neurogastroenterol Motil. 2015;27:363.

15. Villoria A, Azpiroz F, Soldevilla A, Perez F, Malagelada JR. Abdominal accommodation: a coordinated adaptation of the abdominal wall to its content. Am J Gastroenterol. 2008;103(11):2807–15.

16. Barba E, Quiroga S, Accarino A, Lahoya EM, Malagelada C, Burri E, et al. Mechanisms of abdominal distension in severe intestinal dysmotility: abdomino-thoracic response to gut retention. Neurogastroenterol Motil. 2013;25(6):e389–94.

17. Halmos EP, Power VA, Shepherd SJ, Gibson PR, Muir JG. A diet low in FODMAPs reduces symptoms of irritable bowel syndrome. Gastroenterology. 2014;146(1):67–75. e5.
18. Pimentel M, Lembo A, Chey WD, Zakko S, Ringel Y, Yu J, et al. Rifaximin therapy for patients with irritable bowel syndrome without constipation. N Engl J Med. 2011;364(1):22–32.
19. Mego M, Manichanh C, Accarino A, Campos D, Pozuelo M, Varela E, et al. Metabolic adaptation of colonic microbiota to galactooligosaccharides: a proof-of-concept-study. Aliment Pharmacol Ther. 2017;45(5):670–80.
20. Tack J, Broekaert D, Fischler B, Van Oudenhove L, Gevers AM, Janssens J. A controlled crossover study of the selective serotonin reuptake inhibitor citalopram in irritable bowel syndrome. Gut. 2006;55(8):1095–103.
21. Zijdenbos IL, de Wit NJ, van der Heijden GJ, Rubin G, Quartero AO. Psychological treatments for the management of irritable bowel syndrome. Cochrane Database Syst Rev. 2009;1:CD006442.

Essential Reading

Burri E, Barba E, Huaman JW, Cisternas D, Accarino A, Soldevilla A, et al. Mechanisms of postprandial abdominal bloating and distension in functional dyspepsia. Gut. 2014;63(3):395–400. A human mechanistic study showing the similarities between dyspepsia and IBS-associated bloating.

Drossman DA. Functional gastrointestinal disorders: history, pathophysiology, clinical features and Rome IV. Gastroenterology. 2016; A summarized compendium of the latest Rome consensus project (IV) providing the latest classification, features, and diagnostic criteria for the main functional gut disorders.

Malagelada JR, Accarino A, Azpiroz F. Bloating and abdominal distension: old misconceptions and current knowledge. Am J Gastroenterol. 2017;112(8):1221–31. An updated review on the topic describing the various clinical presentations, appropriate diagnostic procedures, and management.

Pimentel M, Lembo A, Chey WD, Zakko S, Ringel Y, Yu J, et al. Rifaximin therapy for patients with irritable bowel syndrome without constipation. N Engl J Med. 2011;364(1):22–32. A controlled trial showing the efficacy of antibiotic rifaximin therapy relieving IBS-associated bloating.

Part III

Chronic Abdominal Pain: Common and Uncommon Causes

Chapter 11
A Diagnostic Approach to Chronic Abdominal Pain

Amrit K. Kamboj and Amy S. Oxentenko

Case Study

A 50-year-old woman presents with a 2-year history of right upper quadrant pain. She describes it as constant and burning with no radiation. Exacerbating factors include sitting or lying on the right side, and she reports no alleviating factors. She denies any other gastrointestinal or systemic symptoms. She has a past medical history of hypertension and hyperlipidemia. She underwent cholecystectomy 3 years ago for biliary colic symptoms. Physical exam is notable for a scar in the right upper quadrant at the site of prior cholecystectomy. Palpation of the right upper quadrant elicits a focal area of tenderness that worsens when the

A. K. Kamboj
Department of Internal Medicine, Mayo Clinic, Rochester, MN, USA

A. S. Oxentenko (✉)
Division of Gastroenterology and Hepatology, Department of Internal Medicine, Mayo Clinic, Rochester, MN, USA
e-mail: oxentenko.amy@mayo.edu

© Springer Nature Switzerland AG 2019
B. E. Lacy et al. (eds.), *Essential Medical Disorders of the Stomach and Small Intestine*,
https://doi.org/10.1007/978-3-030-01117-8_11

209

patient is asked to raise both legs off the examination table. Prior laboratory tests, including complete blood count, electrolyte panel, liver biochemistries, and inflammatory markers, were all unremarkable. A right upper quadrant ultrasound and computed tomography abdomen performed within the last year were both normal without any abnormalities detected. She is becoming increasingly concerned and worried about her pain given its duration and the lack of a formal diagnosis. What is the most likely etiology of this patient's abdominal pain, and how would you manage this patient?

Objectives

- Categorize the broad differential diagnoses for chronic abdominal pain.
- Define a stepwise approach to the work-up of a patient with chronic abdominal pain.
- Review treatment options for unspecified chronic abdominal pain.

Epidemiology

Chronic abdominal pain is commonly encountered throughout medicine, especially in primary care and gastroenterology clinics. In fact, abdominal pain impacts close to 22% of the adult population, affecting slightly more women than men [1]. While there is no formal criterion regarding duration of symptoms that defines chronic abdominal pain, most experts agree that symptoms are generally present for at least 6 months [2, 3]. Chronic abdominal pain can affect patients of all age groups, ethnicities, and backgrounds, although women and those from lower socioeconomic groups are at higher risk. The symptoms can vary from one individual to another and range in intensity from mild with no associated morbidity to severe with major limitations in daily activities.

The disease course and prognosis are variable and depend on the underlying etiology. Functional disorders associated with abdominal pain, including functional dyspepsia and irritable bowel syndrome (IBS), are present in approximately one-fourth of the general population [4]. In patients with symptoms secondary to functional gastrointestinal disorders, approximately 40% had no further symptoms, 20% had the same symptoms, and 40% had different symptoms at 1-year follow-up [5]. A frequently overlooked cause of chronic idiopathic abdominal pain is abdominal wall pain, which accounts for up to 10% of such cases [6]. Chronic abdominal pain can present a diagnostic challenge for clinicians given the broad differential it encompasses and frustration for patients who often have a negative diagnostic work-up and high healthcare costs. Also, there can be an unawareness of exam maneuvers to make specific diagnoses, such as abdominal wall pain. Chronic pain accounts for increased healthcare utilization, with a total financial cost of approximately $600 billion annually, with a significant portion due to abdominal pain [7].

Etiology

Chronic abdominal pain has a wide array of underlying etiologies, including both organic and functional disorders. Organic disorders occur secondary to structural or physiologic causes, while functional disorders have no clear explanation.

The organic etiologies associated with chronic abdominal pain can be captured using a location-based approach, depending on whether the pain occurs predominantly in the right upper quadrant (RUQ), epigastric region, left upper quadrant (LUQ), or lower abdominal region (Fig. 11.1). The organs present in each of these regions help to narrow the

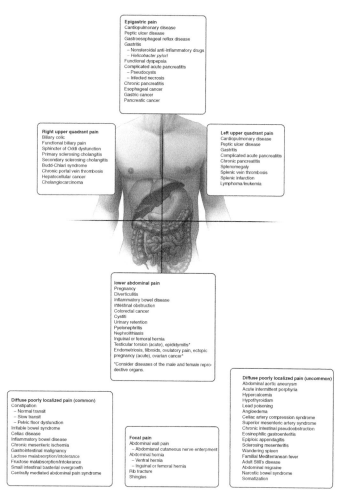

FIGURE 11.1 A location-and character-based approach to etiologies of chronic abdominal pain. (Used with permission of Mayo Foundation for Medical Education and Research, all rights reserved)

differential diagnoses. Right upper quadrant pain is most commonly associated with liver, gallbladder, or biliary tree pathology. Epigastric and LUQ pain can occur secondary to disorders of the esophagus, stomach, duodenum, pancreas, or spleen. In particular, it is important to exclude cardiopulmonary causes of epigastric or LUQ pain, as these can potentially be life-threatening. For example, angina pectoris can have an atypical presentation in women, the elderly, and those with diabetes. Lower abdominal pain may occur secondary to disorders of the small or large intestine, appendix, or genitourinary system. In women, the ovaries and uterus may be responsible for lower abdominal pain, while scrotal or inguinal pathology can cause similar pain in men.

Certain organic etiologies cannot be easily captured using a quadrant-based approach but, rather, can be considered using a character-based approach (focal vs. diffuse) (Fig. 11.1). Focal abdominal pain may occur secondary to musculoskeletal issues, nerve entrapment, or irritation of the parietal peritoneum. Diffuse abdominal pain has a broad differential and can occur secondary to inflammatory, ischemic, metabolic, neoplastic, or malabsorptive etiologies. In cases where the history, physical exam, and diagnostic testing reveal no obvious structural cause of abdominal pain, functional bowel disorders should be considered. The three most common functional disorders associated with abdominal pain include functional dyspepsia, IBS (constipation-predominant, diarrhea-predominant, and mixed-pattern subtypes), and functional abdominal pain syndrome [4]. New developments in our understanding of visceral and central pain led the Rome IV committee to change the term functional abdominal pain syndrome to centrally mediated abdominal pain syndrome (CAP), reflecting the importance of glial and nerve cells [3]. Other common functional bowel disorders include functional constipation, functional diarrhea, functional abdominal bloating, narcotic bowel syndrome, and opioid-induced constipation [8].

Pathophysiology

The pathophysiology of disorders that result in chronic abdominal pain is extensive and wide-ranging. Inflammation can occur throughout the gastrointestinal tract and can present with chronic abdominal pain. Examples of inflammatory conditions include esophagitis due to gastroesophageal reflux disease (GERD), gastritis due to nonsteroidal anti-inflammatory drug (NSAID) use or *Helicobacter pylori* infection, eosinophilic gastroenteritis, chronic pancreatitis due to alcohol abuse, and enteritis or colitis due to inflammatory bowel disease (IBD). The gut microbiome plays a fundamental role in metabolism and immunity, and alterations in gut flora may play a part in various gastrointestinal disorders, including inflammatory conditions, malignancy, and functional bowel disorders [9–12]. Additionally, small intestinal bacterial overgrowth can occur when the normal enteric flora is disrupted, often due to reduced gastric acid production, altered small bowel anatomy, or small intestinal dysmotility [13]. Ischemia occurs when the blood flow to an organ becomes reduced, and patients with mesenteric ischemia are classically elderly with cardiovascular disease, or may occur in those with underlying thromboembolic or hypercoagulable conditions. Chronic mesenteric ischemia presents with postprandial pain, sitophobia, and weight loss and occurs when atherosclerosis is present in at least two of the three mesenteric vessels (celiac artery, superior mesenteric artery, and inferior mesenteric artery) [14]. Mechanical obstruction of the alimentary system, biliary tree, and urinary tract classically presents with acute abdominal pain; however, partial or intermittent obstruction can result in chronic or recurrent symptoms. Similarly, while perforation of gastrointestinal organs such as the stomach, small bowel, or colon typically presents with peritonitis and acute abdominal pain, smaller perforations may heal spontaneously and present with late complications, such as abscesses and fistulae. Medications can result in inflammation and injury (e.g., NSAIDs, bisphosphonates, doxycycline), altered bowel motility with constipation (e.g., opioids, antihistamines, calcium, iron supplements) or diarrhea (e.g., metformin, selective serotonin reuptake inhibitors, proton pump inhibitors, magnesium), and visceral hyperalgesia (opioids). Functional gastrointestinal disorders can be explained using a biopsychosocial model, which includes genetic predisposition, psychological factors, gastrointestinal dysfunction, and central sensitization due to alterations in the brain-gut axis [4].

Symptoms

Chronic abdominal pain is often a nonspecific complaint that can involve discomfort anywhere from the lower chest to the pelvis. The quality, description, location, and radiation of the pain depend on the organ system(s) involved. While patients with chronic abdominal pain may present with isolated abdominal pain, they may also have other concomitant symptoms (Table 11.1). In patients with multiple symptoms, it is important to elucidate the most distressing symptom through a careful history, review of systems, and physical exam. Identifying the primary symptom can provide useful clues to the underlying diagnosis.

Cardiopulmonary causes (e.g., ischemia, pericarditis, pulmonary embolus) must be strongly considered and ruled out if chest pain and shortness of breath are present, especially if these are exertional or inspirational in nature. Alarm features suggestive of a serious underlying issue include fevers, unintentional weight loss, anemia, dysphagia, persistent vomiting, sudden change in bowel habits, hematemesis, melena, hematochezia, or a family history of gastrointestinal cancer. In particular, unintentional weight loss, especially greater than 10% of ideal body weight, should raise the suspicion for malignancy, particularly in elderly patients.

In many patients, abdominal pain can be associated with constipation or diarrhea. The Bristol stool form scale can help provide useful information regarding stool form and consistency [15]. Other patients may complain of bloating or a sensation of increased abdominal pressure with or without visible distention [16]. Heartburn, regurgitation, nausea, and chronic cough may be suggestive of GERD. Melena or black, tarry stool is indicative of an upper gastrointestinal bleed and may be a clue to peptic ulcer disease in the patient presenting

TABLE 11.1 Symptoms to assess in patients presenting with chronic abdominal pain

Constitutional symptoms

Fevers, chills, night sweats

Changes in weight (weight loss/gain)

Malaise, anorexia

Lymphadenopathy

Gastrointestinal symptoms

Dysphagia, odynophagia

Heartburn, reflux

Belching, bloating, distention, flatulence

Nausea, vomiting

Changes in bowel habits (constipation, diarrhea)

Change in bowel color (melena, hematochezia, clay-colored stools)

Non-gastrointestinal symptoms

HEENT[a]: Scleral icterus, oral ulcers, tongue swelling (glossitis)

Endocrine: Heat/cold intolerance, polyuria, polydipsia, polyphagia, abnormal hair growth, nail changes

Cardiovascular: Chest pain, palpitations, orthopnea, paroxysmal nocturnal dyspnea, lower extremity edema, claudication

Pulmonary: Cough, shortness of breath, wheezing, hemoptysis

Genitourinary: Dysuria, increased urinary frequency, nocturia, hematuria, tea-colored urine, testicular pain, urethral or vaginal discharge, vaginal bleeding, dyspareunia, dysmenorrhea, change in menses

Musculoskeletal: Arthralgias, myalgias

TABLE 11.1 (continued)

Skin: Jaundice, rashes, tender nodules, necrotic/deep ulcers, cyanosis, pruritis

Neuropsychiatric: Headache, muscle weakness, ataxia, depression, anxiety

[a]HEENT, head, eye, ear, nose, and throat

with epigastric pain, while hematochezia is more typical of lower gastrointestinal bleeding and may occur in those with abdominal pain due to ischemia or inflammation. Hepatomegaly, jaundice, scleral icterus, clay-colored stools, and tea-colored urine are suggestive of hepatobiliary or pancreatic pathology. Genitourinary disorders should be suspected in patients with dysuria, increased urinary frequency, hematuria, nocturia, or pain in the suprapubic, testicular, or flank regions. Patients with coexisting depression and anxiety are more likely to have a functional disorder compared to the normal population.

Diagnostic Evaluation

The diagnostic evaluation of a patient with chronic abdominal pain begins with a thorough history and comprehensive physical exam (Table 11.2). The history should focus on eliciting the pain description, quality, location, radiation, and intensity, along with exacerbating and alleviating factors. An exhaustive review of systems should be performed to identify concomitant symptoms (Table 11.1) as these may provide clues to the underlying diagnosis. The past medical, family, and social history can be useful in identifying risk factors for certain disorders. Given the chronicity of the pain, the clinician should review prior laboratory and imaging studies along with previous procedures in order to understand the work-up to date and to avoid repeating tests when possible. The physical exam should include a complete abdominal and

TABLE 11.2 Important history and physical exam elements to obtain in a patient presenting with chronic abdominal pain

I. History of present illness

Onset, frequency, and duration (acute vs. chronic)

Description and quality (sharp, dull, achy, stabbing, burning, pressure)

Location and radiation

Intensity (scale 1–10)

Exacerbating and alleviating factors

Previous episodes

Relationship to food

Bowel habits

Review of symptoms (see Table 11.1)

II. Review medical and surgical history

Past medical history (including gastrointestinal and cardiopulmonary diseases)

Past surgical history (including previous abdominal surgeries)

Prior procedures (endoscopy, colonoscopy, ERCP[a])

Prior imaging studies (ultrasound, CT[b], MRI[c])

Menstrual history (including last menstrual period)

Psychosocial assessment (abuse, PTSD[d], depression, anxiety, somatization)

III. Review medication list (including NSAIDs[e], immunosuppressive agents, narcotics)

IV. Review family history (including colon cancer, IBD[f], autoimmune disorders)

V. Review social history

Alcohol, tobacco, recreational drug use

Sexual history (history of STDs[g], new sexual partners)

TABLE 11.2 (continued)

Use of contraception

Dietary habits

VI. Physical exam

Vital signs (stable vs. unstable)

General appearance

Abdominal examination

Inspection (patient position, prior scars, skin changes)

Auscultation (bowel sounds)

Percussion (tympanic vs. dullness)

Palpation (tenderness, organomegaly, masses)

Specialized tests (Carnett's sign, Murphy's sign)

Rectal examination (fecal impaction, evidence of bleeding, features of pelvic floor dysfunction, masses)

Focused physical exam (including pelvic exam) as guided by patient history

[a]ERCP, endoscopic retrograde cholangiopancreatography
[b]CT, computed tomography
[c]MRI, magnetic resonance imaging
[d]PTSD, post-traumatic stress disorder
[e]NSAIDs, nonsteroidal anti-inflammatory drugs
[f]IBD, inflammatory bowel disease
[g]STDs, sexually transmitted diseases

rectal exam. While auscultating for bowel sounds, gentle pressure may be applied to the stethoscope; classically, abdominal tenderness lessens in patients with functional bowel disorders when they become distracted, while the pain may worsen in those with structural bowel disorders. Carnett's sign (Fig. 11.2), a clinical test that can help identify abdominal wall pain, should be routinely performed in patients presenting with chronic abdominal pain that is focal in nature [17]. The remainder of the physical exam should be guided by the patient's history.

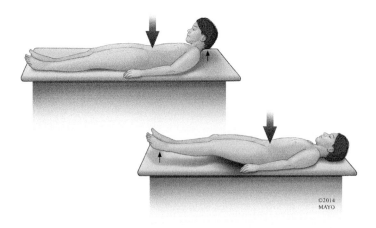

FIGURE 11.2 Carnett's sign can help identify abdominal wall pain. **Step 1**: The clinician identifies and palpates the point of maximal abdominal tenderness (resting supine position). **Step 2**: The patient raises both legs off the examination table (tense position) while the clinician palpates the abdomen. Alternatively, the patient can raise their head and shoulders off the bed, tensing the abdominal wall. **Positive Carnett's sign**: Palpation of abdominal muscles in the tense position elicits the same or more tenderness as the rest position → musculoskeletal source (abdominal wall pain). (Used with permission of Mayo Foundation for Medical Education and Research, all rights reserved)

The next step in the evaluation of chronic abdominal pain consists of obtaining standard laboratory tests, as indicated (Fig. 11.2). For most patients, this may include some or all of the following: complete blood count, electrolyte panel, calcium, creatinine, liver biochemistries, lipase, C-reactive protein, and thyroid-stimulating hormone. IgA-tissue transglutaminase antibody should be considered in those with bloating, diarrhea, weight loss, or other manifestations of celiac disease. In women who are sexually active and of childbearing age, pregnancy should be ruled out. Patients younger than 60 years of age with dyspepsia and without alarm symptoms should be evaluated for *H. pylori* infection with a stool antigen or breath test [18]. In patients with microcytic anemia, iron studies including iron, total iron binding capacity, and ferritin should be obtained. If IBD is suspected, fecal calprotectin may be helpful; the prevalence of IBD is less than 1% when the C-reactive protein and fecal calprotectin are low [4]. Patients with abdominal pain associated with nausea, hypotension, skin hyperpigmentation, hyponatremia, or hyperkalemia should have a morning cortisol level checked to rule out adrenal insufficiency. Additional laboratory testing should be guided by the history and physical exam.

If the testing above reveals an underlying etiology for the patient's symptoms, disease specific medical management should be initiated. However, if no underlying etiology is identified, patients should be stratified into low-risk and high-risk categories based on age and alarm features. Patients less than 60 years of age and without alarm features may be considered low-risk and should be offered empiric pharmacotherapy and/or psycho-behavioral therapy based on their principal symptom. Many low-risk patients may have a functional etiology of their chronic abdominal pain. Patients aged 60 years and older or with alarm features are more likely to have organic disease and may require additional evaluation. For both low-risk and high-risk patients, close follow-up is necessary to verify the diagnosis and assess treatment response.

Ultrasound is the imaging modality of choice for RUQ pain to exclude gallstone-related disorders or biliary obstruction; Doppler evaluation can be added to assess the portal, hepatic, and mesenteric veins, as indicated [19]. A computed tomography of the abdomen (with or without pelvis) is the imaging modality of choice for evaluation of mid, diffuse, or lower abdominal pain when the diagnosis is unclear from the history, physical exam, and laboratory results. Oral contrast is used for bowel visualization, while IV contrast is used for visualization of vascular structures and solid organs [20]. In a pregnant patient, ultrasound and magnetic resonance imaging are the modalities of choice to minimize ionizing radiation exposure. An esophagogastroduodenoscopy should be performed when a patient presents with epigastric pain, heartburn, nausea/vomiting, dysphagia, or features of upper

GI bleeding, to allow for visualization of the esophagus, stomach, and duodenum. A colonoscopy may provide useful diagnostic information in the evaluation of chronic abdominal pain in the presence of lower GI bleeding, iron-deficiency anemia, chronic diarrhea, or new-onset constipation and should be offered to all patients who are due for colorectal cancer screening or surveillance [21].

Treatment

An effective patient-physician interaction is essential in the management of patients with chronic abdominal pain. Given the chronicity of symptoms, many patients are frustrated and unsatisfied with their health and healthcare providers. Therefore, it is essential to build a strong rapport with these patients in order to gain their trust and develop a therapeutic relationship. This not only improves compliance with recommended tests and treatments but also improves outcomes and patient satisfaction. Clinicians should approach patients with empathy and listen to their symptoms carefully. Even when a prior evaluation has been unrevealing or other providers have dismissed patient symptoms as functional or patients believe their abdominal pain is "all in their head," clinicians should be systematic in their approach to avoid anchoring bias [22]. Instead, a diagnostic algorithm, as outlined in Fig. 11.3, should be followed.

The treatment of chronic abdominal pain also depends on whether an underlying etiology is found. When a specific cause is identified, it should be treated using standard medical management. For example, if a patient is found to have celiac disease, a gluten-free diet should be instituted. Similarly, if a patient is found to have *H. pylori* infection, she should be treated with appropriate therapy, and testing should be performed to confirm eradication [18]. Those with classic biliary colic or gallstone-related complications usually benefit from cholecystectomy. A trigger point injection may offer effective pain control for patients with abdominal wall pain [23].

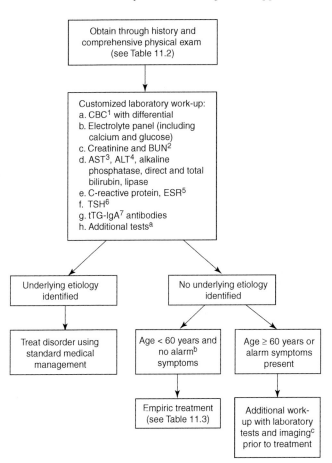

¹CBC: Complete blood count; ²BUN: Blood urea nitrogen ³AST: Aspartate transaminase; ⁴ALT: Alanine trasaminase; ⁵ESR: Erythrocyte sedimentation rate; ⁶TSH: Thyroid stimulating hormone; ⁷tTG-IgA: Tissue transglutaminase antibody.
ªAdditional tests should be obtained guided by patient history and physical exam and may include a pregnancy test, urinalysis, fecal calprotectin, *Helicobacter pylori stool* or breath test, glucose breath test, stool pathogen panel and ova/parasite exam, AM cortisol, Human immunodeficiency virus screen, and iron studies (iron, total iron binding capacity, and ferritin).
ᵇAlarm symptoms include fever, unintentional weight loss, dysphagia, persistent vomiting, sudden change in bowel habits, hematemesis, melena hematochezia, and family history of gastrointestinal cancer.
ᶜImaging modalities may include esophagoduodenoscopy, colonoscopy, computed tomography, magnetic resonance imaging, or ultrasound.

FIGURE 11.3 Diagnostic algorithm to evaluate patients with chronic abdominal pain

If no underlying etiology can be identified, patients can be treated empirically with pharmacotherapy and/or psycho-behavioral counseling based on their principal symptom. Patients may benefit from dietary and medication modifications if these factors are felt to be causally related to the pain. Over-the-counter medications tailed to patient symptoms can be initiated (Table 11.3). Prescription medications, such as tricyclic antidepressants or other neuromodulating agents, may be required and can be used in conjunction with behavioral and/or psychological therapies, if necessary [4]. In general, serotonin-norepinephrine reuptake inhibitors are more effective than selective serotonin reuptake inhibitors for the treatment of chronic visceral pain [24]. Cognitive behavioral therapy (CBT) helps patients identify maladaptive thoughts and behaviors and is the most effective psychological therapy for functional abdominal pain [4]. Continued and escalating doses of opioids can lead to worsening abdominal pain and should be avoided. In refractory cases, a multidisciplinary pain management program that combines physical therapy, occupational therapy, and CBT can prove useful [4].

Case Study: Follow-Up

This patient's chronic abdominal pain was secondary to abdominal wall pain. As with our patient, other patients with abdominal wall pain may not have any abnormalities on laboratory or imaging studies. This diagnosis is primarily based on the physical exam, specifically Carnett's sign. With this examination technique, the clinician first palpates the area of maximal abdominal tenderness with the patient lying supine and relaxing the abdominal wall. The patient is then asked to lift both legs off the examination table or raise their upper torso in an "abdominal crunch," with both maneuvers designed to tense the abdominal wall muscles. Carnett's sign is considered positive when there is increased tenderness to palpation with tensing of the abdominal wall muscles and is strongly suggestive of abdominal wall pain. In contrast, those with visceral

TABLE 11.3 Treatment of unspecified chronic abdominal pain

I. Establish an effective and robust patient-physician relationship

Approach patient with empathy

Listen to the patient carefully to assess and understand their symptoms

Validate patient fears and concerns, when appropriate

II. Implement lifestyle changes, dietary modifications, and medication adjustments

III. Offer pharmacotherapy based on principal symptom or associated features

Constipation: Dietary fiber, osmotic laxatives, stimulant laxatives, secretagogues (e.g., lubiprostone, linaclotide, plecanatide), suppositories, or biofeedback

Diarrhea: Antidiarrheal agents (loperamide), anticholinergic agents, bile salt sequestrants (cholestyramine), probiotics

Gastroesophageal reflux: Antacids, H_2-receptor antagonists, PPIs[a]

Nausea and vomiting: Antihistamine agents (promethazine), serotonin 5-HT_3 receptor antagonists (ondansetron), phenothiazines (prochlorperazine)

Dyspepsia: *Helicobacter pylori* eradication treatment, PPIs, TCAs[b], prokinetics (metoclopramide), buspirone, FDgard

Delayed gastric emptying (gastroparesis): Prokinetics (metoclopramide), macrolide antibiotics (erythromycin, for acute episodes only), antiemetics

Depression or anxiety: Antidepressants (SNRIs[c], SSRIs[d], TCAs)

Visceral pain: Smooth muscle antispasmodics (dicyclomine), peppermint oil, antidepressants (SNRIs, SSRIs, TCAs)

Abdominal wall pain: Trigger point injection (local anesthetic +/− corticosteroids)

(continued)

TABLE 11.3 (continued)

Narcotic bowel syndrome: Stop narcotics and control withdrawal symptoms (clonidine, benzodiazepines, antidepressants)

IV. Offer psychological and behavioral interventions (cognitive behavioral therapy) based on symptoms, functional impairment, and psychological distress

V. If pain remains refractory, consider referral to a multidisciplinary pain rehabilitation program (physical and occupational therapy, cognitive behavioral therapy)

[a]PPIs, proton pump inhibitors
[b]TCAs, tricyclic antidepressants
[c]SNRIs, serotonin-norepinephrine reuptake inhibitors
[d]SSRIs, selective serotonin reuptake inhibitors

abdominal pain have amelioration of their abdominal tenderness as the tensed musculature protects the abdominal viscera. The positive and negative likelihood ratios for Carnett's sign in the diagnosis of abdominal wall pain are 2.62 and 0.23, respectively [25]. This patient underwent a right upper quadrant trigger point injection with 2 ml of 1% lidocaine and 0.5 ml of betamethasone at the site of maximal tenderness, with dramatic improvement in her pain. At a follow-up visit 6 months later, she remained free of pain.

Clinical Pearls

- The diagnostic evaluation of a patient with chronic abdominal pain requires a thorough history, comprehensive physical exam, and individualized laboratory testing.
- If the diagnostic evaluation does not reveal an underlying etiology, patients should be stratified into low-risk and high-risk categories based on age and alarm symptoms.
- Carnett's sign is a physical exam maneuver that can identify abdominal wall pain and should be routinely

performed in the evaluation of patients with focal chronic abdominal pain.

- Low-risk patients (age <60 years and without alarm symptoms) may be treated empirically with pharmacotherapy and/or psycho-behavioral therapy based on their principal underlying symptom, whereas high-risk patients (age ≥60 years or with alarm features) may require additional evaluation prior to treatment.

Self-Test

Question 1. A 40-year-old woman presents with a 4-year history of epigastric burning and fullness that typically occurs 1 hour after eating. She has a prior history of fibromyalgia and depression. Prior work-up, including an esophagogastroduodenoscopy, *Helicobacter pylori* stool antigen, and right upper quadrant ultrasound, have all been negative or normal. She denies any constipation, diarrhea, heartburn, or weight loss and has found no relief with over-the-counter antacid medications.

What is the most likely diagnosis?

(a) Irritable bowel syndrome
(b) Functional dyspepsia
(c) Gastroesophageal reflux disease
(d) Peptic ulcer disease
(e) Biliary colic

Question 2. A 70-year-old man presents with a 4-month history of worsening abdominal pain. He notes that his abdominal pain starts within 30 min of eating and resolves over the next 2 hours. He has developed a fear of eating and has lost 15 pounds of weight during this time. He has a history of hypertension, hyperlipidemia, and 40-pack-year tobacco use. He denies a history of alcohol use. He underwent coronary angiogram with drug-eluting stent placement to his left anterior descending artery 6 months ago for unstable angina. His medications include aspirin, clopidogrel, atorvastatin, metoprolol, and lisinopril. He denies diarrhea, melena, or hematochezia. A complete blood count and fasting glucose are within normal limits. An esophagogastroduodenoscopy was performed 6 months ago in the evaluation of nausea, around the time of his coronary angiogram, and was found to be normal.

What is the most likely diagnosis?

(a) Gastric malignancy
(b) Medication side effect
(c) Chronic mesenteric ischemia
(d) Chronic pancreatitis
(e) Peptic ulcer disease

Question 3. A 61-year-old man presents with a 6-month history of epigastric pain. He describes the pain as burning and achy. It starts several hours after eating a meal and lasts for 1–2 hours. The pain also awakens him from sleep. He has lost 10 pounds of weight unintentionally during this time. He denies any melena or hematochezia. His past medical history is notable for osteoarthritis and benign prostatic hypertrophy. His only medications are over-the-counter analgesics for joint pain. His complete blood count reveals a microcytic anemia. His last colonoscopy at age 60 was unremarkable.

What is the next best step in management?

(a) Computed tomography of the abdomen
(b) Colonoscopy
(c) Abdominal ultrasound
(d) *Helicobacter pylori* stool antigen
(e) Esophagogastroduodenoscopy

Question 4. A 30-year-old woman presents with a 3-year history of diffuse abdominal pain. She has a lifelong history of constipation with one bowel movement per week. She also describes a sense of incomplete evacuation, excessive straining, and occasional bloating. Several times per month, she has to manually evacuate stool using her fingers. She has seen two providers previously for the same complaint, and an esophagogastroduodenoscopy, colonoscopy, and computed tomography scan of the abdomen and pelvis have been unremarkable. She consumes 60 ounces of water daily and has found no benefit with fiber supplementation, which tends to worsen symptoms of chronic bloating. Her menstrual periods are regular, and her past medical history is unremarkable other than two uneventful vaginal deliveries. Abdominal examination reveals mild diffuse tenderness, and rectal examination reveals limited perineal descent and paradoxical contraction on simulated defecation, with hard stool palpable in the rectal vault.

What is the next best step in management?

(a) Anorectal manometry with balloon expulsion
(b) Increasing doses of stimulant laxatives
(c) Defecating proctogram
(d) Colonic transit study
(e) Subtotal colectomy

References

1. Sandler RS, Stewart WF, Liberman JN, Ricci JA, Zorich NL. Abdominal pain, bloating, and diarrhea in the United States: prevalence and impact. Dig Dis Sci. 2000;45(6):1166–71.
2. Tolba R, Shroll J, Kanu A, Rizk MK. The epidemiology of chronic abdominal pain. In: Chronic abdominal pain. New York: Springer New York; 2015. p. 13–24.
3. Schmulson MJ, Drossman DA. What Is New in Rome IV. J Neurogastroenterol Motil. 2017;23(2):151–63.
4. Bharucha AE, Chakraborty S, Sletten CD. Common functional gastroenterological disorders associated with abdominal pain. Mayo Clin Proc. 2016;91(8):1118–32.
5. Halder SLS, Locke GR, Schleck CD, Zinsmeister AR, Melton LJ, Talley NJ. Natural history of functional gastrointestinal disorders: a 12-year longitudinal population-based study. Gastroenterology. 2007;133(3):799–807.

6. Srinivasan R, Greenbaum DS. Chronic abdominal wall pain: a frequently overlooked problem. Practical approach to diagnosis and management. Am J Gastroenterol. 2002;97(4):824–30.

7. Gaskin DJ, Richard P. The economic costs of pain in the United States. J Pain. 2012;13(8):715–24.

8. Lacy BE, Mearin F, Chang L, Chey WD, Lembo AJ, Simren M, et al. Bowel disorders. Gastroenterology. 2016;150(6):1393–407.

9. Fischer H, Holst E, Karlsson F, Benoni C, Toth E, Olesen M, et al. Altered microbiota in microscopic colitis. Gut. 2015;64(7):1185–6.

10. Harris JK, Fang R, Wagner BD, Choe HN, Kelly CJ, Schroeder S, et al. Esophageal microbiome in eosinophilic esophagitis. PLoS One. 2015;10(5):e0128346.

11. Guarner F, Malagelada J-R. Gut flora in health and disease. Lancet. 2003;361(9356):512–9.

12. Mayer EA, Savidge T, Shulman RJ. Brain–gut microbiome interactions and functional bowel disorders. Gastroenterology. 2014;146(6):1500–12.

13. Dukowicz AC, Lacy BE, Levine GM. Small intestinal bacterial overgrowth: a comprehensive review. Gastroenterol Hepatol (N Y). 2007;3(2):112–22.

14. Hohenwalter EJ. Chronic mesenteric ischemia: diagnosis and treatment. Semin Intervent Radiol. 2009;26(4):345–51.

15. Blake MR, Raker JM, Whelan K. Validity and reliability of the Bristol Stool Form Scale in healthy adults and patients with diarrhoea-predominant irritable bowel syndrome. Aliment Pharmacol Ther. 2016;44(7):693–703.

16. Kamboj AK, Oxentenko AS. Workup and management of bloating. Clin Gastroenterol Hepatol. 2018;16:1030.

17. Sharpstone D, Colin-Jones DG. Chronic, non-visceral abdominal pain. Gut. 1994;35:833–6.

18. Kamboj AK, Cotter TG, Oxentenko AS. Helicobacter pylori: the past, present, and future in management. Mayo Clin Proc. 2017;92(4):599–604.

19. Yarmish GM, Smith MP, Rosen MP, Baker ME, Blake MA, Cash BD, et al. ACR appropriateness criteria right upper quadrant pain. J Am Coll Radiol. 2014;11(3):316–22.

20. Rawson JV, Pelletier AL. When to order a contrast-enhanced CT. Am Fam Physician. 2013;88(5):312–6.

21. Rex DK, Boland CR, Dominitz JA, Giardiello FM, Johnson DA, Kaltenbach T, et al. Colorectal cancer screening: recommendations for physicians and patients from

the U.S. Multi-Society Task Force on Colorectal Cancer. Gastroenterology. 2017;153(1):307–23.

22. Saposnik G, Redelmeier D, Ruff CC, Tobler PN. Cognitive biases associated with medical decisions: a systematic review. BMC Med Inform Decis Mak. 2016;16(1):138.

23. Nazareno J, Ponich T, Gregor J. Long-term follow-up of trigger point injections for abdominal wall pain. Can J Gastroenterol. 2005;19(9):561–5.

24. Sobin WH, Heinrich TW, Drossman DA. Central neuromodulators for treating functional GI disorders: a primer. Am J Gastroenterol. 2017;112(5):693–702.

25. Takada T, Ikusaka M, Ohira Y, Noda K, Tsukamoto T. Diagnostic usefulness of Carnett's test in psychogenic abdominal pain. Intern Med. 2011;50(3):213–7.

Essential Reading

Bharucha AE, Chakraborty S, Sletten CD. Common functional gastroenterological disorders associated with abdominal pain. Mayo Clin Proc. 2016;91(8):1118–32. This article provides a comprehensive review of functional gastrointestinal disorders associated with abdominal pain.

Lacy BE, Mearin F, Chang L, Chey WD, Lembo AJ, Simren M, et al. Bowel disorders. Gastroenterology. 2016;150(6):1393–407. This article also provides a comprehensive review of functional bowel disorders that includes their epidemiology, clinical evaluation, physiologic and psychosocial features, and treatment.

Srinivasan R, Greenbaum DS. Chronic abdominal wall pain: a frequently overlooked problem. Practical approach to diagnosis and management. Am J Gastroenterol. 2002;97(4):824–30. This article discusses diagnosis and management of chronic abdominal wall pain.

Chapter 12
Vascular Disorders

David A. Tendler

Case Study

A 64-year-old female presents to her internist's office complaining of escalating abdominal pain. The pain is difficult to
localize and has been present, to a lesser extent, for the past
several months. She has found that the pain seems to inten-
sify approximately 20 min after eating and then gradually
subsides. The pain does not radiate and is associated with
mild nausea. Her bowel movements have not changed appre-
ciably and she denies blood in the stool. Today, she awoke
from sleep with more persistent, intense pain. Her medical
history is notable for hypertension, hyperlipidemia, and sleep
apnea. She is a former smoker. Her family history is notable
for her brother having had a myocardial infarction at age 65.
Additional history reveals a weight loss of 20 pounds over the
past several months, attributed to a desire to avoid pain
provocation. She has also had mild diarrhea over that time
span. Physical exam notes an afebrile woman in mild-
moderate distress. Vital signs include a blood pressure of

D. A. Tendler (✉)
Duke University, Durham, NC, USA
e-mail: David.Tendler@duke.edu

© Springer Nature Switzerland AG 2019   233
B. E. Lacy et al. (eds.), *Essential Medical Disorders
of the Stomach and Small Intestine*,
https://doi.org/10.1007/978-3-030-01117-8_12

140/90 and heart rate of 98 beats per minute. Her abdominal exam reveals a mildly distended but soft abdomen without appreciable tenderness, rebound, or guarding. Her bowel sounds are hypoactive. The remainder of the exam is unremarkable. After obtaining a complete blood count and comprehensive metabolic panel, she is sent to the local radiologist for an abdominal plain film, which reveals a mild ileus with scattered air-fluid levels and some prominent loops of bowel without a transition point. What do you do next?

Objectives

1. Heighten awareness of the risk factors, signs, and symptoms of intestinal ischemia, paramount to obtaining prompt and appropriate care.
2. Understand the various forms of intestinal ischemia and their clinical manifestations.
3. Review the diagnostic modalities and therapeutic options for patients with intestinal ischemia.

Intestinal Ischemia

Epidemiology

Acute Mesenteric Ischemia

Acute mesenteric ischemia is an uncommon condition with incidence estimates of acute thromboembolic ischemia of 2–7.3 per 100,000 in the general population, although it may account for up to 10% of emergency department admissions for an acute abdomen among patients over 70 years of age [1, 2]. The proportion of cases attributed to each form of acute mesenteric ischemia varies among population studies, as follows [3]:

- – Acute embolic mesenteric ischemia: 50%
- – Acute thrombotic mesenteric ischemia: 15–25%

- Nonocclusive mesenteric ischemia: 5–30%
- Acute mesenteric venous ischemia: 2–10%

The risk factors for developing intestinal ischemia vary according to the specific cause; however, conditions that are generally associated with an increased risk for vascular disease also predispose to intestinal ischemia (Table 12.1). This includes a history of cardiac disease (e.g., atherosclerosis, valvular abnormalities, arrhythmias, or myocardial dysfunction), a history of peripheral artery disease, a history of cardiac or aortic surgery, a history of hemodialysis and/or other hypovolemic states, a history of vasculitis, vasoconstricting medications and drugs, hypercoagulable states, and anatomical anomalies that may lead to bowel strangulation (e.g., hernias, volvulus) or extrinsic compression of the superior mesenteric artery.

Acute embolic mesenteric ischemia occurs most commonly among patients with a history of cardiac arrhythmia (i.e., atrial fibrillation), cardiac valvular disease, recent myocardial infarction, ventricular or aortic aneurysm, and/or history of aortic atherosclerosis. *Acute and/ or chronic thrombotic mesenteric ischemia* occurs most often among patients with a history of peripheral vascular disease, atherosclerosis, advanced age, and/or low cardiac output states. *Nonocclusive mesenteric ischemia* is typically seen among critically ill patients and/or patients with risk factors for acute reduction in intestinal perfusion. Examples include cardiogenic shock, sepsis, cardiac arrhythmia, dialysis, cardiopulmonary bypass, and drug use (e.g., alpha-adrenergic blockers, digoxin, and cocaine). *Acute mesenteric venous thrombosis* risk factors include hereditary hypercoagulable states, oral contraceptive use, myeloproliferative disorders, acute inflammatory conditions of the abdomen (e.g., pancreatitis, diverticulitis), malignancy, recent abdominal surgery, or abdominal trauma.

Mortality rates from acute arterial mesenteric ischemia exceed 65% [4], owing largely to challenges in obtaining rapid diagnosis and therapy, in conjunction with common

TABLE 12.1 Mesenteric ischemia risk factors

Acute embolic mesenteric ischemia

    Atrial fibrillation

    Valvular heart disease

    Recent myocardial infarction

    Aortic or ventricular aneurysm

    Aortic atherosclerosis

    Endocarditis

Acute or chronic thrombotic mesenteric ischemia

    Peripheral vascular disease

    Atherosclerosis

    Advanced age

    Congestive heart failure/low cardiac output state

Mesenteric vein thrombosis

    Hereditary thrombophilia

    Personal or family history of venous thromboembolism

    History of malignancy

    Myeloproliferative disorder

    Oral contraceptive use

    Recent abdominal surgery or trauma

    Acute gastrointestinal inflammation (i.e., pancreatitis, diverticulitis, inflammatory bowel disease)

    Cirrhosis with portal hypertension

    Abdominal mass with venous compression

Acute nonocclusive ischemia

    Critically ill patients

    Cardiogenic shock

TABLE 12.1 (continued)

| Sepsis |
| Acute aortic valvular insufficiency |
| Cardiac arrhythmia |
| Cardiopulmonary bypass |
| Dialysis |
| Drugs (i.e., cocaine, alpha-adrenergic blockers, digoxin) |
| History of vasculitis (i.e., polyarteritis nodosa) |

comorbidities in this population of patients. Among patients with acute nonocclusive mesenteric ischemia, the mortality rates range from 70% to 90% [4]. Patients with acute mesenteric venous thrombosis tend to fare somewhat better, having overall mortality rates of 10–45% [4].

Chronic Mesenteric Ischemia

Approximately 18% of individuals over age 65 will have evidence of having a significant stenosis of the celiac artery or superior mesenteric artery, a minority of whom exhibit related symptoms [5]. Risk factors for symptomatic disease include age over 60, female gender, history of cigarette smoking, a history of coronary artery disease, cerebrovascular disease, or peripheral vascular disease.

Pathophysiology

Intestinal ischemia manifests when blood flow to a segment of bowel is insufficient to meet its metabolic needs and adequate intestinal perfusion cannot be maintained by the collateral circulation. The arterial blood supply of the small intestine is provided mainly by the superior mesenteric artery (SMA); however, extensive collaterals exist between the SMA and celiac artery, as well as between the SMA and inferior mesenteric artery (IMA) (Fig. 12.1). These collaterals serve to protect the small bowel from transient periods of compromised perfusion, although these vessels typically undergo vasoconstriction in the setting of prolonged reductions in splanchnic blood flow, resulting in ischemia. Because collateralization of the mesenteric vasculature often becomes more developed in patients with preexisting mesenteric vascular disease, as is the case in patients with chronic mesenteric ischemia, symptoms related to mesenteric thrombosis may be more insidious than those of acute embolic mesenteric ischemia. Generally, high-grade stenosis (>70%) of at least two of the major mesenteric arteries is necessary for patients to develop ischemic symptoms because of the collateral circulation [6]. In the case of nonocclusive ischemia, acute arterial hypoperfusion results in generalized mesenteric vasoconstriction and intestinal ischemia. Intestinal ischemia due to mesenteric venous thrombosis occurs as a result of occlusion of the superior mesenteric vein (SMV) and impaired venous drainage of the small intestine. The resulting increases in venous pressure leads to fluid efflux and pronounced bowel wall edema. This, in turn, results in systemic hypovolemia, hypotension, and mesenteric arterial vasoconstriction and vasospasm, which further exacerbate the ischemic insult. The distal small intestine is most often affected, with the majority of cases involving the ileum and/ or jejunum [7].

Clinical Presentation

Abdominal pain out of proportion to abdominal tenderness is classically described, related to the fact that, prior to infarction, intestinal ischemia is not an inflammatory event that produces peritoneal inflammation. The abdominal pain is typically acute and severe, in the case of acute embolic ischemia and acute nonocclusive ischemia. It is often periumbilical but can be hard for patients to precisely

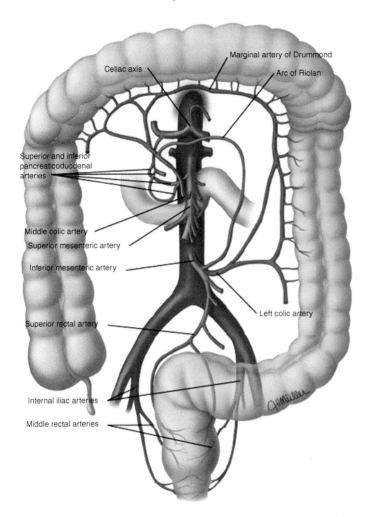

FIGURE 12.1 An extensive collateral blood supply between the celiac artery and SMA (via the superior and inferior pancreaticoduodenal arteries) and the SMA and IMA (via the arc of Riolan and marginal artery of Drummond) helps to protect the bowel from transient periods of diminished perfusion

localize. Nausea, vomiting, and distention are common associated symptoms. Because patients with acute thrombotic ischemia often have an antecedent history of chronic mesenteric ischemic symptoms, the pain may be indolent, subacute, or acutely severe. Those patients, who commonly have cardiovascular disease risk factors, may report a history of having the classic triad of chronic mesenteric ischemic symptoms, comprised of postprandial abdominal pain ("intestinal angina"), sitophobia (aversion to eating due to anticipated pain), and weight loss [8]. Diarrhea may also be an associated symptom. One study revealed that the probability of having chronic mesenteric ischemia was 60% if these four symptoms were all present vs. 13% if they were absent [9]. The pain may be dull or cramping, epigastric, or periumbilical and usually starts within an hour of eating and subsides over the course of the ensuing 2 h. Large or high-fat content meals are more likely to provoke symptoms. Patients with mesenteric venous thrombosis generally have a more insidious, escalating history of pain, typically developing over the course of 5–14 days, although acute pain may occur [10]. The pain is often initially colicky and periumbilical and is also out of proportion to abdominal tenderness at the beginning of the episode. Abdominal distention may be present, related both to bowel wall edema and ileus. Pertaining to the unique risk factors involved in mesenteric venous thrombosis, patients tend to be somewhat younger (mean 45–60) than those suffering from thromboembolic ischemia and do not necessarily have a history of cardiovascular disease [11]. Because patients with acute nonocclusive ischemia are most often severely ill with acute precipitating events, as described previously, symptoms and clinical signs may be unreliable, particularly among those intubated and/or sedated. In addition to abdominal pain, which may be absent in up to 25% of patients, distention and mental status changes may also be appreciated [12]. As all forms of ischemia progress to infarction, noted findings often include abdominal distention, tenderness with the development of peritoneal signs, absent bowel sounds, occult or gross blood in the stool, and the development of a feculent odor to the breath.

Diagnostic Evaluation

Rapid diagnosis, which remains the critical determinant of outcome, relies on the clinician having a high degree of clinical suspicion. Laboratory studies are generally not helpful in diagnosing *chronic* mesenteric ischemia, making it paramount that clinicians have a high index of suspicion in the appropriate clinical setting. Among patients with *acute* intestinal ischemia, laboratory studies are generally nonspecific. Patients may exhibit a leukocytosis, increased hematocrit from hemoconcentration, metabolic acidosis, and/or elevated lactate level. It is important to note that none of these laboratory findings are sufficiently sensitive or specific as individual tests for diagnosing intestinal ischemia, particularly prior to the development of bowel infarction and necrosis. Similarly, abdominal plain films are neither sufficiently sensitive nor specific for diagnosing intestinal ischemia; however, suggestive findings may include ileus, bowel wall thickening, "thumb-printing" due to bowel wall edema, and pneumatosis intestinalis in cases of more advanced ischemia. CT angiography without oral contrast (which can obscure the mesenteric vessels) is typically advised as the initial study of choice for most patients with suspected mesenteric ischemia. In addition to a high sensitivity and specificity among experienced radiologists, it also allows for the exclusion of other conditions that may present similarly (e.g., mechanical bowel obstruction, complicated diverticulitis, Crohn's disease) [13]. While MR angiography is highly accurate for diagnosing intestinal ischemia, its use is limited by cost, available, and speed of obtaining the exam. Among patients without signs of bowel infarction, conventional angiography is generally then recommended, as it allows for both definitive diagnosis and potential therapeutic intervention.

Conventional angiography also is the diagnostic modality of choice for patients with suspected acute nonocclusive mesenteric ischemia, which can be missed by either CT angiography or MR angiography. It also allows for intra-arterial infusion of a vasodilator, if deemed appropriate. Among patients with peritoneal signs or other clinical or radiographic signs of bowel infarction, surgical exploration should be pursued without delay (Fig. 12.2).

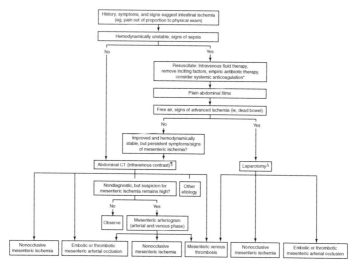

FIGURE 12.2 Diagnosis and initial management of acute mesenteric ischemia

CT: computed tomography

 * Patients ultimately identified with nonocclusive mesenteric ischemia will not benefit from anticoagulation, at which point it can be discontinued

 ¶ Imaging signs associated with mesenteric ischemia include focal or segmental bowel wall thickening, intestinal pneumatosis, portal vein gas, portomesenteric thrombosis, mesenteric arterial calcification, and mesenteric artery occlusion

 Δ Medically fit patients

Treatment

Acute Mesenteric Ischemia

The management of intestinal ischemia is tailored to the specific etiology. Acutely, patients should be given nothing per mouth, placed on supplemental oxygen, and treated with empiric broad-spectrum antibiotics and should undergo nasogastric decompression. Intravenous fluids are important to maintain adequate blood volume and prevent further vasoconstriction. Unless contraindicated, antithrombotic therapy with unfractionated heparin to limit thrombus propagation is advised.

In patients with acute thromboembolic intestinal ischemia, prompt restoration of mesenteric blood flow may be achieved with either surgical laparotomy with embolectomy and/or mesenteric bypass or endovascular intervention [14, 15]. The latter may include catheter-based thrombus aspiration, thrombolysis, or balloon angioplasty (with or without stent placement). The decision of whether to pursue surgical or endovascular therapy is determined by both the clinical status of the patient and the expertise of the managing institution. Patients who have clinical signs of advanced ischemia or infarction or are hemodynamically unstable should be promptly taken to surgery, which has the additional advantage of assessing the viability of the involved segment of bowel visually or with the assistance of intraoperative Doppler imaging, angiography, or intravenous fluorescein dye injection. Nonviable bowel segments are resected, and a "second-look" laparotomy may be planned 24–48 h later to resect any additional nonviable bowel.

Patients who are hemodynamically stable, without contraindications to thrombolysis, do not have signs of advanced ischemia, or are poor-risk surgical candidates may be considered for endovascular therapy, if managed in a hospital with appropriate expertise. Highly selected patients who are hemodynamically stable, without signs of advancing bowel ischemia, and have good collateral perfusion demonstrated on vascular imaging may be initially managed on heparin anticoagulation with close monitoring and serial imaging. Surgical or endovascular therapy may then be pursued nonemergently or urgently if signs of clinical progression become apparent. Long-term management includes the use of anticoagulation and antiplatelet agents with careful surveillance of mesenteric artery patency.

The treatment of patients with nonocclusive intestinal ischemia consists of identifying and treating inciting factors (e.g., hypotension, heart failure, sepsis, vasoconstricting medications), in addition to the general management measures discussed previously. The use of anticoagulation in this population remains controversial given a lack of supporting outcome data. Similarly, there is a dearth of outcome data regarding intra-arterial vasodilator therapy. Nonetheless, this is commonly pursued to treat splanchnic vasoconstriction when felt to be a contributing insult [16]. Similar to patients with acute thromboembolic ischemia, emergent surgical exploration with resection of infarcted bowel should be pursued when clinical or radiographic signs of advanced ischemia are present.

The initial management of patients with acute or subacute mesenteric venous thrombosis involves systemic anticoagulation, bowel rest, intravenous fluids, intravenous antibiotics, and careful monitoring, including an assessment for possible variceal bleeding. Surgery is initially reserved for patients with evidence of bowel infarction, in which case second-look operations to reassess the viability of non-resected bowel is often necessary. In selected patients with acute mesenteric venous thrombosis, transvenous or trans-arterial (SMA) catheter-based thrombolysis may be pursued when bowel necrosis is not apparent and systemic anticoagulation does not result in an adequate response [17, 18]. Long-term management includes excluding a hypercoagulable state among patients with no identifiable cause, as well as anticoagulation. The length of anticoagulation is determined by the presence or absence of correctable risk factors.

Chronic Mesenteric Ischemia

The management of asymptomatic patients with incidentally discovered mesenteric occlusive disease is supportive, including management of hypertension, dyslipidemia, obesity, diabetes, and smoking cessation, as appropriate. Antiplatelet therapy is typically advised. Patients with symptomatic disease should be considered for either surgical or endovascular revascularization. The latter may include percutaneous transluminal angioplasty (PTCA) with or without stent placement. Generally, restenosis rates are higher in those patients who receive angioplasty alone. Surgical reconstruction appears to have superior initial patency rates with lower rates of symptomatic restenosis, although endovascular therapy appears to have lower periprocedural morbidity and mortality rates and no difference in overall survival [19]. As such, endovascular therapy is generally advised as a first-line option for patients with significant comorbidities, provided technical expertise is available [20]. Regular monitoring of patency with duplex ultrasound, CT angiography, or MR angiography (depending on institutional expertise) should be performed [21].

Miscellaneous Disorders of the Mesenteric Vasculature

Median Arcuate Ligament Syndrome

The median arcuate ligament syndrome, also known as celiac artery compression syndrome or celiac axis syndrome, is caused by compression of the celiac artery by the median arcuate ligament of the diaphragm. The median arcuate ligament is a fibrous band that bridges the crura of the diaphragm, typically above the level of the celiac axis. Variations in either the branch point of the celiac axis off of the aorta or in the position of the median arcuate ligament may lead to compression of the celiac artery, which becomes more pronounced during expiration. Compression of the adjacent celiac nerve plexus may also contribute to symptoms attributable to the syndrome [22]. The syndrome tends to affect women disproportionally than men, particularly those with a thin body habitus, and is most often diagnosed between the ages of 40 and 60 [23]. Symptoms may include postprandial abdominal pain, unintentional weight loss, nausea, bloating, and diarrhea. An abdominal bruit may be appreciated on exam. The pain may be attenuated by leaning forward or bending the knees to the chest [24]. While the symptom complex may be similar to those of chronic mesenteric ischemia, the conditions differ with respect to risk factors, which may aid in pursuing appropriate diagnostic testing. Cross-sectional imaging with CT angiography or MR angiography may reveal celiac artery compression. The diagnosis is then confirmed with vascular imaging with respiratory maneuvers. Both duplex ultrasonography and conventional angiography are capable of revealing diagnostic changes in respiration-induced flow velocities, with the modality of choice often determined by institutional expertise [25]. In symptomatic patients, surgical decompression of the celiac artery by release of the median arcuate ligament is advised, usually with concomitant ganglionectomy [22]. Intraoperative vascular assessment may help to identify patients who do not respond adequately to surgical decompression and may benefit from revascularization.

Superior Mesenteric Artery (SMA) Syndrome

An uncommon cause of proximal small bowel obstruction occurs when the angle between the superior mesenteric artery and aorta is excessively narrowed, resulting in compression of the third portion of the duodenum. It is most often a result of marked weight loss that leads to loss of the mesenteric fat pad that ordinarily helps to preserve the normal SMA-aortic angle [26]. Symptoms include nausea, vomiting, postprandial abdominal pain, and weight loss. The diagnosis may be suggested by upper GI barium series or CT scan with oral contrast, which may demonstrate dilation of the stomach and proximal duodenum, transitioning to normal caliber bowel at the level of the third portion of the duodenum [27]. Initial management involves nutritional and caloric support with the goal of weight gain. Positional changes to a prone or left lateral decubitus position may help to alleviate pressure on the duodenum. Surgical decompression with duodenojejunostomy is pursued when symptoms persist despite conservative measures [26].

Case Study: Follow-Up

Our 64-year-old patient, a women with vascular disease risk factors, presents with the classic symptom complex of chronic mesenteric ischemia (postprandial abdominal pain, food avoidance, weight loss, and diarrhea), present for several months prior to a more acute history of escalating abdominal pain. Her history should raise suspicion for acute thrombotic mesenteric ischemia. Because acute occlusive ischemia is associated with very high morbidity and mortality rates, an expedited evaluation is paramount. An urgent CT angiography revealed high-grade atherosclerotic disease of the celiac artery and superior mesenteric artery with a superimposed thrombus at the origin of the superior mesenteric artery. She was placed on oxygen, IV fluids, unfractionated heparin, and empiric broad-spectrum antibiotics. A nasogastric tube was placed, and consultations with interventional (vascular) radiology, general surgery, and vascular surgery were obtained. Because neither peritoneal signs nor radiographic signs of advanced ischemia were present, she was deemed an appropriate candidate for angiographic intervention. The thrombus was successfully aspirated, and angioplasty with stenting was performed for management of the underlying high-grade stenoses of the celiac and superior mesenteric arteries. She was carefully monitored and was eventually discharged to home on aspirin, warfarin, and statin therapy.

Clinical Pearls

- Evaluation for chronic mesenteric ischemia should be pursued in patients with cardiovascular disease risk factors with a history of postprandial abdominal pain, food aversion, and weight loss.
- Evaluation for acute mesenteric ischemia with urgent CT angiography should be rapidly pursued in patients with subacute or acute abdominal pain "out of proportion to the physical exam findings," particularly when cardiovascular disease risk factors or thrombophilia risk factors are present.

Self-Test

Question 1. Which of the following is a true statement pertaining to acute mesenteric ischemia?

A. Patients with a history of myocardial infarction or atrial fibrillation are at increased risk for acute mesenteric venous thrombosis.

B. Patients with acute mesenteric thrombosis rarely have gastrointestinal symptoms preceding the acute event.

C. The mortality rates of acute mesenteric ischemia due to mesenteric venous thrombosis are more favorable than other forms of acute mesenteric ischemia.

D. Barium upper gastrointestinal exam is helpful in making the diagnosis of mesenteric ischemia.

Question 2. Patients with chronic mesenteric ischemia classically present with which of the following symptom complexes?

A. Abdominal pain and bloating relieved by defecation

B. Postprandial abdominal pain, aversion to eating, and weight loss

C. Night sweats, chills, and bloody diarrhea

D. Abdominal distention, confusion, and hematemesis

Question 3. A patient presenting with a proximal small bowel obstruction due to SMA syndrome is most likely to have experienced which of the following?

A. Recent use of oral contraceptive pills
B. A family member with a history of pulmonary embolism
C. Prior umbilical hernia repair
D. Significant weight loss following several courses of chemotherapy

References

1. Kärkkäinen JM, Lehtimäki TT, Manninen H, et al. Acute mesenteric ischemia is a more common cause than expected of acute abdomen in the elderly. J Gastrointest Surg. 2015;19:1407.
2. Bjorck M, Koelemay M, Acosta S, et al. Management of diseases of the mesenteric arteries and veins- clinical practice guidelines of the European Society of Vascular Surgery. Eur J Vasc Endovasc Surg. 2017;53:460–510.
3. Cappell MS. Intestinal (mesenteric) vasculopathy. I Acute superior mesenteric arteriopathy and venopathy. Gastroenterol Clin North Am. 1998;27:783.
4. Schoots IG, Koffeman GI, Legemate DA, et al. Systematic review of survival after acute mesenteric ischaemia according to disease aetiology. Br J Surg. 2004;91:17.
5. Wilson DB, Mostafavi K, Craven TE, et al. Clinical course of mesenteric artery stenosis in elderly Americans. Arch Intern Med. 2006;166:2095.
6. Boley SJ, Brandt LJ, Sammartano RJ. History of mesenteric ischemia. The evolution of a diagnosis and management. Surg Clin North Am. 1997;77:275.
7. Clavien PA, Dürig M, Harder F. Venous mesenteric infarction: a particular entity. Br J Surg. 1988;75:252.
8. White CJ. Chronic mesenteric ischemia: diagnosis and management. Prog Cardiovasc Dis. 2011;54:36.
9. ter Steege RW, Sloterdijk HS, Geelkerken RH, et al. Splanchnic artery stenosis and abdominal complaints: clinical history is of limited value in detection of gastrointestinal ischemia. World J Surg. 2012;36:793.

10. Rhee RY, Gloviczki P, Mendonca CT, et al. Mesenteric venous thrombosis: still a lethal disease in the 1990s. J Vasc Surg. 1994;20:688.

11. Morasch MD, Ebaugh JL, Chiou AC, et al. Mesenteric venous thrombosis: a changing clinical entity. J Vasc Surg. 2001;34:680.

12. Finucane PM, Arunachalam T, O'Dowd J, Pathy MS. Acute mesenteric infarction in elderly patients. J Am Geriatr Soc. 1989;37:355.

13. Ofer A, Abadi S, Nitecki S, et al. Multidetector CT angiography in the evaluation of acute mesenteric ischemia. Eur Radiol. 2009;19:24.

14. Acosta S, Björck M. Modern treatment of acute mesenteric ischaemia. Br J Surg. 2014;101:e100.

15. Arthurs ZM, Titus J, Bannazadeh M, et al. A comparison of endovascular revascularization with traditional therapy for the treatment of acute mesenteric ischemia. J Vasc Surg. 2011;53:698.

16. Habboushe F, Wallace HW, Nusbaum M, et al. Nonocclusive mesenteric vascular insufficiency. Ann Surg. 1974;180:819.

17. Kim HS, Patra A, Khan J, et al. Transhepatic catheter-directed thrombectomy and thrombolysis of acute superior mesenteric venous thrombosis. J Vasc Interv Radiol. 2005;16:1685.

18. Hollingshead M, Burke CT, Mauro MA, et al. Transcatheter thrombolytic therapy for acute mesenteric and portal vein thrombosis. J Vasc Interv Radiol. 2005;16:651.

19. Cai W, Li X, Shu C, et al. Comparison of clinical outcomes of endovascular versus open revascularization for chronic mesenteric ischemia: a meta-analysis. Ann Vasc Surg. 2015;29:934.

20. Pecoraro F, Rancic Z, Lachat M, et al. Chronic mesenteric ischemia: critical review and guidelines for management. Ann Vasc Surg. 2013;27:113.

21. Baker AC, Chew V, Li CS, et al. Application of duplex ultrasound imaging in determining in-stent stenosis during surveillance after mesenteric artery revascularization. J Vasc Surg. 2012;56:1364.

22. Jimenez JC, Harlander-Locke M, Dutson EP. Open and laparoscopic treatment of median arcuate ligament syndrome. J Vasc Surg. 2012;56:869.

23. Reilly LM, Ammar AD, Stoney RJ, Ehrenfeld WK. Late results following operative repair for celiac artery compression syndrome. J Vasc Surg. 1985;2:79.

24. Kim EN, Lamb K, Relles D, et al. Median arcuate ligament syndrome-review of this rare disease. JAMA Surg. 2016;151:471.

25. Gruber H, Loizides A, Peer S, Gruber I. Ultrasound of the median arcuate ligament syndrome: a new approach to diagnosis. Med Ultrason. 2012;14:5.
26. Merrett ND, Wilson RB, Cosman P, Biankin AV. Superior mesenteric artery syndrome: diagnosis and treatment strategies. J Gastrointest Surg. 2009;13:287.
27. Unal B, Aktaş A, Kemal G, et al. Superior mesenteric artery syndrome: CT and ultrasonography findings. Diagn Interv Radiol. 2005;11:90.

Essential Reading

Bala M, Kashuk J, Moore EE, et al. Acute mesenteric ischemia: guidelines of the world Society of Emergency Surgery. World J Emerg Surg. 2017;12:38.
Bjorck M, Koelemay M, Acosta S, et al. Management of diseases of the mesenteric arteries and veins- clinical practice guidelines of the European Society of Vascular Surgery. Eur J Vasc Endovasc Surg. 2017;53:460–510.
Fidelman N, AbuRhama AF, Cash BD. ACR appropriateness criteria radiological management of mesenteric ischemia. J Am Coll Radiol. 2017;14:S266–71.

Chapter 13
Centrally Mediated Abdominal Pain Syndrome

Imran Aziz, Hans Törnblom, and Magnus Simrén

Case Study

A 40-year-old female house cleaner is referred to a gastroenterologist for a second opinion because of severe chronic abdominal pain during the last 3 years. She has previously consulted several doctors and also visited the emergency room in view of her constant symptoms. Her clinical history dates back to her teenage years, where during stressful periods (such as having to

I. Aziz (✉) · H. Törnblom
Department of Internal Medicine and Clinical Nutrition, Institute of Medicine, Sahlgrenska Academy, University of Gothenburg, Gothenburg, Sweden
e-mail: imran.aziz@sth.nhs.uk; hans.tornblom@gu.se

M. Simrén
Department of Internal Medicine and Clinical Nutrition, Institute of Medicine, Sahlgrenska Academy, University of Gothenburg, Gothenburg, Sweden

Center for Functional Gastrointestinal and Motility Disorders, University of North Carolina, Chapel Hill, NC, USA
e-mail: magnus.simren@medicine.gu.se

© Springer Nature Switzerland AG 2019   253
B. E. Lacy et al. (eds.), *Essential Medical Disorders of the Stomach and Small Intestine*,
https://doi.org/10.1007/978-3-030-01117-8_13

move school, being bullied, and finding it difficult to make new friends), she used to experience episodic lower abdominal pain and constipation; she remembers at this point being diagnosed with irritable bowel syndrome. However, over the years, her symptoms of central abdominal pain have become almost constant. She no longer reports bowel disturbances, and the abdominal pain is not related to eating or menses. She has no alarm symptoms. Extensive investigations over the last few years including blood tests, abdominal imaging (X-rays, ultrasounds and CT scans), upper gastrointestinal endoscopy, colonoscopy, and laparoscopy have been normal. As her abdominal pain is increasingly dominating her life, she has had to take time off work and also suffered a relationship breakdown. She has become increasingly depressed and been prescribed an SSRI by the family doctor.

Objectives

1. Understand the epidemiology of CAPS.
2. Recognise the clinical presentation of CAPS and its diagnostic criteria.
3. Appreciate the management strategy of CAPS.
4. Understand the basic principles of neuromodulators.

Epidemiology

CAPS is less common than other functional gastrointestinal disorders, such as irritable bowel syndrome or functional dyspepsia [1]. Historically, the prevalence of CAPS was reported as being between 0.5% and 2.1% [1, 2], although a recent large population-based survey performed across 3 English speaking countries using the Rome IV criteria reported only 1 case of CAPS from almost 6000 adults (0.02%) [3]. The discrepancy in prevalence may be due to the increasing stringency of current diagnostic criteria and also because previous surveys did not incorporate all of the criteria required for CAPS, such as whether the pain limited some aspects of daily function. The condition of CAPS affects women more than men, with a ratio of 1.5 to 2, and has a peak age of onset in the fourth decade, which then decreases with age [2].

CAPS has a significant impact on work presenteeism and absenteeism. Subjects with CAPS miss approximately 12 days of work per year, which is threefold higher compared to those without abdominal pain. Moreover, around 11% feel "too sick to go to work", again threefold higher compared to those without abdominal pain [2].

There is also increased healthcare utilisation in subjects with CAPS, with approximately 80% having previously consulted a physician, of which half see a physician between one and three times per year specifically for abdominal pain [2, 4]. A significant proportion of patients with CAPS are referred to secondary and tertiary gastro-enterology care. Even in this setting, they can experience consultations with different physicians (even within the same specialty) and potentially undergo unnecessary and repetitive investigations. A 7-year follow-up study from the United Kingdom reported that patients with CAPS were on average seen by 5.7 consultants, underwent 6.4 endo-scopic or radiological procedures, and had 2.7 surgical interventions (commonly hysterectomy and exploratory laparotomy) with little symptom benefit [5]. Moreover, a substantial proportion are misinformed that their symp-toms are related to adhesions although there is no good evidence to suggest adhesions cause the chronic and unre-lenting pain that is associated with CAPS; rather the symp-toms of adhesions are different and related to acute or subacute obstruction [1].

Aetiology

CAPS is a functional gastrointestinal disorder character-ised by a disturbance of brain-gut interaction in the absence of any organic pathology to explain the symptoms [1]. It was previously termed functional abdominal pain syndrome [6, 7]. The pathophysiology of CAPS is incompletely understood but considered to be due to a combination of genetic, environmental, and behavioural factors, with aversive early life events and psychosocial stressors having a strong association. This can modulate the endogenous pain system, whereby the development of central sensitisation with disinhibition of pain signals, rather than increased peripheral excitability, leads to constant or near-constant abdominal pain [1, 6, 7].

An altered brain structure has also been observed in somatic and visceral pain disorders, although this has yet to be sufficiently explored in CAPS. In the context of irritable bowel syndrome, an increased thickness of the somatosensory cortex, and decreased cortical thickness in regions of pain processing (e.g. the anterior cingulate cortex and the insula), have been noted. Moreover, IBS symptom severity was negatively correlated with cingulate cortex thickness, suggesting that a loss of neural density may be implicated in symptom generation. It has been speculated that similar structural brain changes may exist in CAPS given the severity and chronicity of pain. However, it remains to be determined whether such brain manifestations are a cause or a consequence of the pain [1].

Symptoms

The diagnosis of CAPS can be made in accordance with the Rome IV criteria (Table 13.1) [1]. The cardinal symptom is constant or near-constant abdominal pain, which tends to be widespread. The pain is chronic in nature and largely independent from physiological events such as eating, defecation, or menses. The pain is not feigned, cannot be explained by an alternate condition, and limits some aspect of daily functioning such as the ability to work, perform household activities, or attend social events.

There are other clinical features of CAPS which, despite lacking specificity, may aid the clinician towards framing the diagnosis of CAPS (Fig. 13.1). For example, patients may become tearful in clinic when they describe their symptoms and often use verbal and non-verbal methods to express the severity of their pain and its detrimental impact on daily life. They also tend to report symptoms with a sense of urgency, play down the role of psychosocial factors, have associated somatisation, and frequently request additional investigations and opiates. They tend to focus on complete recovery and have a history of seeing multiple healthcare providers, who they feel have not been able to empathise or improve their symptoms; this may have also led to previous litigation attempts and a general loss of confidence with the healthcare system. Finally, they may give a history of another functional gastrointestinal disorder, such as irritable bowel syndrome, which has transitioned towards CAPS as the central component begins to dominate.

TABLE 13.1 The Rome IV diagnostic criteria for CAPS

Must include all of the following:

1. Continuous or nearly continuous abdominal pain

2. No or only occasional relationship of pain with physiological events (e.g. eating, defecation, or menses)

3. Pain limits some aspect of daily functioning (e.g. impairments in work, intimacy, social/leisure, family life, and caregiving for self and others)

4. The pain is not feigned

5. Pain is not explained by another structural or functional gastrointestinal disorder or other medical conditions

6. The criteria must be fulfilled for the last 3 months with symptom onset at least 6 months before diagnosis

Used and modified with permission [1]

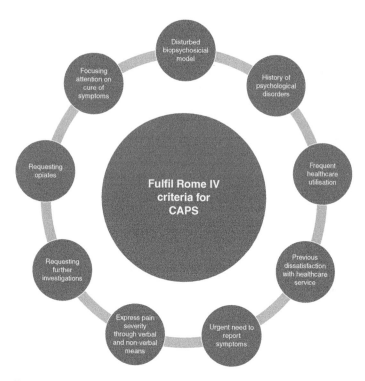

FIGURE 13.1 The characteristic phenotype of patients with CAPS. The inner circle represents that patients must fulfil the Rome IV criteria for CAPS. The outer circles represent some of the characteristics features of CAPS, although these are not sensitive or specific to CAPS

Diagnostic Evaluation

There is currently no diagnostic biomarker for CAPS. Hence, the diagnosis is based upon recognising the characteristic symptoms as outlined by the Rome IV committee (Table 13.1) and excluding organic pathology in a judicious and cost-effective manner. The workup towards excluding organic pathology comprises:

A. A thorough clinical history enquiring for alarm symptoms, such as weight loss or rectal bleeding.

B. Performing an abdominal examination, to check for lymphadenopathy and abdominal masses. Some patients will exhibit *erythema ab igne* suggesting that heat provides relief of symptoms, although there is no direct evidence to support this. A positive Carnett's test (i.e. increasing abdominal pain with tensing of the abdominal musculature) suggests a component of abdominal wall pain. However, anecdotal experience from expert centres suggests that patients with CAPS may also report increasing abdominal pain during a Carnett's test, presumably as a consequence of hypervigilance [6, 7].

C. Baseline laboratory investigations, which include checking for anaemia, celiac disease, and inflammation.

D. Further investigations, such as endoscopies and/or CT abdomen, should be reserved only for those with alarm features as detected by the aforementioned clinical history, examination, and limited laboratory tests.

In the absence of alarm features, or negative further investigations in those with alarm symptoms, a firm diagnosis of CAPS should be made. Unfortunately, it is common to see patients with CAPS who have not been informed of their diagnosis and who are subjected to unnecessary invasive investigations, particularly before they have reached the attention of a specialist in functional gastrointestinal disorders.

Treatment

There is a lack of evidenced-based data evaluating the treatment strategies for CAPS, although the principles are similar to those adopted in treatment of the abdominal pain component of severe irritable bowel syndrome. At the cornerstone of any successful treatment plan is to develop and foster a strong patient-physician relationship. This can then lead to an explanation and acceptance of the diagnosis, a clear understanding that in the absence of a cure (like in many other functional gastrointestinal diseases), the treatment goals are based upon reducing symptoms and improving function whilst living with abdominal pain, followed by implementing therapeutic strategies which comprise centrally acting pharmacological and/or behavioural therapy (Fig. 13.2). Importantly, this provision of care should be maintained with close follow-up [1].

As a physician, it is essential not to view these patients as being "difficult" but rather try and enjoy the clinical challenge they pose. This is pertinent given that they are likely to have experienced a troublesome and disillusioned journey with the healthcare system thus far. Hence, it should be viewed as an opportunity to restore their confidence, with the

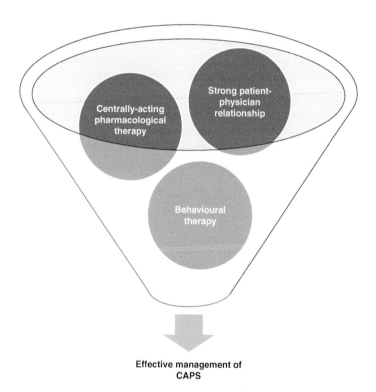

Centrally-acting pharmacological therapy

Strong patient-physician relationship

Behavioural therapy

Effective management of CAPS

Figure 13.2 The strategy to effectively manage CAPS

aims of consultation being to establish trust and to understand the patients' needs by use of the multidimensional biopsychosicial model. This is best achieved through allocating sufficient clinic time, initially asking open questions, listening, and showing empathy, followed by appropriately targeted closed questions.

Following this, a positive diagnosis of CAPS should be made. Patients should be informed that the pain being experienced within the abdomen is not due to an organic pathology in that region, but rather due to the brain not inhibiting endogenous pain signals (i.e. central sensitisation). It should be relayed that CAPS is an unfortunate manifestation of the adverse events within their biopsychosocial model. This will aid towards patient understanding and acceptance that further investigations of the abdomen are not necessary and that they carry appreciable risks.

Treatment strategies should be discussed whilst emphasising the importance of patient responsibility. It should be made clear that CAPS is unlikely to be cured and that the aim of treatment is therefore to reduce symptoms, improve function, and restore a sufficient quality of life. Opiates are contraindicated as they can precipitate drug dependence and in some cases also narcotic bowel syndrome (also known as opioid-induced gastrointestinal hyperalgesia). Instead, the treatment options available are centrally acting pharmacological and/or behavioural therapies [1, 8, 9]. Given that centrally acting pharmacological therapies are widely available, they are usually adopted first line and comprise either tricyclic antidepressants (TCAs) or serotonin noradrenergic reuptake inhibitors (SNRIs), rather than selective serotonin reuptake inhibitors (SSRIs). The reasons for opting for a TCA or an SNRI are due to their serotonergic and also noradrenergic properties, which help towards improving mood and pain, respectively. In contrast, SSRIs possess serotonergic but lack noradrenergic properties, meaning that they improve mood but not pain (Table 13.2) [1, 8, 9]. Due to familiarity, gastroenterologists tend to favour TCAs although their use can be restricted by anti-muscarinic (dry eyes, dry mouth, constipation) and antihistaminic side effects (lethargy, weight gain); in such instances, patients can then be switched to an SNRI although there is a relative paucity of randomised controlled trials evaluating their clinical effectiveness in functional gastrointestinal disorders. Importantly, these medications are started at low doses and titrated upwards, which contrasts with the high-dose treatment required for depression – this concept can be used to reassure patients who hold reservations that they are being treated for a psychiatric disorder. Indeed, recent consensus suggests that one way of further reducing the stigma attached to antidepressants is to refer to them as neuromodulators instead.

In those who fail to respond to the aforementioned medication, the next step would be augmentation therapy, i.e. the use, usually at lower dosages, of two or more treatments that act on different receptor sites or areas of the brain to enhance the therapeutic effect [1, 8, 9]. This includes not only TCAs, SSRIs, and SNRIs but also atypical antipsychotics (such as quetiapine), 5-HT1a agonists (such as buspirone), and tetracyclic antidepressants (such as mirtazapine). Importantly these neuromodulators work on different receptors than TCAs, SNRIs, and SSRIs and hence augment the overall pharmacological effect. Augmentation therapy should be coordinated by physicians who are familiar with the side effects and risks of these drugs and can be done in collaboration with a psychiatrist. A referral to a psychiatrist also allows for further consultation and the addition of certain neuromodulators which gastroenterologists may largely be unaccustomed to prescribing. Moreover, it paves the way for considering behavioural therapies which have been shown to be of benefit in other functional gastrointestinal disorders such as IBS. These include cognitive behavioural therapy, hypnotherapy, mindfulness, and psychodynamic interpersonal therapy which also could be viewed upon as augmenting treatment options for patients already on treatment with neuromodulators with incomplete effects [1].

TABLE 13.2 Action of neuromodulators on receptor sites [1, 8, 9]

	Serotonin	Norepinephrine	Histamine	Acetylcholine
Tricyclic antidepressants (TCA)	✓	✓	✓	✓
Serotonin and norepinephrine reuptake inhibitors (SNRI)	✓	✓	–	–
Selective serotonin reuptake inhibitors (SSRI)	✓	–	–	–

Case Study

The patient was given a diagnosis of CAPS and the nature of the condition was relayed. She understood that given the (a) chronicity of her symptoms, (b) absence of alarm features, and (c) negative abdominal investigations, further investigations were not needed as an organic cause of her symptoms had been adequately excluded. Her SSRI was continued as the dose prescribed was being used to treat depression. However, to improve her pain, she was commenced on a TCA at a low dose of 25 mg each night, which was increased after 4 weeks to 50 mg each night. At follow-up, she felt some improvement in clinical symptoms although her quality of life remained poor. At this stage she was referred for a psychiatry consult. During this visit the provider was able to gather further details on her biopsychosicial history and explore her symptoms and goals, with the end result that quetiapine was initiated. Later in the course of her condition, she also underwent hypnotherapy. The culmination of augmentation therapy led to a sufficient improvement in clinical symptoms and ability to return back to work. She continues to be managed by the gastroenterologist and psychiatrist in collaboration.

Clinical Pearls

- CAPS is a consequence of central sensitisation, with disinhibition of endogenous nociceptive input.
- The basis of effectively managing CAPS is to establish a strong patient-physician relationship.
- Opiates should be avoided as they can precipitate drug dependence and the paradox of narcotic bowel syndrome (opioid-induced gastrointestinal hyperalgesia); instead centrally acting pharmacological and/or behavioural therapies are the valid treatment options for CAPS.

Self-Test

Question 1. Which of the following statements regarding CAPS is true?

A. CAPS is characterised by chronic constant or near-constant abdominal pain that is commonly associated with altered bowel habit.
B. CAPS is associated with chronic constant or near-constant abdominal pain with relative independence from gastrointestinal physiological events.
C. CAPS is always exacerbated by eating.

Question 2. Which of the following receptor sites do tricyclic antidepressants (TCA) work on?

A. Norepinephrine, serotonin, and histamine but not acetylcholine
B. Norepinephrine, serotonin, and acetylcholine but not histamine
C. Norepinephrine, serotonin, acetylcholine, and histamine

Question 3. Which of the following neuromodulators would not be considered as first-line therapy for CAPS?

A. Selective serotonin reuptake inhibitors (SSRI)
B. Serotonin norepinephrine reuptake inhibitors (SNRI)
C. Tricyclic antidepressants (TCA)

References

1. Keefer L, Drossman DA, Guthrie E, et al. Centrally mediated disorders of gastrointestinal pain. Gastroenterology. 2016;150(6):1408–19.
2. Drossman DA, Li Z, Andruzzi E, et al. U.S. householder survey of functional gastrointestinal disorders. Prevalence, sociodemography, and health impact. Dig Dis Sci. 1993;38(9):1569–80.
3. Aziz I, Palsson OS, Törnblom H, Sperber AD, Whitehead WE, Simrén M. The prevalence and impact of overlapping Rome IV-diagnosed functional gastrointestinal disorders on somatization, quality of life, and healthcare utilization: a cross-sectional

general population study in three countries. Am J Gastroenterol. 2018;113(1):86–96.

4. Koloski NA, Talley NJ, Boyce PM. Epidemiology and health care seeking in the functional GI disorders: a population-based study. Am J Gastroenterol. 2002;97(9):2290–9.

5. Maxton DG, Whorwell PG. Use of medical resources and attitudes to health care of patients with chronic abdominal pain. Br J Med Econ. 1992;2:75–9.

6. Drossman DA. Functional abdominal pain syndrome. Clin Gastroenterol Hepatol. 2004;2(5):353–65.

7. Sperber AD, Drossman DA. Review article: the functional abdominal pain syndrome. Aliment Pharmacol Ther. 2011;33(5):514–24.

8. Sobin WH, Heinrich TW, Drossman DA. Central neuromodulators for treating functional GI disorders: a primer. Am J Gastroenterol. 2017;112(5):693–702.

9. Drossman DA, Tack J, Ford AC, Szigethy E, Törnblom H, Van Oudenhove L. Neuromodulators for functional gastrointestinal disorders (disorders of gut-brain interaction): a Rome foundation working team report. Gastroenterology. 2018;154(4):1140–1171.e1141.

Essential Reading

Drossman DA, Tack J, Ford AC, Szigethy E, Törnblom H, Van Oudenhove L. Neuromodulators for functional gastrointestinal disorders (disorders of gut-brain interaction): a Rome foundation working team report. Gastroenterology. 2018;154(4):1140–1171. e1141. This article provides an advanced and comprehensive review of the use of neuromodulators in clinical practice.

Keefer L, Drossman DA, Guthrie E, et al. Centrally mediated disorders of gastrointestinal pain. Gastroenterology. 2016;150(6):1408–19. This article provides an authoritative overview on Rome IV defined centrally mediated abdominal pain syndrome.

Sobin WH, Heinrich TW, Drossman DA. Central neuromodulators for treating functional GI disorders: a primer. Am J Gastroenterol. 2017;112(5):693–702. This article is a primer to help gastroenterologists understand how best to use central neuromodulators to optimise patient care.

Chapter 14
Postcholecystectomy Pain

Enrico Stefano Corazziari and Nadia Pallotta

Case Study

A 46-year-old female teacher is referred to a gastroenterologist for eight episodes of severe epigastric pain over a 24-month period. The episodes occurred at 2–4-month intervals; in between these episodes, she did not have any symptoms. On each occasion, the pain built up to a steady level, lasted for 45–60 min, and then resolved spontaneously. On three occasions the pain was so severe as to require evaluation in the emergency room. On six occasions the pain radiated to the right subscapular region and the right shoulder, while on five occasions, the pain was associated with nausea and vomiting. The pain was not relieved by bowel movements, antacids, or postural changes. The patient's past

E. S. Corazziari (✉)
Department of Gastroenterology, Clinical Institute Humanitas,
Rozzano, Italy
e-mail: enrico.corazziari@humanitas.it

N. Pallotta
Department of Internal Medicine and Medical Specialties,
Department of Gastroenterology A, University La Sapienza,
Rome, Italy
e-mail: nadia.pallotta@uniroma1.it

© Springer Nature Switzerland AG 2019   267
B. E. Lacy et al. (eds.), *Essential Medical Disorders*
of the Stomach and Small Intestine,
https://doi.org/10.1007/978-3-030-01117-8_14

surgical history was notable for a cholecystectomy 10 years earlier after several episodes of right upper quadrant biliary colic that resembles the recent pain except for the current location of pain in the epigastrium. An elevated (three times the upper limit of normal) AST and ALT were reported in the three available emergency room records. On all of these occasions, serum amylase and lipase were normal. A recent abdominal ultrasound was reported as unremarkable; the CBD diameter was 8 mm. The patient inquires as to the cause of her pain and whether other tests are necessary.

Objectives

- Understand the epidemiology of postcholecystectomy pain.
- Appreciate the physiology of postcholecystectomy pain.
- Understand the diagnostic algorithm of postcholecystectomy pain.
- Review treatment options for postcholecystectomy pain.

Epidemiology

Laparoscopic cholecystectomy is considered one of the most effective, safe, and commonly performed surgical procedures. Nonetheless, it is not devoid of postsurgical morbidity (1.6–5.3%), mortality (0.08–0.14%), and persistent postcholecystectomy symptoms [1]. As discussed below, a number of different symptoms may develop after cholecystectomy, one of the most common of which is abdominal pain. Flatulence is the most common de novo symptom reported by up to 62% of patients [2]. It is worth pointing out that symptoms of either diarrhea or constipation commonly develop after cholecystectomy; however, when these symptoms are present prior to cholecystectomy, they are likely to persist after removal of the gallbladder in up to 85% and 76% of patients, respectively.

Cholecystectomy is frequently performed in patients with non-specific abdominal pain; gallstones may or may not be coincidentally present in some of these patients. Indeed, it is not uncommon to encounter patients in clinic with irritable bowel syndrome (IBS) or functional dyspepsia who have previously undergone cholecystectomy [3]. In these patients, a prior cholecystectomy is unlikely the cause of long-term postsurgical symptoms. However, even considering patients with more specific biliary pain as an indication for cholecystectomy, abdominal pain persists or arises de novo in up to 33% and 14% of patients, respectively, after surgery [2].

In the EPISOD study, more than half of patients referred for sphincterotomy for postcholecystectomy biliary pain had previously undergone cholecystectomy for a "poorly functioning gallbladder" (e.g., acalculous functional gallbladder disorder or gallbladder dyskinesia) without improvement in their symptoms [4]. The prevalence of postcholecystectomy pain is highly variable in published reports, from 1% to 37%, with rates highest in patients without gallstones, those without specific (e.g., biliary-type) abdominal symptoms, and those referred for elective surgery [5]. Thus, the most common cause of postcholecystectomy pain, even with a biliary-like presentation, is an overlooked non-biliary disorder. Retained or recurrent common bile duct stones have been reported to range from 1.2% to 14%, being symptomatic in only approximately 0.3%. Stones that spill out into the peritoneum have been reported to range from 0.1% to 20% but are rarely symptomatic [5]. The prevalence of sphincter of Oddi dysfunction (SOD) in postcholecystectomy patients has not been sufficiently investigated and ranges from 1.5% in a householder survey to 14% in a selected group of patients investigated with sphincter of Oddi (SO) manometry [6].

Pathophysiology

Nature and Characterization of Postcholecystectomy Biliary Pain

Biliary pain (Table 14.1) lacks a precise localization, is nonspecific in nature, and is identical to that triggered by the many

TABLE 14.1 Rome IV diagnostic criteria for biliary pain

Pain located in the epigastrium and/or right upper quadrant and all of the following are required:

Pain builds up to a steady level and lasts at least 30 min

Occurs at intervals and does not occur daily

Severe enough to interfere with daily activities and/or leads to an emergency department evaluation

Rarely (<20%) related to bowel movements

Rarely (<20%) relieved by postural change

Rarely (<20%) relieved by acid suppression

Supportive criteria:

The pain may be associated with:

Nausea and vomiting

Radiation to the back and/or right subscapular region

Waking from sleep

and diverse functional and structural alterations of the organs that share the same innervation. During distension of the bile duct, the pain is localized to the epigastrium alone or radiates to the back, right upper quadrant, and midline in 47%, 18%, and 16% of cases, respectively [7]. The non-specific nature of the pain is highlighted by the fact that the same type of pain may occur during distension of the esophagus, duodenum, ileum, and colon. The biliary tract is highly innervated by afferent nerves that convey mechanical and noxious stimuli to several dorsal root ganglia and to multiple segments of the spinal cord. Such diffuse innervation explains how viscero-somatic nerve connections may account for the localization of biliary pain in different areas of the abdomen and thorax and even the right shoulder. In addition, autonomic extrinsic nerves and enteric plexi regulate and connect the terminal choledochus and the SO to the duodenum, pancreas, and stomach, each of them sharing with the other several reflex patterns.

Pathophysiology of Postcholecystectomy Biliary Pain

One mechanism leading to biliary-like pain after cholecystectomy is a sudden pressure increase in the bile duct following any obstruction to bile flow, in the absence of the gallbladder, which serves as reservoir. This sudden increase in pressure may occur in the presence of residual or recurrent stone(s) in the bile duct or when the SO is stenosed or strictured. In both of these situations, there may be evidence of secondary bile duct dilatation. In absence of a structural obstruction to bile flow, more complex mechanisms have been hypothesized on the basis of experimental evidence in animals. After resection of the gallbladder and, thus, of the nerves connecting the gallbladder to the SO, the cholecysto-SO reflex, which normally inhibits the sphincter in response to gallbladder distension, disappears, and abnormal SO contractions may cause intraductal pressure to increase leading to the development of abdominal pain [5]. Under normal conditions, cholecystokinin inhibits SO contractility via a neural pathway; however, in postcholecystectomy patients with SOD, cholecystokinin instead causes a paradoxical excitatory contraction of the sphincter [8], which can cause abdominal pain. In the absence of any structural or SO motor alterations that may account for increased bile duct pressure, a pure sensory mechanism for pain has been advocated. It is likely that in genetically predisposed subjects, episodes of biliary pain (e.g., due to cholecystitis) activate and increase the sensitivity of the afferent nociceptive pathway which subsequently undergoes neuroplastic changes. Such sensitivity persists after the noxious trigger has been removed (e.g., at the time of cholecystectomy), and even minor increases in choledochal pressure can elicit pain. Similar to other functional gastrointestinal disorders, nociceptive sensitization may occur at one or more levels of the nociceptive nervous pathway from neurons in the dorsal root ganglia to a number of different regions in the brain. Another possible mechanism that might explain post-

cholecystectomy pain in the absence of any structural alteration is the process of cross-sensitization. In this situation, a
noxious stimulus from a neighboring organ (e.g., pancreas or
duodenum, both of which share similar afferent nervous system pathways) can be experienced by some patients as
biliary-like pain [9]. Likewise it seems plausible that nociceptive sensitization of an adjacent organ can elicit biliary-like
pain by cross-sensitization.

Symptoms

In patients with recurrent pain after cholecystectomy, the
greatest challenge is in determining the source of the pain,
even if the pain characteristics are consistent with "typical"
biliary pain which, according to the Rome IV consensus statement (Table 14.1), is usually referred to the epigastric region or
right upper quadrant, rises rapidly to reach its maximal severity, and then remains steady and severe for 30 min or longer, a
pattern easily distinguishable from the waxing and waning pain
of renal colic or intestinal obstruction [5]. For the most part,
"typical" biliary pain is intermittent (not daily) and infrequent,
although in some people, it may be continuous, with episodic
flares [2]. The pain may radiate to the back or right shoulder
and be accompanied by nausea and vomiting. Food or narcotics may precipitate the pain. The pain may awaken the patient
from sleep, interrupt a patient's daily activities, or lead to an
emergency room visit. The pain is not relieved by bowel movements, postural changes, or acid suppressive agents. The pain
may begin several years after a cholecystectomy and may be
similar to the pain leading to the cholecystectomy.

Diagnostic Evaluation

The initial diagnostic approach relies on a careful history and
physical examination. In many patients, the correct diagnosis
for the reported abdominal pain is functional dyspepsia, irri-

table bowel syndrome, or a musculoskeletal disorder [5]. Non-biliary findings are more likely when the pain is atypical and long-standing and is associated with other less specific abdominal symptoms and when cholecystectomy was performed in the absence of gallstones. Regular use of narcotics should be carefully investigated as these agents can affect receptors in the bile duct and SO and because chronic use may lead to narcotic bowel syndrome. Postoperative complications, such as bile duct strictures, retained or recurrent common bile duct stones, acid-related diseases, pancreatitis, and fatty liver disease should be excluded. Upper endoscopy is useful to exclude peptic ulcer disease and esophagitis. Increased serum liver and pancreas enzymes, which peak within hours of typical biliary pain, may indicate SO obstruction and/or SOD. Bile duct imaging is mandatory to rule out choledocholithiasis and operative bile duct injury and to evaluate bile duct size even if the finding of a "dilated bile duct" is difficult to interpret [10]. Although ultrasound may be used initially, magnetic resonance cholangiopancreatography (MRCP) and endoscopic ultrasound (EUS) both provide more complete information regarding the pancreatobiliary system [5]. EUS is considered the preferred method to rule out a retained bile duct stone and to evaluate abnormalities of the papilla [5].

In some patients, the reported pain can arise secondary to organic biliary pathology (e.g., a stone in the common bile duct or a stenotic sphincter). SOD is suspected when the pain is typical and when other conditions have been excluded. A major issue in this context is the lack of a diagnostic gold standard. Historically, patients with SOD have been classified into three subgroups: type I (abdominal pain plus both serum liver chemistries (> twice normal) on at least two occasions and bile duct ≥9 mm), type II (abdominal pain plus one of the two objective data measures), and type III (abdominal pain only without any objective measures) [11]. However, the results of randomized trials have determined that most type I SOD patients respond favorably to endoscopic sphincterotomy, thus suggesting a fibrotic structural pathology as the cause of their symptoms [10, 11]. In contrast, symptoms in type III SOD patients, without objective findings of bile obstruction or abnormalities in the papilla, do not respond to sphincterotomy [10, 11]. Importantly, type I and III SOD patients do not require any specific invasive investigation as they can be diagnosed by a combination of symptoms, MRCP, and laboratory tests as described above. Thus, the term SOD should be reserved solely for patients with postcholecystectomy biliary pain and one of the objective findings of bile flow obstruction (e.g., type II SOD) [5] (Table 14.2).

Hepatobiliary scintigraphy is a noninvasive measure of biliary drainage that has been shown to be abnormal in patients with SOD [11–14]. Clinical research studies have demonstrated that scintigraphy accurately differentiates between patients that do, and do not, have other objective evidence of biliary obstruction [11]. Accordingly, abnormal hepatic hilum to duodenum transit times decrease after sphincterotomy in patients with evidence of biliary obstruction [13] (Fig. 14.1). Its accuracy in the diagnosis of SOD

TABLE 14.2 Rome IV diagnostic criteria for functional biliary sphincter of Oddi disorder

All the following criteria must be included:
Typical biliary pain
Elevated liver enzymes or dilated bile duct
Absence of bile duct stones or other structural abnormalities
Supportive criteria:
Normal amylase/lipase
Abnormal sphincter of Oddi manometry
Abnormal Hepatobiliary scintigraphy

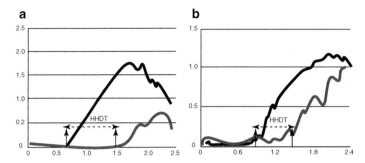

FIGURE 14.1 Hepatobiliary scintigraphy in a patient with postcholecystectomy biliary pain and SOD submitted to sphincterotomy. Hepatic hilum (blue) and duodenum (red) time-activity curves are shown. Hepatobiliary scintigraphy performed before SO sphincterotomy (**a**) and after SO sphincterotomy (**b**). The prolonged hepatic hilum-duodenum transit (HHDT) time normalizes after sphincterotomy

remains less clear. Furthermore, this test is not widely available in the United States. In contrast, SO manometry (SOM) allows direct measurement of biliary and pancreatic sphincter pressures in addition to evaluation of phasic wave amplitudes, duration, frequency, and propagation pattern. To date, only the basal pressure measurement has been shown to correlate with clinical outcome following sphincterotomy [5, 15]. Sphincter of Oddi manometry is recommended in patients with suspected type II SOD because it has been shown that, in these patients, biliary manometry predicts the response to biliary sphincterotomy [5,15]. Pancreatic sphincter assessment should be avoided in patients with biliary pain to reduce the risk of pancreatitis. SOM, however, is also not widely available. Endoscopic retrograde cholangiopancreatography (ERCP) is recommended only for patients who need SO manometry (i.e., previous type II SOD) or for those with strong evidence of biliary obstruction (e.g., previous type I SOD or retained bile duct stones) and, therefore, need endoscopic treatment. Figure 14.2 shows a diagnostic algorithm for patients with postcholecystectomy pain.

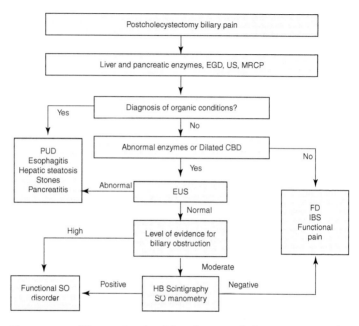

FIGURE 14.2 Diagnostic algorithm for postcholecystectomy pain. After exclusion of structural conditions, patients without dilated bile ducts or elevated liver enzymes can no longer be considered affected by sphincter of Oddi dysfunction. In the presence of a high level of objective evidence for biliary obstruction, patients should undergo sphincterotomy at a center of excellence. If the evidence is less convincing further tests may be helpful. EGD esophagogastroduodenoscopy, US ultrasound, MRCP magnetic resonance cholangiopancreatography, CBD common bile duct, PUD peptic ulcer disease, EUS endoscopic ultrasound, FD functional dyspepsia, IBS irritable bowel syndrome, SO sphincter of Oddi, HB hepatobiliary

Treatment

The spectrum of treatments for suspected SOD ranges from traditional pharmacologic management to sphincter ablation to complementary and alternative medicine approaches. The value of current treatments for management of patients with suspected functional SOD is difficult to prove and predict in an individual patient. The placebo effect of intervention is high, with about one-third of sham-treated patients claiming long-term benefit in blinded randomized studies [5].

Because of the risks and uncertainties involved with invasive approaches, it is important to explore conservative management initially. Psychosocial stress has been shown to affect SOD, but does not cause SO stenosis, highlighting the importance of holistic patient management. Smooth muscle antispasmodics and relaxants including nitrates, calcium channel blockers, phosphodiesterase type V inhibitors, trimebutine, hyoscine butylbromide, octreotide, and nitric oxide have been shown to reduce basal sphincter pressures in SOD patients and asymptomatic volunteers during standard SO manometry [5, 11]. As alluded to earlier, because of the frequent overlap with functional bowel disorders, such as IBS and functional dyspepsia, psychotropic neuromodulating agents may be useful. A trial of duloxetine was found to improve symptoms in one study [16]. Amitriptyline has also been successfully used. While there have been some trials reporting clinical success [5, 11] of pharmacologic therapy for suspected SOD, it has been limited by the lack of long-term outcomes data and the potential for adverse effects. Nevertheless, this approach should be considered because some studies have shown that medical therapy may decrease the need for more aggressive treatments in about 50% of cases [17, 18]. Importantly, none of these drugs are specific to the SO and may also be useful in patients with non-biliary functional disorders. It is interesting that the efficacy of these agents is highest in the previous SOD type III group classification and lowest in the previous SOD type I [17, 18], highlighting the low sensitivity of these diagnostic criteria.

Transcutaneous electrical nerve stimulation (TENS) and acupuncture also have been shown to reduce SO pressure in patients with biliary dyskinesia [5]; however, their long-term efficacy has not been evaluated. Endoscopic biliary sphincterotomy has been widely used to treat suspected SOD, and retrospective studies have reported a high rate of success

[5, 11] and relief of clinical symptoms independent of SO motility results [19, 20]. The evidence for biliary sphincterotomy in patients with SOD, however, is not strong as most studies have been retrospective and unblinded and did not use objective assessments [21]. The most convincing data come from three small, randomized studies which showed that sphincterotomy was more effective than a sham procedure in patients with elevated basal biliary sphincter pressures [5, 15, 22]. There is concern about the use of sphincterotomy in patients without clear evidence for SO obstruction due to the potential for serious complications including pancreatitis in 10–15% of patients, bleeding and retroduodenal perforation (~1% of cases), and late restenosis [5]. According to Rome IV consensus recommendations [5], only patients with definite evidence of SO obstruction (type I SOD) should be treated with endoscopic sphincterotomy without prerequisite SO manometry. Patients with a history of increased serum liver chemistries associated with attacks of abdominal pain are likely to respond favorably to sphincterotomy (e.g., a type II SOD patient) [23]. On the contrary, patients with attacks of abdominal pain but normal laboratory and imaging findings did not benefit from endoscopic sphincterotomy (biliary or dual) compared to a sham group after 5 years of follow-up. Normal pancreatic manometry, delayed gastric emptying, daily opioid use, and age younger than 40 years all predict poor outcomes [24]. Patients are more likely to respond if their pain was not continuous and was accompanied by nausea and vomiting and there had been a pain-free interval of at least 1 year after cholecystectomy [24].

Case Study: Follow-Up

Although the clinical presentation of the pain was consistent with biliary-like pain, an upper endoscopy was performed to rule out other possible causes of epigastric pain such as reflux esophagitis or peptic ulcer disease and was normal; gastric biopsies did not show evidence of *Helicobacter pylori*. To exclude the presence of retained common bile duct stones or other abnormalities of the biliary tract, an MRCP was performed and was normal. This confirmed the absence of significant CBD dilatation that could justify the presence of a fixed obstruction at the choledocho-duodenal junction. The elevated levels of liver enzymes temporally related to the episodes of abdominal pain on three separate occasions, however, strongly supported the clinical suspicion of type II SOD. Due to the risks of a diagnostic ERCP with SO manometry, the patient underwent a quantitative hepatobiliary scintigraphy study, which confirmed a marked delay of bile flow from the liver to the duodenum. This scintigraphic finding prompted referral to a center of excellence to perform endoscopic biliary sphincterotomy. At 2-year follow-up, the patient reported that the pain had not recurred.

Self-Test

Question 1. Which one of the following answers (A–D) most accurately completes the following statement?
Biliary pain builds up to a steady level, lasts 30 min or longer, and:

A. Is located in the right upper quadrant
B. Is similar to the pain triggered by distension of the esophagus
C. Radiates to the back in almost all cases
D. Mainly occurs after eating a fatty meal

Question 2. After cholecystectomy, in the absence of structural pathology of the biliary tract and/or sphincter of Oddi, the pathophysiological mechanism(s) leading to biliary pain relies mainly on which one of the following:

A. Increased resistance to bile outflow and subsequent rise in intrabiliary pressure
B. Loss of the physiological cholecysto-sphincteric reflex

C. Paradoxical response to cholecystokinin after cholecystectomy

D. Complex interaction among altered innervation of the SO, persistent activation of nociceptive neurons, and cross-sensitization with neighboring organs

Question 3. The term "suspected" SO dysfunction (SOD) should be used for patients with which one of the following:

A. Postcholecystectomy biliary pain and one of the objective findings of bile flow obstruction

B. Postcholecystectomy biliary pain in the absence of structural pathology of the biliary tract as assessed by EUS

C. Postcholecystectomy biliary pain and at least two objective findings of bile flow obstruction

D. Postcholecystectomy biliary pain and objective findings of abnormal SO manometry and/or hepatobiliary scintigraphy

References

1. Pucher PH, Brunt LM, Davies N, et al., SAGES Safe Cholecystectomy Task Force. Outcome trends and safety measures after 30 years of laparoscopic cholecystectomy: a systematic review and pooled data analysis. Surg Endosc. 2018;32:2175–83.

2. Lamberts MP, Lugtenberg M, Rovers MM, et al. Persistent and de novo symptoms after cholecystectomy: a systematic review of cholecystectomy effectiveness. Surg Endosc. 2012;27:709–18.

3. Corazziari E, Attili AF, Angeletti C, et al. A. Gallstones, cholecystectomy and irritable bowel syndrome (IBS) MICOL population-based study. Dig Liver Dis. 2008;40:944–50.

4. Cotton PB, Pauls Q, Keith J, et al. The EPISOD study: long-term outcomes. Gastrointest Endosc. 2018;87:205–10.

5. Cotton PB, Elta GH, Carter CR, et al. Gallbladder and sphincter of Oddi disorders. Gastroenterology. 2016;150:1420–9.

6. Drossman DA, Li Z, Andruzzi E, et al. U.S. householder survey of functional gastrointestinal disorders. Prevalence, sociodemographic and health impact. Dig Dis Sci. 1993;38:1569–80.

7. Doran FS. The sites to which pain is referred from the common bile-duct in man and its implication for the theory of referred pain. Br J Surg. 1967;54:599–606.

8. Luman W, Williams AJ, Pryde A, et al. Influence of cholecystectomy on sphincter of Oddi motility. Gut. 1997;41:371–4.

9. Desautels SG, Slivka A, Hutson WR, et al. Postcholecystectomy pain syndrome: pathophysiology of abdominal pain in sphincter of Oddi type III. Gastroenterology. 1999;116:900–5.

10. Leung WD, Sherman S. Endoscopic approach to the patient with motility disorders of the bile duct and sphincter of Oddi. Gastrointest Endosc Clin N Am. 2013;23:405–34.

11. Tarnasky PR. Post-cholecystectomy syndrome and sphincter of Oddi dysfunction: past, present and future. Expert Rev Gastroenterol Hepatol. 2016;10:1359–72.

12. Corazziari E, Cicala M, Scopinaro F, et al. Scintigraphic assessment of SO dysfunction. Gut. 2003;52:1655–6.

13. Corazziari E, Cicala M, Habib FI, et al. Hepatoduodenal bile transit in cholecystectomized subjects. Relationship with sphincter of Oddi function and diagnostic value. Dig Dis Sci. 1994;39:1985–93.

14. Cicala M, Habib FI, Vavassori P, et al. Outcome of endoscopic sphincterotomy in post cholecystectomy patients with sphincter of Oddi dysfunction as predicted by manometry and quantitative choledochoscintigraphy. Gut. 2002;50:665–8.

15. Toouli J, Roberts-Thomson IC, Kellow J, et al. Manometry based randomised trial of endoscopic sphincterotomy for sphincter of Oddi dysfunction. Gut. 2000;46:98–102.

16. Pauls Q, Durkalski-Mauldin V, Brawman-Mintzer O, et al. Duloxetine for the treatment of patients with suspected sphincter of Oddi dysfunction: a pilot study. Dig Dis Sci. 2016;61:2704–9.

17. Vitton V, Delpy R, Gasmi M, et al. Is endoscopic sphincterotomy avoidable in patients with sphincter of Oddi dysfunction? Eur J Gastroenterol Hepatol. 2008;20:15–21.

18. Kalaitzakis E, Ambrose T, Phillips-Hughes J, et al. Management of patients with biliary sphincter of Oddi disorder without sphincter of Oddi manometry. BMC Gastroenterol. 2010;10:124.

19. Viceconte G, Viceconte GW, Pietropaolo V, et al. Endoscopic sphincterotomy: indications and results. Br J Surg. 1981;68:376–80.

20. Thatcher BS, Sivak MV, Tedesco FJ, et al. Endoscopic sphincterotomy for suspected dysfunction of the sphincter of Oddi. Gastrointest Endosc. 1987;33:91–5. 101.

21. Petersen BT. An evidence-based review of sphincter of Oddi dysfunction: part I, presentations with "objective" biliary findings (types I and II). Gastrointest Endosc. 2004;59:525–34.
22. Geenen JE, Hogan WJ, Dodds WJ, et al. The efficacy of endoscopic sphincterotomy after cholecystectomy in patients with sphincter-of-Oddi dysfunction. N Engl J Med. 1989;320:82–7.
23. Lin OS, Soetikno RM, Young HS. The utility of liver function test abnormalities concomitant with biliary symptoms in predicting a favorable response to endoscopic sphincterotomy in patients with presumed sphincter of Oddi dysfunction. Am J Gastroenterol. 1998;93:1833–6.
24. Freeman ML, Gill M, Overby C, et al. Predictors of outcomes after biliary and pancreatic sphincterotomy for sphincter of oddi dysfunction. J Clin Gastroenterol. 2007;41:94–102.

Part IV

Demystifying the Challenging Post-operative Patient

Chapter 15
Common Upper Gastrointestinal Operations

Steven P. Bowers

Case Study

A 40-year-old male, current smoker with a two-drink-per-day alcohol history, awoke from sleep with acute, generalized abdominal pain. He had no history of illicit drug use or nonsteroidal anti-inflammatory agent (NSAID) use and no prior medical history. When seen in the emergency room, he had a rigid abdomen with diffuse peritoneal signs of guarding and rebound tenderness. Abdominal CT scan revealed findings of free air and fluid in the abdominal cavity, consistent with acute perforation of a hollow viscus (Fig. 15.1). The patient was given intravenous fluid and antibiotics and promptly prepared for the operating room.

The operation performed was exploratory laparoscopy with closure of a perforated duodenal ulcer and creation of a Graham patch. A laparoscopic cannula was placed by open Hasson technique in the base of the umbilicus, and laparoscopic exploration revealed copious bilious fluid and a 5-mm perforation in the anterior duodenal bulb (Fig. 15.2). The perforation was closed with absorbable sutures. Upper endoscopy was performed to confirm the location of the perforation in the duodenal bulb and to exclude pyloric obstruction

S. P. Bowers (✉)
Mayo Clinic Florida, Jacksonville, FL, USA
e-mail: bowers.steven@mayo.edu

© Springer Nature Switzerland AG 2019
B. E. Lacy et al. (eds.), *Essential Medical Disorders of the Stomach and Small Intestine*,
https://doi.org/10.1007/978-3-030-01117-8_15

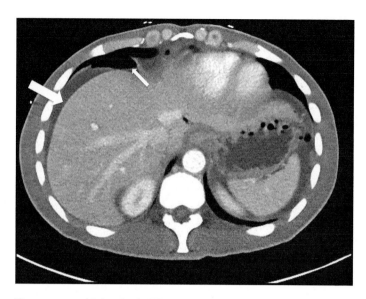

FIGURE 15.1 Abdominal CT scan showing free abdominal fluid (large arrow) and pneumoperitoneum (small arrow)

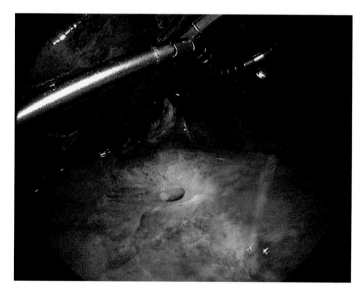

FIGURE 15.2 Intraoperative photo during laparoscopic exploration revealing anterior duodenal perforated ulcer

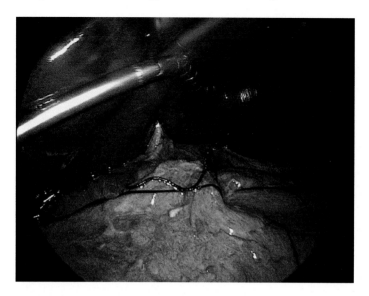

FIGURE 15.3 Intraoperative photo showing Graham patch closure of perforated anterior duodenal bulb ulcer. Sutures have not been secured over omental pedicled flap

or a concomitant posterior duodenal ulcer. A tongue of omentum was mobilized and sutured to patch the ulcer closure site (Fig. 15.3). The abdomen was cleansed with copious irrigation and suction of fluid.

The patient remained on antibiotics for 24 h and underwent upper GI contrast study to confirm patency of the duodenum and absence of an ongoing leak (Fig. 15.4). He was then started on a liquid diet and discharged on postoperative day 3, with treatment for presumed *Helicobacter pylori* infection.

Objectives

1. Describe indications for, and technical details of, the most common elective upper gastrointestinal operations performed in the United States.
2. Describe indications for, and technical details of, the most common emergency upper gastrointestinal operations performed in the United States.

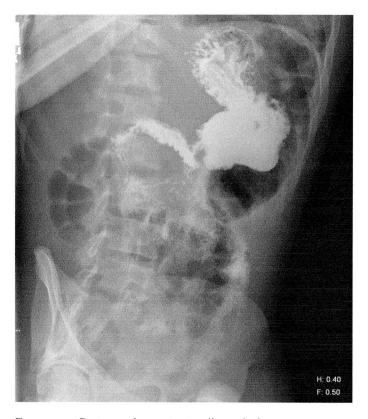

FIGURE 15.4 Postoperative contrast radiograph shows no extravasation of contrast and patency of the duodenal bulb

Epidemiology

Table 15.1 lists the most common upper gastrointestinal operations performed in the United States. The ranking of most common operations changes every few years, as different disease processes attain greater prominence in the population. Currently, the United States is in the midst of an obesity epidemic, and bariatric or weight loss operations are generally available in most communities. Thus, bariatric

TABLE 15.1 Most common elective upper gastrointestinal operations in the United States

Operation type	Operation	Estimated incidence (per 100,000 per year)
Bariatric surgery		
	Sleeve gastrectomy	28.4
	Roux-en-Y gastric bypass	18.9
Antireflux surgery		
	Hiatal hernia repair, fundoplication	8.3
	Esophagogastric myotomy	0.8
Gastrectomy		
	Distal gastrectomy	0.7
	Total gastrectomy	0.5
	Wedge gastrectomy	0.8
Esophagectomy		
	Distal esophagectomy	0.4
	Near-total esophagectomy	0.2
Pancreatectomy		
	Whipple procedure	0.4
	Distal pancreatectomy	0.2

Data extracted from reports utilizing the National Inpatient Sample of hospital admissions [1–7]

operations have the highest annual incidence among upper gastrointestinal operations. Proton pump inhibitors (PPIs) have been effective in reducing the need for antireflux surgery over the last decade, and gastric cancer resection continues to decline, but operations for esophageal and pancreatic malignancy have been steadily rising in incidence.

TABLE 15.2 Most common emergency upper gastrointestinal operations in the United States

Operation type	Operation	Estimated incidence (per 100,000 per year)
Peptic ulcer bleeding		13.2
	Oversew bleeding	
	Vagotomy and pyloroplasty	
	Antrectomy +/− vagotomy	
Peptic ulcer perforation		2.9
	Graham patch closure	
Symptomatic hiatal hernia		2.4
	Paraesophageal hernia repair	

Data extrapolated from reports utilizing the National Inpatient Sample of hospital admissions [3]

Table 15.2 lists the most common emergency upper gastrointestinal operations performed [2, 3]. Despite the increase in utilization of interventional endoscopy techniques for acute upper gastrointestinal hemorrhage, the incidence of emergency operations for control of peptic ulcer bleeding remains relatively high. Emergency operations for the control of upper gastrointestinal perforation have not decreased substantially either with widespread use of antiacid secretory medications. Additionally, with the aging population, the incidence of emergency operations for acutely symptomatic hiatal hernia has been rising.

Bariatric Operations

Etiology/Pathophysiology

Obesity is the accumulation of fat mass due to surplus ingested calories, with its metabolic and physiologic consequences. Obesity is multifactorial, and its causes derive from decreased relative metabolism or increased relative caloric ingestion or absorption. Because massive weight reduction is extraordinarily rare with dietary therapy alone, bariatric operations have emerged as the only viable option for massive weight loss in morbidly obese patients, defined by the National Institutes of Health as those with body mass index (BMI) of greater than 35 kg/m^2 with obesity-related cardiovascular risk factors or with a BMI of greater than 40 kg/m^2.

Bariatric operations as a whole have been increasing, with the increase over the last 5–10 years due almost exclusively to the rise of the sleeve gastrectomy as an option for most patients [1]. This rise is based on the ability of most surgeons to perform the procedure via a minimally invasive technique and the lower rate of subsequent operations – at least in the short term. Sleeve gastrectomy has thus largely supplanted the adjustable gastric band as the bariatric surgery option for the most risk-averse patient. The Roux-en-Y gastric bypass remains the default revisional operation of choice because of its effectiveness in challenging situations, and the Roux-en-Y gastric bypass is considered the procedure of choice for patients with pre-existing gastroesophageal reflux and insulin-dependent diabetes mellitus.

There are three major mechanisms of weight loss for the sleeve gastrectomy. One, sleeve gastrectomy creates the greatest restriction of all bariatric operations; early after the operation, food regurgitation is common for dietary indiscretions, thus limiting intake. Two, resecting the fundus reduces ghrelin levels which leads to a loss of the sensation of ravenous hunger in sleeve gastrectomy patients. Three, removing the fundus leads to rapid gastric emptying which induces a moderate incretin effect. This is responsible for the antidiabetic effect of the sleeve gastrectomy. Because there is no metabolic consequence of softer high-calorie density food in sleeve gastrectomy patients, weight loss is less than that seen in Roux-en-Y patients, and weight regain is more common.

The Roux-en-Y gastric bypass creates a small gastric pouch with a restrictive outlet into the jejunum (see Fig. 15.5).

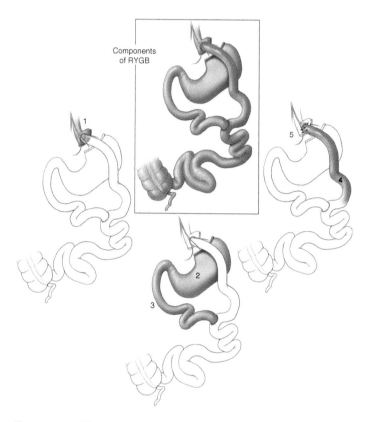

FIGURE 15.5 The components of the Roux-en-Y gastric bypass operation (RYGB) include (1) the proximal gastric pouch, (2) the remnant stomach, (3) the duodenum and biliopancreatic limb, (4) the alimentary limb, and (5) the gastrojejunostomy anastomosis. (Used with permission of Mayo Foundation for Medical Education and Research, all rights reserved)

There is less restriction than seen in the sleeve gastrectomy, but a greater incretin effect due to the rapid entry of food into the distal bowel. The substantial hindgut incretin effect of the Roux-en-Y is responsible for the higher rates of resolution of diabetes after the Roux-en-Y when compared to sleeve gastrectomy. The gastrojejunostomy causes rapid gastric emptying of high-calorie density foods into the jejunum and leads to dumping syndrome, which serves as a behavioral repellant toward the ingestion of high-calorie density foods. By 2 years, however, the dumping syndrome is an effective deterrent in less than 20% of Roux-en-Y patients.

Operative Description

Sleeve gastrectomy is performed by mobilizing the greater curve of the stomach from the distal antrum to the angle of His at the gastroesophageal junction (GEJ; see Fig. 15.6). Surgical staplers are used to divide the stomach in a vertical fashion with removal of the greater curvature at a point 2–6 cm from the pylorus. A bougie dilator (36–48 Fr) is used to ensure that the outflow tract from the stomach is not too restrictive. Hiatal hernias identified during the sleeve gastrectomy operation should be repaired to minimize postoperative gastroesophageal reflux.

The Roux-en-Y gastric bypass operation is performed by first transecting the proximal stomach to create a proximal rectangular gastric pouch approximately 5 cm by 3 cm. Then the jejunum is divided and reconstructed in a "Y" configuration such that the biliopancreatic limb is attached well downstream of the proximal alimentary limb. The alimentary limb is then connected to the proximal gastric pouch. The gastrojejunostomy anastomosis can be created by suture, surgical stapler, or a combination of stapled and sutured anastomosis. A standard proximal gastric bypass will have a biliopancreatic limb length between 40 and 60 cm (range of 25–100 cm) and an alimentary limb length between 80 and 150 cm (at least 40 cm required to prevent alkaline reflux). A long-limb gastric bypass is defined as having an alimentary limb of greater than 150 cm length, and this is now a common practice.

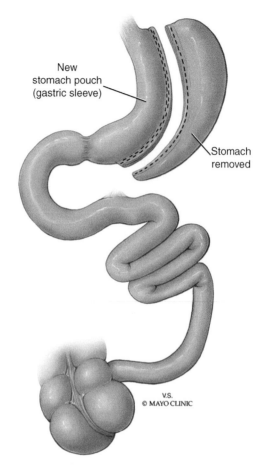

FIGURE 15.6 The laparoscopic sleeve gastrectomy – variations in technique involve the proximity to the pylorus of the gastric staple line and the size dilator used to size the sleeve. (Used with permission of Mayo Foundation for Medical Education and Research, all rights reserved)

Complications of Operation

Complications after bariatric operations can be classified as early or late, based on the timing of presentation. The major early (perioperative) complications are pulmonary embolus (PE) and proximal gastric or anastomotic leak, presenting in most cases in the hospital or shortly after discharge. Leak and pulmonary embolus can both present with tachycardia, tachypnea, and hemodynamic collapse and can be life-threatening. Prompt resuscitation, CT angiography to rule out PE, and percutaneous or surgical drainage of peritoneal soilage are essential to patient survival. Leak after Roux-en-Y gastric bypass generally presents within the first week after operation, but leak after sleeve gastrectomy is often seen between weeks 1 and 3 (see Chap. 16 for further details).

Sleeve gastrectomy increases the likelihood of gastro-esophageal reflux, due to gastric restriction and transection of gastric sling fibers in the lower esophageal sphincter mechanism. Recurrence of hiatal hernia is not uncommon, and severe reflux in the setting of hiatal hernia after sleeve gastrectomy often requires reoperation with conversion to Roux-en-Y gastric bypass. Stenosis of the restrictive portion of the sleeve resection may require endoscopic dilation, but rarely requires reoperation.

Nutritional deficiencies are common without monitoring and therapy. Patients should be on multivitamins and calcium starting at operation, and the clinician should have a low threshold for administering thiamine to any patient with persistent postoperative emesis. Vitamin B12 should be administered or levels monitored, and all menstruating women should receive supplemental iron. Approximately 7–10% of patients after gastric bypass will require subsequent cholecystectomy.

Clinical Pearls

- Clinicians should have a low threshold for administering thiamine and vitamin B12 for patients after bariatric surgery.
- Small bowel obstruction or internal hernia can be difficult to diagnose.
- While a leak after gastric bypass often occurs early after the operation (hours to days), leak after sleeve gastrectomy may not occur for up to 3 weeks after operation.

Antireflux Surgery

Etiology/Pathophysiology

Many factors contribute to the development of gastroesophageal reflux disease (GERD) and erosive esophagitis. A large hiatal hernia is the predominant cause of severe GERD; however, abnormalities in lower esophageal sphincter (LES) function and esophageal clearance play a major role in the pathophysiology of reflux. For the vast majority of patients with symptoms of reflux such as heartburn and regurgitation, a PPI will control symptoms. For patients with medically refractory GERD, objective evidence of GERD is mandatory before considering antireflux surgery. Ambulatory esophageal pH testing off all antisecretory medications is the best method to document severe reflux. Because there is an excellent correlation between pH testing and findings on upper endoscopy (EGD) of Barrett's esophagus or severe erosive esophagitis (LA class C or D), pH testing can be omitted in those patients. The combination of pH testing, EGD, high-resolution esophageal motility testing, contrast esophagram/barium swallow, and gastric emptying study (when emesis and nausea are prominent symptoms) allows the surgeon to devise the appropriate antireflux operation.

A paraesophageal hiatal hernia is defined by the finding of a non-reducible hiatal sac in the mediastinum [4]. The finding of the fundus above the gastroesophageal junction (GEJ) in the setting of a hiatal hernia is also consistent with a paraesophageal hernia. Patients with paraesophageal hernia more often present with symptoms of chest pain and dysphagia, and these symptoms are not likely to be managed with antisecretory medications. As hiatal hernias enlarge with more stomach above the hiatus, rotation of the stomach (volvulus) may occur. Organo-axial volvulus denotes rotation of the stomach around an axis formed by the esophageal and pyloric attachments of the stomach, creating an "upside-down U"-shaped stomach. Rotation of the stomach about the axis formed by the mesenteric attachments of the stomach, mesentero-axial volvulus, creates an "N"-shaped stomach. Mesentero-axial volvulus is significantly more likely to present with acute incarceration of the stomach in the mediastinum, requiring emergency decompression of the stomach and prompt operation to avoid gastric necrosis. Borchardt's triad diagnostic of gastric volvulus with incarceration consists of epigastric pain, dry heaving or retching, and inability to pass a gastric tube below the hiatus. Approximately 25% of patients with paraesophageal hernia have anemia due to Cameron's erosions of the stomach.

The fundoplication operation, wrapping the fundus of the stomach around the lower esophagus, prevents reflux by increasing the basal pressure of the LES and by augmenting LES pressure when the stomach is full. Years of experience have determined that the optimal balance between controlling reflux and minimizing dysphagia comes with a short fundoplication (2 cm in length) calibrated around a bougie dilator (16–20 mm diameter). In patients with spastic esophageal disorders or severe ineffective peristalsis, Nissen fundoplication may be contraindicated, and the preferred antireflux operation is a partial fundoplication. The Toupet fundoplication is a 270-degree posterior partial fundoplication, with the pillars of the fundoplication suture fixated to the anterior-lateral esophagus, leaving the anterior 90 degrees uncovered by the stomach. The Toupet fundoplication is associated with less postoperative dysphagia and similar reflux control in most patients.

Operative Description

The fundamental principles of the Nissen fundoplication are mobilization of the fundus of the stomach, dissection of the mediastinal esophagus to create sufficient abdominal esophageal length (greater than 3 cm), closure of the hiatus hernia, and construction of the fundoplication over a bougie dilator. There is an artistic element involved in the creation of the fundoplication, and surgeons employ numerous variations in techniques. Several techniques are used to close the hiatus (e.g., simple interrupted sutures, mattressed sutures with or without buttress material such as Teflon pledgets). Biomaterial mesh may be incorporated into the repair or used as onlay.

The Nissen fundoplication can be structured in fundamentally one of the two ways: the anterior stomach is wrapped around the lower esophagus, with the apex of the fundus fixated to the greater curvature of the fundus and the anterior esophagus. Alternatively, the posterior stomach is pulled around the posterior esophagus, and the anterior stomach pulled around the anterior esophagus, and the two fixated at the patient's right aspect of the esophagus. The latter results in a more symmetric fundoplication wrap as seen at endoscopy, but this technique has proven to be more difficult to teach surgeons in training, and most centers utilize the prior technique.

In the setting of a foreshortened esophagus due to chronic transmural esophageal inflammation and/or hiatal hernia, an esophageal lengthening procedure may be required. In the Collis – or wedge – gastroplasty technique, the surgeon creates a short tube of cardia approximately 3 cm long by resecting a short triangular piece of the stomach at the angle of His. The gastroplasty tube is sized with a bougie dilator and technique of stapling up against the dilator. The surgeon must include the native GEJ in the fundoplication to prevent dilation of the gastroplasty tube over time.

Complications of Operation

The Nissen fundoplication is a unique operation, in that patient symptoms are largely subjective, there exists an art in creating the fundoplication, and patient outcomes are largely subjective. Thus, in-depth knowledge of the foregut physiology and preparation of patient expectations is imperative for good outcomes. Conditions with heightened sensitivity, such as fibromyalgia, are associated with worse outcomes after antireflux surgery. It is essential that postoperative emesis or dry heaving be avoided, particularly in the immediate postoperative period, because acute herniation of the fundoplication can occur with failure of hiatal closure. Dysphagia is common after operation, and patients that cannot progress to swallow solid food by 2 months after operation may benefit from endoscopic dilation of the fundoplication. Aerophagia with frequent belching is a natural consequence of reflux; however, after Nissen fundoplication, aerophagia may cause considerable discomfort. Because of the dynamic effect of the fundoplication, most patients cannot belch swallowed air after a Nissen. The gas bloat syndrome refers to patients debilitated by gaseous distention of the abdomen and who are unable to change their dietary behavior to minimize aerophagia.

Fundoplication failure implies that the fundoplication is anatomically not capable of balancing the control of gastric reflux with the ability to swallow solids. The rate of anatomical fundoplication failure requiring reoperation is estimated at about 1% per year after operation. For patients with large hiatal hernias (greater than 5 cm), the rate of failure of hiatal closure is high, approaching 50% after 5 years. Generally, patients are more likely to be symptomatic if the fundoplication is improperly performed or migrates onto the stomach (the "slipped wrap") than if the hiatal hernia closure fails.

Clinical Pearls

- Objective evidence of reflux is required for consideration of antireflux surgery; this includes positive pH testing or visible evidence during upper endoscopy of esophageal injury.
- Paraesophageal hernia generally does not present with reflux symptoms, but with chest pain or dysphagia, and may cause chronic or acute anemia or acute volvulus with incarceration.
- A complete foregut physiologic evaluation (endoscopy, esophageal manometry, pH testing, contrast esophagram) is deemed essential for good outcomes after fundoplication.

Operations for Peptic Ulcer Disease

Etiology/Pathophysiology

Peptic ulcer disease (PUD) was epidemic in the past and directly related to alcohol use and smoking. Knowledge of – and the ability to detect and eradicate – *Helicobacter pylori* infection of the stomach has dramatically reduced the incidence of PUD. The annual detection of *H. pylori* in the United States peaked in 1998 and has steadily declined since. However, the incidence of complicated PUD has been slower to decline. For example, the prevalence of upper gastrointestinal hemorrhage due to PUD has declined faster than gastric perforation or gastric outlet obstruction due to ulcer disease. *H. pylori* is currently identified in over 50% of adults aged over 50 years, but found in only 5% of people aged less than 25 years. *Helicobacter* infection in the antrum is associated with increased gastric acid production due to hypergastrinemia and secondary hypertrophy of parietal cells; *Helicobacter* infection is associated with decreased duodenal bicarbonate production. Peptic ulcers associated with increased acid production include duodenal bulb and pyloric channel ulcers.

Nonsteroidal anti-inflammatory drugs (NSAIDs) are increasingly responsible for peptic ulcer disease. NSAIDs and aspirin inhibit COX-1 receptors, decreasing the turnover of gastric mucosa. There is a dose-dependent increase in bleeding risk with NSAID or aspirin use, in addition to a synergistic effect with steroids, anticoagulants, and antiplatelet drugs. *Helicobacter* positivity almost triples the risk of developing peptic ulcer in those taking NSAIDs.

Peptic ulcer disease remains the most common cause of upper gastrointestinal (UGI) hemorrhage, and in the Western world, gastric ulcers are now more prevalent than duodenal ulcers as a cause of GI bleeding. Urgent or emergent upper endoscopy is required in patients with a suspected UGI hemorrhage, and in the vast majority of cases, endoscopic therapy can control the bleeding. However, 8–10% of patients undergoing endoscopic therapy will rebleed, and some of these patients will require operation. In addition, because these endoscopic techniques are not universally available on an emergent basis, surgical control of life-threatening bleeding is the most common emergency upper GI operation. Based on population outcome studies, the operation for acute control of peptic ulcer bleeding with the lowest postoperative mortality is oversewing of the ulcer with vagotomy with drainage [5, 6].

Perforated peptic ulcer most commonly occurs (in 60% of cases) in the anterior duodenal bulb, with the remainder split between the prepyloric antrum and gastric body. Nonoperative management of perforated peptic ulcer is acceptable in young patients without tachycardia, peritonitis, or large pneumoperitoneum (greater than the L1 vertebral body height on upright chest radiograph). Management includes broad-spectrum antibiotics, gastric decompression, a negative test for extravasation of contrast, and subsequent treatment of *H. pylori*. The expectation should be that 30% of patients initially managed nonoperatively will require operation.

The operation for perforated peptic ulcer disease should address the perforation, the ulcer and risk of subsequent ulcer disease, and the peritonitis. For patients with a perforated ulcer who are negative for *H. pylori* and are not taking ulcerogenic drugs, the surgeon should consider definitive ulcer surgery. For patients taking ulcerogenic drugs in whom therapy can be changed or those in whom *H. pylori* status is unknown, secure closure of the ulcer alone can be undertaken. The Graham patch closure of perforated peptic ulcer is highly effective for perforations less than 2 cm in size. For perforations involving the pyloric channel, a pyloroplasty incorporating the perforation, along with truncal vagotomy, is effective. Resection is indicated for perforations of giant ulcers.

Refractory peptic ulcers are exceedingly uncommon in the *H. pylori* era and should alert the clinician to the possibility of a gastric cancer. EGD should be repeated at 3-month intervals with systematic biopsy of ulcer edges to document the absence of a malignancy. Confirmation of eradication, avoidance of ulcerogenic drugs, and smoking cessation are paramount prior to consideration of operation. Truncal vagotomy and pyloroplasty are the simplest and lowest risk procedure. Vagotomy and antrectomy with reconstruction eliminate basal acid secretion and reduce stimulated acid production by 80%, and subtotal gastrectomy eliminates the gastric antrum and reduces parietal cell mass. Highly selective vagotomy (or posterior truncal vagotomy and anterior seromyotomy) preserves pyloric function (decreasing the risk of postoperative dumping syndrome) but is the least effective of all definitive ulcer operations in preventing recurrence.

Operative Description

For acute ulcer hemorrhage requiring operation, the first step in management must be control of hemorrhage. For this the surgeon must identify the site of hemorrhage with certainty.

For a posterior duodenal bulb-penetrating ulcer, an anterior duodenotomy is made, and the surgeon oversews the ulcer with a series of stitches to ligate the gastroduodenal artery proximally (superiorly) and distally (inferiorly) and ligate the pancreaticoduodenal branch with a "U" stitch across the ulcer bed. A decision is then made for simple closure of the duodenotomy, incorporation of the duodenotomy into pyloroplasty with accompanying truncal vagotomy, or resection distal to the duodenotomy to allow antrectomy.

The vagotomy and pyloroplasty operation consists of division of both anterior and posterior vagus nerves at the hiatus, along with Heineke-Mikulicz pyloroplasty. The so-called V&P operation is the most versatile and common of the anti-ulcer operations. The pyloroplasty incision can be used as exposure to the posterior duodenal bulb to oversew posterior penetrating duodenal ulcers, can be incorporated into the perforation in case of perforated anterior duodenal bulb or pyloric channel ulcers, and is effective for most gastric outlet obstruction due to ulcer disease. The operation can be performed by either laparoscopic technique for elective procedures or more commonly via an open approach for emergent procedures [7].

Antrectomy is performed for giant duodenal ulcers and for all non-healing gastric ulcers to exclude occult malignancy. The operation is performed by mobilizing the distal stomach, dividing the gastroepiploic arcade and the right gastric arcade, and dividing the duodenum flush with the pancreas. Pathology to confirm duodenal Brunner's glands should confirm that no antrum has been left behind. After antrectomy, there are many reconstructive options. The Billroth I reconstruction is now antiquated, because of greater complication rates and chronically delayed emptying, but consists of anastomosis of gastric antrum to the duodenal bulb. The Billroth II gastrojejunostomy is by far the most common. The jejunum is not divided, but brought up to the stomach as a loop, with the gastrojejunostomy performed by stapled or sutured technique. A consequence of the Billroth II procedure is alkaline reflux gastritis, and, if necessary, there are several options for bile diversion (e.g., Braun enteroen-terostomy, uncut Roux-en-Y reconstruction, or Roux-en-Y gastroenterostomy reconstruction).

For perforated peptic ulcer, Graham patch closure of a duo-denal ulcer is the standard operation. The ulcer can be closed with an absorbable suture, and a tongue of omentum can be created such that the omentum buttresses the ulcer closure site. Sutures are placed to tightly fix the omental buttress in place. The abdomen must be thoroughly cleansed with irrigation and all foodstuff and exudate removed if possible. The author pre-fers to perform intraoperative endoscopy to confirm closure and exclude posterior "kissing ulcers" as a potential cause of obstruction or postoperative hemorrhage. With perforated gastric ulcers, the surgeon should consider resection if the ulcer is large or located in an atypical site (other than the lesser curve antrum). For prepyloric ulcers without obstruction on EGD, Graham patch closure is also acceptable.

Complications of Operation

The most serious complication of peptic ulcer disease is leak-age from the duodenal stump after antrectomy. Typically occurring from 5 to 8 days after operation, duodenal stump blowout can be accompanied by sepsis and hemodynamic collapse. Wide drainage is essential for survival. Leakage of gastrojejunostomy is less likely than leakage of gastroduode-nostomy in Billroth I or duodenal stump leakage. The affer-ent loop syndrome refers to obstruction of the afferent limb of Billroth II gastrojejunostomy. This presents with pain relieved with bilious emesis and can be associated with duo-denal stump blowout if undiagnosed. Small bowel obstruc-tion risk is roughly 10% lifelong due to intestinal aspects of operation. Rebleeding after oversewing of a posterior pene-trating ulcer is rare, particularly after definitive antiulcer operation, but can be managed by arterial embolization therapy by interventional radiology.

For recurrent ulcers after definitive ulcer operation, pathologic evidence of complete vagotomy and antrectomy is important to confirm that the operation was performed as planned. Gastrinoma should be excluded, as well as ulcerogenic drugs and smoking. Dumping syndrome is related to the intake of high-calorie density foods and can be debilitating in up to 10% of patients in the first year. Post-vagotomy diarrhea may occur but can generally be controlled medically.

Clinical Pearls

- Vagotomy and pyloroplasty are the most safe and effective antiulcer operation and can be used in most clinical situations.
- Refractory gastric ulcers should arouse suspicion of malignancy until healed or resected.
- Endoscopic therapy, where available, is the best first option for hemorrhage control.
- Ulcerogenic drugs are emerging as the major cause of peptic ulcer disease.

Gastrectomy for Malignancy

Etiology/Pathophysiology

Gastric adenocarcinoma is classified by the Lauren classification as being intestinal type or diffuse type. Intestinal-type cancers are related to *H. pylori* infection (particularly Cag A strains) and result from a progressive sequence of inflammatory changes in the stomach, from atrophic gastritis to intestinal metaplasia. Intestinal-type cancers are generally located in the distal stomach and are decreasing in incidence with greater eradication of *H. pylori*.

Diffuse-type cancers are so named because they do not form glands but rather exist as individual cells. This trait is due to the core molecular abnormality of loss of the ability to form intercellular adhesions (due to loss of expression of the E-cadherin molecule). Diffuse gastric cancer is associated with greater early metastatic potential and infiltration of the gastric wall, leading to the linitis plastica syndrome. Diffuse gastric cancer is more likely to occur in the proximal stomach and is more prevalent than intestinal-type cancer in the Western world.

Patients with gastric cancer may present with iron deficiency, bleeding, or gastric obstruction, and these symptoms generally indicate locally advanced disease. Staging of gastric cancer is of vital importance to plan therapy. Imaging (CT scan with contrast) is used to exclude obvious metastatic disease, and endoscopic ultrasound is best at determining depth of tumor invasion. Early gastric cancer, limited to the gastric submucosa, may be amenable to endoscopic resection, or surgical resection without complete regional lymphadenectomy, as lymphatic metastasis is less likely. For locally advanced gastric cancer, optimal patient survival is with multimodality therapy, consisting of chemotherapy prior to resection or chemoradiation after resection [8]. Regarding resection of locally advanced gastric cancer, survival at all stages is increased with the extent of lymphatic resection, and the surgeon must balance the morbidity of greater lymphadenectomy with the favorable prognosis that greater lymphadenectomy brings.

Resection of the stomach is based on the need for nodal resection and sampling and resection of an adequate margin of normal stomach. In early gastric cancer, wedge resection with local lymphatic basin resection may be appropriate when endoscopic resection is not possible or available. Wedge gastrectomy is appropriate for local removal of tumors where the resultant shape of the stomach is not critically distorted. This includes most lesions of the greater curvature of the stomach and excludes lesions in the prepyloric antrum and cardia of the stomach. If preoperative staging is not definitive of status of tumor invasion, local resection is discouraged due to the greater survival with greater lymphadenectomy in locally advanced gastric cancer. For locally advanced gastric cancer, subtotal gastrectomy is most appropriate for all gastric cancers where a 5-cm proximal margin of normal stomach can be obtained. For cancers where the proximal extent of the mass is within 5 cm of the GEJ, a total gastrectomy should be undertaken. Extended total gastrectomy or esophagectomy is used when the tumor abuts or includes the GEJ.

Gastrointestinal stromal tumors (GIST) of the stomach are increasingly being referred for gastric resection. GIST is a tumor derived from the interstitial cells of Cajal; the c-kit oncogene is diagnostic of GIST. Because metastasis to regional lymph nodes is very rare, the majority of GIST lesions can be resected with a small margin of normal stomach, provided the capsule of the tumor is resected intact. Neoadjuvant therapy with the tyrosine kinase inhibitor imatinib is indicated in some patients.

Operative Description

Wedge gastrectomy is guided by intraoperative endoscopy, and the boundaries of required resection are marked. The stomach specimen is then staple resected or resected and the lumen closed with suture or stapled techniques. Staple resection is more often used in lesions of the greater curvature or exophytic GIST lesions, and occasionally intragastric techniques may be required for endophytic GIST lesions or lesions of the lesser curve. Frozen section pathology is indicated to ensure clear and adequate margins of resection. Operation can be performed by open or laparoscopic technique.

The subtotal gastrectomy operation consists of resection of the distal stomach from the duodenum to the proximal stomach. The duodenal margin is stapled flush with the pancreas at 2 cm distal to the pylorus. The proximal resection margin should be assessed based on the location of the proximal extent of the tumor, guided by intraoperative endoscopy if needed. This includes lymphadenectomy of three of the four major lymphovascular basins of the stomach (subpyloric and gastroepiploic nodes, hepatic and right gastric nodes, left gastric and gastrohepatic nodes). The short gastric and splenic/peripancreatic nodes are additionally resected in the total gastrectomy operation, and distal mediastinal nodes are resected in the extended total gastrectomy operation. At least 15 resected nodes are required for gastrectomy operation to be considered adequate.

Esophagojejunostomy after total gastrectomy is performed via stapled technique or sutured techniques. Importantly with esophagojejunostomy, there is a higher postoperative anastomotic complication rate than seen in gastrojejunostomy, so drainage of the field and routine use of feeding jejunostomy at the time of operation play a greater role in management.

Complications of Operation

Leakage of esophagojejunostomy anastomosis can occur in up to 5% of operations; routine testing of anastomotic integrity with a contrast esophagram is indicated prior to initiation of feeding. Contingency planning including drainage and jejunal feeding is preferred as well. Leakage of the duodenal stump occurs in up to 3% of gastric resections. Leakage of gastrojejunostomy after subtotal gastrectomy is rare. Wedge gastrectomy is complicated more often by staple line bleeding than leakage, with inverted staple lines more prone to bleeding than everted staple lines. Afferent loop syndrome is a possibility with Billroth II reconstruction, whereas small bowel obstruction due to an internal hernia is possible with Roux-en-Y reconstruction. Roux stasis, a syndrome of delayed emptying of the alimentary limb of the Roux-en-Y reconstruction, can cause chronic nausea. As with any small intestinal operation, the risk of subsequent bowel obstruction is approximately 10% lifetime after operation.

Clinical Pearls

- Endoscopic ultrasound and axial imaging are optimal for preoperative staging of gastric cancer.
- Multimodality therapy optimizes survival for locally advanced gastric cancer.
- The number of resected lymph nodes has a major effect on survival stage for stage.

Pancreatectomy for Malignancy

Etiology/Pathophysiology

Pancreatic ductal adenocarcinoma (PDAC) is the leading cause of cancer-related deaths due to upper gastrointestinal malignancy and second only to colon cancer as the cause of gastrointestinal cancer death. It is a highly malignant disease, where the only hope for survival lies in surgical resection. Most pancreatic cancer arises in the proximal pancreas, and the most common presenting symptom is jaundice due to biliary obstruction. Elevation of the tumor marker CA 19–9 is correlated with poor survival, and lymph node-positive cancer portends a dismal prognosis. A small number of pancreatic cancer patients have a familial lineage that includes pancreatic cancer, but most PDAC is sporadic and related to smoking, obesity, and binge drinking or chronic pancreatitis. Intraductal papillary mucinous neoplasm (IPMN) lesions are associated with progression to PDAC, with main duct-type IPMN highly likely to be associated with PDAC. Smaller branch-duct IPMNs without worrisome features can be observed.

Because distal PDAC does not cause any herald symptoms such as jaundice, distal pancreatic cancers are more likely to be unresectable at presentation due to vascular invasion or metastatic disease. Those patients with suspected PDAC without metastatic disease at presentation should undergo staging with endoscopic ultrasound (with or without confirmatory FNA) and axial imaging (dedicated pancreas protocol CT scan or MRI). Based on staging tests assessing the extent of tumor involvement of the nearby superior mesenteric and celiac vascular pedicles, patients can be classified as resectable, borderline resectable, or unresectable. Although there is no proven survival benefit for neoadjuvant combination chemotherapy for borderline resectable patients, this therapeutic approach is becoming the standard. There is ample evidence that adjuvant chemotherapy after resection is associated with survival benefit, and adjuvant chemoradiation is offered to patients with margin-positive or node-positive disease. Because of the risk of morbidity of the pancreaticoduodenectomy operation, improved overall outcomes are observed in centers with established surgeon and care team expertise and a volume-outcome relationship are seen.

Operative Description

The traditional Whipple operation consists of en bloc resection of the gastric antrum, duodenum, and head of the pancreas with common bile duct (see Fig. 15.7a, b). Pylorus-preserving pancreaticoduodenectomy allows retention of the gastric antrum and proximal 2–3 cm of duodenal bulb (see Fig. 15.7b). This has no effect on survival but may improve patient satisfaction by decreasing dumping syndrome and risks of subsequent marginal ulceration. The gallbladder is removed to prevent biliary complications later; this facilitates reconstruction at the cystic duct-hepatic duct confluence. Reconstruction consists of reconstitution of pancreatic drainage, biliary drainage, and gastric drainage, generally via sequential anastomoses to a single loop of the jejunum.

Distal pancreatectomy is commonly performed for suspected malignancy by first mobilizing and then removing the spleen. Palpation aided by intraoperative ultrasound is used

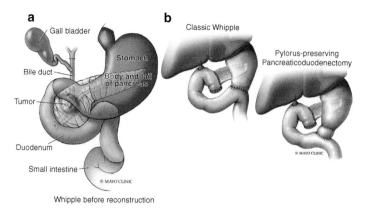

FIGURE 15.7 (**a**) Resection of the cancer of the pancreatic head cancer with reconstruction via (**b**) Whipple operation or pylorus-preserving pancreaticoduodenectomy. (Used with permission of Mayo Foundation for Medical Education and Research, all rights reserved)

to identify the lesion and appropriate margins. The pancreatic parenchyma can be staple transected with the splenic vein and the splenic artery in most cases.

Subtotal distal pancreatectomy indicates division of the pancreatic gland at the neck of the pancreas. In these cases, dissection of the anterior SMV and portal vein is performed, and the splenic vein and artery are individually ligated and divided. Resection then proceeds similarly to distal pancreatectomy. Drainage of distal pancreatectomy is by surgeon discretion.

Complications of Operation

Pancreatic leak occurs in approximately 10–15% of pancreas resection cases but is increased in soft gland (20–25%) and decreased in firm gland cases (3–5%). A small pancreatic duct is associated with an increased risk of leak, along with obesity and preoperative level of jaundice. Technically, pancreas fistula is defined by drain amylase greater than three times the upper limit of normal serum value on the third day after operation. Pancreas leaks can be asymptomatic and require no additional treatment (Grade A), can require antibiotics and parenteral nutrition of drainage procedures (Grade B), or can be associated with sepsis and hemorrhage or require operative control (Grade C). Because of the proximity of the pancreaticojejunostomy to the gastroduodenal artery ligation, pseudoaneurysm is not uncommon with uncontrolled pancreatic leak and can be a fatal complication without prompt identification and embolization by interventional radiology.

Delayed gastric emptying (DGE) is the most common complication after pancreaticoduodenectomy. Because DGE is frequently associated with pancreatic leak, axial imaging is indicated in patients with signs of delayed gastric emptying to assess for concomitant peripancreatic fluid collection. Nutritional support may be necessary in patients with a persistent delay in gastric emptying.

In patients anticipated to undergo splenectomy, vaccination for encapsulated bacterial pathogens should be performed at least 2 weeks prior to operation or failing that at least 2 weeks following operation. These vaccinations (to protect against *Streptococcus pneumoniae*, *Neisseria meningitidis*, and *Haemophilus influenzae* type b) effectively prevent overwhelming post-splenectomy sepsis.

Clinical Pearls

- Pancreaticoduodenectomy should be performed in centers and by surgeons with advanced experience with the procedure.

The majority of patients with pancreatic cancer will not be candidates for resection, but surgical resection is the only hope for long-term survival.

Esophagectomy

Etiology/Pathophysiology

There has been a dramatic change in the epidemiology of esophageal cancer over the last 30 years in the Western world. Squamous cell carcinoma of the esophagus, associated with smoking and binge drinking, is now decreasing in incidence, while esophageal adenocarcinoma (EAC) is the most rapidly increasing cancer in the Western world. EAC arises from progression of Barrett's metaplasia – dysplasia sequence – and is associated with GERD, male gender, Caucasian race, and central obesity. Barrett's esophagus is identified in approximately 20% of patients after the healing of erosive esophagitis. Non-dysplastic Barrett's esophagus has an annual risk of progression to EAC of 0.3% per year. The risk of progression of Barrett's with low-grade dysplasia is approximately 10% over 5 years, and risk of progression with high-grade dysplasia may be as high as 60% over 3 years, if left untreated.

Early esophageal cancer is defined as cancer that can be definitively treated with endoscopic resection techniques, provided clear resection margins can be obtained. In lesions that are believed amenable to endoscopic mucosal resection (EMR), EMR should be attempted. Lymphovascular invasion, poorly differentiated lesions, and involvement of the submucosa are predictors of failure of endoscopic resection therapy, and these patients should be considered for esophagectomy. Endoscopic ultrasound is the most accurate test to assess for involvement of regional lymph nodes, but positron emission tomography (PET) scan is indicated to assess for metastatic spread. Patients who undergo EMR may be counseled for esophagectomy or may be entered into surveillance program. Fit patients with superficial tumors who are not candidates for EMR should undergo esophagectomy as primary therapy.

Patients with locally advanced esophageal cancer receive a survival benefit from multimodality therapy, consisting of combination neoadjuvant chemoradiation therapy, followed by esophagectomy [9]. Patients with squamous cancer have approximately a 55% chance of complete pathologic response with chemoradiation therapy, and if no lesion is detected on endoscopy after chemoradiation, these patients may be entered into a surveillance program. EAC patients have lower rates of complete response with neoadjuvant therapy (25–30%), and complete response can only be confirmed at pathologic exam of the resection specimen.

The extent of resection of esophagectomy is based on the proximal extent of tumor, with the goal of achieving a 5-cm proximal margin. For distal lesions this is most often achieved with the Ivor-Lewis esophagectomy procedure, with abdominal and right chest exposure and two-field lymphadenectomy. For more proximal tumors, a near-total esophagectomy can be performed with esophagogastric anastomosis in the left neck, via transhiatal esophagectomy technique or three-field technique (the McKeown procedure).

Operative Description

The Ivor-Lewis procedure consists of abdominal exposure via open incision or laparoscopy, with mobilization of the entire greater curvature of the stomach, preserving the gastroepiploic arcade (see Fig. 15.8a). The duodenum is mobilized via Kocher maneuver such that the pylorus can reach the midline. The left gastric pedicle is divided with hepatic and posterior gastric lymphadenectomy. The hiatus is dissected and the esophagus mobilized into the mediastinum. The gastric conduit is created by surgical stapler starting below the incisura, with the goal of creating a conduit 4–5 cm in width based on the greater curve of the stomach (see Fig. 15.8b). A pyloromyotomy is performed to minimize delayed gastric emptying. A jejunal feeding tube is placed on surgeon discretion.

Right thoracic access is by open thoracotomy or video-assisted thoracic surgery (VATS) technique. With the lung retracted anteriorly, the distal esophagus is encircled and dis-

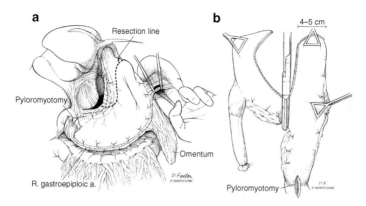

FIGURE 15.8 (**a**) Mobilization of the stomach for use in gastric conduit reconstruction for esophagectomy. (**b**) Stapling of the conduit 4–5 cm in width for optimal conduit blood supply and emptying. (Used with permission of Mayo Foundation for Medical Education and Research, all rights reserved)

sected from the mediastinal structures, and the specimen (with the proximal aspect of gastric conduit attached) was removed through the thoracic incision. Esophagogastric anastomosis can be performed by stapled technique or sutured technique. Chest drains are left to reexpand the lung and drain the pleural space.

In the transhiatal esophagectomy, the abdominal portion of operation is initially similar to the Ivor-Lewis resection; however, simultaneous dissection of the left cervical field is performed through an anterior sternocleidomastoid incision. This allows circumferential dissection of the esophagus at the hiatus and at the thoracic inlet.

Postoperative care starts with maximizing oxygen delivery to the patient and conduit. When a jejunal tube has been placed, nutrition is started with the goal to increase to nutritional goals on or about postoperative day 5. Generally, centers will obtain routine contrast esophagram to confirm conduit drainage and exclude esophageal anastomotic leakage prior to initiating oral intake [10].

Complications of Operation

Pneumonia is the most serious complication and is the driver of mortality after esophagectomy. Minimally invasive surgical approach, regional anesthetic block, early mobilization of postoperative patients, anesthesia protocols to avoid fluid overload, and nutritional strategies to minimize aspiration contribute to reduce pneumonia rates. Atrial fibrillation occurs in up to 30% of patients after major thoracic operation and requires immediate rate control and often requires chemical cardioversion. Atrial fibrillation is associated with other complications such as pneumonia and esophageal anastomotic leakage.

Anastomotic leakage rates are approximately 4–6% for intrathoracic anastomosis and 18–25% for cervical esophageal anastomosis. Most patients with anastomotic leakage are managed with drainage and/or endoscopic procedures such as self-expandable metallic stent or intraluminal vacuum-assisted closure, but major reoperation is required in up to 20% of leaks due to conduit ischemia. In case where leak has been controlled with drainage, anastomotic stricture is not uncommon.

Clinical Pearls

- Barrett's esophagus patients should be enrolled in surveillance programs to detect dysplastic changes before progression to adenocarcinoma.
- Squamous cell cancer of the esophagus is on the decline, but has a more favorable response to chemoradiation.
- Efforts to reduce pneumonia after esophagectomy will reduce mortality.

Self-Test

Question 1. A 70-year-old male presents to the emergency room with acute epigastric abdominal pain. He has tachycardia and a rigid and tender abdomen, and upright chest radiograph reveals a large pneumoperitoneum. He has a history of prior peptic ulcer disease and was previously found to be negative for *Helicobacter* infection. He has not been on ulcerogenic medications. Which of the following is the optimal therapy for his condition, based on the intraoperative finding?

- A. Observation and no operation, with nasogastric drainage and intravenous antibiotics, as he has no risks factors for failure of medical therapy
- B. Prompt operation with Graham patch closure of large pyloric channel ulcer, without intraoperative endoscopy
- C. Prompt operation, with intraoperative endoscopy to confirm location of ulcer, inclusion of anterior duodenal bulb perforated ulcer into pyloroplasty incision, Heineke-Mikulicz closure of pyloroplasty, and truncal vagotomy, for definitive ulcer therapy
- D. Prompt operation with Graham patch closure of large perforation of a high greater curve gastric ulcer, with endoscopy scheduled for 8 weeks after discharge
- E. Resuscitation and initial nonoperative management, with scheduled operation the next available operative day for vagotomy and antrectomy with Billroth II reconstruction

References

1. Nguyen NT, Vu S, Kim E, Bodunova N, Phelan MJ. Trends in utilization of bariatric surgery, 2009–2012. Surg Endosc. 2016;30:2723–7.
2. Boudourakis LD, Wang TS, Roman S, Desai R, Sosa JA. Evolution of the surgeon-volume, patient-outcome relationship. Ann Surg. 2009;250:159–65.
3. Scott JW, Olufajo OA, Brat GA, Rose JA, Zogg CK, Haider AH, Salim A, Havens JM. Use of national burden to define operative emergency general surgery. JAMA Surg. 2016;151:e160480. https://doi.org/10.1001/jamasurg.2016.0480.
4. Schlottmann F, Strassle PD, Allaix ME, Patti MG. Paraesophageal hernia repair in the USA: trends of utilization stratified by surgical volume and consequent impact on perioperative outcomes. J Gastrointest Surg. 2017;21:1199–205.
5. Crofts TJ, Park KGM, Steele RJC, Chung SSC, Li AKC. A randomized trial of nonoperative treatment for perforated peptic ulcer. NEJM. 1989;320:970–3.
6. Robles R, Parrila P, Lujan JA, Torralba JA, Cifuentes J, Liron R, Pinero A. Long-term follow-up of bilateral truncal vagotomy and pyloroplasty for perforated duodenal ulcer. Br J Surg. 1995;82:665.
7. Schlottmann F, Strassle PD, Patti MG. Comparative analysis of perioperative outcomes and costs between laparoscopic and open antireflux surgery. J Am Coll Surg. 2017;224:327–33.
8. Sarvepalli S, Garg SK, Sarvepalli SS, Anugwom C, Wadhwa V, Thota PN, Sanaka MR. Hospital utilization in patients with gastric cancer and factors affecting in-hospital mortality, length of stay and costs. J Clin Gastroenterol. 2018. https://doi.org/10.1097/MCG.0000000000001016.
9. Schlottman F, Strassle PD, Charles AG, Patti MG. Esophageal cancer surgery: spontaneous centralization in the US contributed to reduce mortality without causing health disparities. Ann Surg Oncol. 2018;25:1580–7.
10. Al-Refaie WB, Muluneh B, Zhong W, Parsons HM, Tuttle TM, Vickers S, Hebermann EB. Who receives their complex cancer surgery at low volume hospitals? J Am Coll Surg. 2012;214:81–7.

Essential Reading

Boudourakis LD, Wang TS, Roman S, Desai R, Sosa JA. Evolution of the surgeon-volume, patient-outcome relationship. Ann Surg. 2009;250:159–65. This article sets standards for annual surgeon volume where perioperative clinical outcomes are measurably better when compared to low-volume surgeons. This volume-outcome relationship is relevant for gastrectomy, esophagectomy, and pancreatectomy operations, and there is reduced mortality for esophagectomy when performed by a high-volume surgeon.

Chapter 16
Complications of Gastrointestinal Surgery

Amar Mandalia and Allison R. Schulman

Case Study

Mr. F is a 60-year-old male who presented to the emergency room with 2 days of melena and generalized weakness. He denied other gastrointestinal symptoms. Notably, he was diagnosed with stage III colon cancer 1 year prior. He underwent neoadjuvant chemotherapy and a subsequent total colectomy. He remained in remission until approximately 3 months prior to presentation when surveillance imaging revealed a metastatic deposit within the mesentery and adherent to the proximal jejunum. He underwent an uncomplicated partial small bowel resection with end-to-end anastomosis 6 weeks prior to presentation. His other past medical history includes coronary artery disease. His medications include aspirin, atenolol, and atorvastatin. He does not have any allergies. His family history is notable for a first-degree relative (mother) with colon cancer diagnosed at age 53. He was a former smoker of 20 pack years and quit several years ago but recently restarted smoking due to the stress from his cancer diagnosis. He does not drink alcohol or use

A. Mandalia · A. R. Schulman (✉)
Division of Gastroenterology and Hepatology, University of Michigan, Ann Arbor, MI, USA
e-mail: amandali@med.umich.edu; arschulm@med.umich.edu

© Springer Nature Switzerland AG 2019   321
B. E. Lacy et al. (eds.), *Essential Medical Disorders of the Stomach and Small Intestine*,
https://doi.org/10.1007/978-3-030-01117-8_16

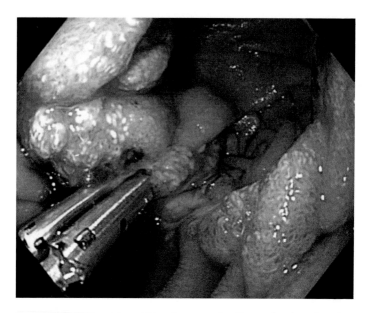

FIGURE 16.1   Placement of two hemostatic clips at the site of oozing within the anastomotic ulcer bed

illicit drugs. On physical exam, he was hemodynamically stable and had a benign abdominal exam. Rectal exam yielded dark tarry stool which was guaiac positive. Labs were notable for a hemoglobin of 6.0 grams/deciliter (g/dL) which was down from 8.2 g/dL 1 week prior to presentation. The inpatient gastroenterology team was consulted. A subsequent push enteroscopy revealed a slowly oozing anastomotic ulcer. Epinephrine was injected, and two hemostatic clips were placed with effective hemostasis (Fig. 16.1).

Objectives

Gastrointestinal surgery in the upper gastrointestinal tract is commonly performed for various indications. There are a number of unique complications that arise in this patient population and require specific knowledge for proper management. Our chapter will focus on the epidemiology, pathophysiology, diagnosis, and management of various structural and motility-related complications following the most commonly performed upper gastrointestinal interventions. When relevant, endoscopic management will be highlighted.

Anastomotic Ulceration

Anastomotic (marginal) ulcers occur at the resection margin of the intestinal wall (Fig. 16.2). This complication is reported in up to 8.6% of patients who have undergone partial or total gastrectomy and between 5% and 27% of patients undergoing pancreaticoduodenectomy [1]. The rate of marginal ulceration following Roux-en-Y gastric bypass (RYGB) ranges from 0.6% to 16%; however, this is likely underreported as patients may be asymptomatic [2–4].

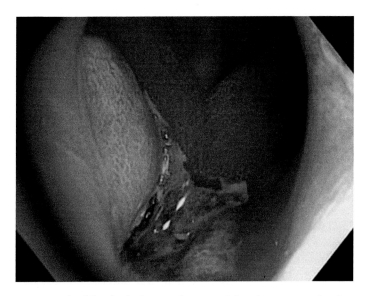

FIGURE   16.2 Marginal ulcer at the gastrojejunal anastomosis after Roux-en-Y gastric bypass

TABLE 16.1 Predisposing risk factors for anastomotic ulcerations	Smoking
	Medications (nonsteroidal anti-inflammatory drugs, steroids)
	Diabetes mellitus
	History of peptic ulcer disease
	Presence of foreign body (i.e., staples, sutures)

The underlying mechanisms contributing to the development of anastomotic ulcerations are not fully delineated, although reduced local blood flow and anastomotic tension may contribute. There are several known risk factors for the development of marginal ulceration shown in Table 16.1. Of note, nicotine stimulates basal acid output and inhibits nitric oxide synthesis, thereby leading to a reduction of angiogenesis in the mucosa and resultant ischemia. In RYGB anatomy, the Roux limb is not protected by the buffering alkaline fluid that is typically transmitted from the duodenum, thus exposing the anastomosis to acid secretion from the gastric pouch. Additional risk factors that have been proposed in RYGB include the location and size of the gastric pouch, foreign material such as staples or sutures, and the presence of a gastrogastric fistula. The impact of *Helicobacter pylori* (*H. pylori*) infection is controversial [3, 5]. Jejunojejunal anastomotic ulcers are rarely reported.

Anastomotic ulcers can occur anytime postoperatively. Clinical presentation ranges from being asymptomatic to having severe pain, obstruction, gastrointestinal bleeding, and, rarely, perforation. Anemia has been reported in 10.6% of patients [6].

Prevention of anastomotic ulcers includes cessation of smoking and avoidance of nonsteroidal anti-inflammatory drugs (NSAIDs). The benefit of postoperative prophylaxis with proton pump inhibitor (PPI) therapy is controversial and not routinely prescribed [7, 8].

Diagnosis is made by upper endoscopy. Figure 16.3 outlines an algorithm for the diagnosis and management of marginal

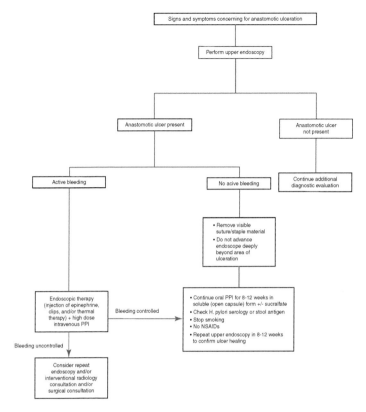

FIGURE 16.3 Diagnostic and management algorithm of anastomotic ulceration

ulceration. If hemostasis is required, endoscopic management includes injection of hemostatic agents (i.e., epinephrine), use of cautery, and/or through the scope (TTS) or cap-mounted hemostatic clips. Furthermore, foreign body material should be removed with forceps, loop cutters, or endoscopic scissors to reduce local irritation and tension. The majority of patients respond to medical therapy with PPIs, with sucralfate added for adjunctive therapy when desired. In patients with RYGB, PPIs should be prescribed in an open capsule (soluble) form, as studies have demonstrated improvement in healing time, fewer endoscopic surveillance procedures, and an overall decrease in healthcare utilization. Repeat upper endoscopy should be performed every 8–12 weeks following ulcer diagnosis to assess for healing. Endoscopic suturing may have a role in the treatment of recalcitrant marginal ulcers. Surgical revision may be required for patients in whom ulcers persist despite maximum medical therapy.

Postoperative Bleeding

Postoperative gastrointestinal (GI) bleeding can range from minimal oozing to life-threatening hemorrhage. The incidence varies depending on the surgical procedure performed with rates of 0.4% following resection of gastric cancer [9], 1.6–12.3% following pancreaticoduodenectomy [10], and 0.3–0.9% following bariatric surgery [11]. The incidence of bleeding following RYGB is higher compared to other bariatric surgeries and most commonly occurs at the gastrojejunal anastomosis.

Anastomotic Leaks

Leaks occur on the margin of an anastomosis and can lead to the formation of fistulas to other parts of the GI tract, intra-abdominal structures, or skin. Leaks are reported in 10.6% of patients undergoing esophagectomies for esophageal cancer [12] and 1.5–1.8% of patients undergoing gastrectomy for gastric cancer [13, 14]. The incidence of leaks following RYGB and sleeve gastrectomy (SG) is 0.5–8.3% and 0.3–7.0%, respectively [15–18]. Risk factors for the development of leaks are shown in Table 16.2. Oxygen dependence, hypertension, and hypoalbuminemia have also been implicated in SG and RYGB.

Diagnosis is typically made by cross-sectional imaging which demonstrates the presence of a fluid collection in an extraluminal space. CT scan is more sensitive and specific for

TABLE 16.2 Risk factors for anastomotic leaks

Anastomotic tension
Ischemia
Distal obstruction
Surgical technique
Diabetes mellitus
Medications (nonsteroidal anti-inflammatory drugs, steroids)
Infection

diagnosis than upper GI (UGI) series. Physical examination may reveal hemodynamic instability, abdominal tenderness, or peritoneal signs. Laboratory findings may include leukocytosis, metabolic acidosis, or elevated C-reactive protein. It is imperative to diagnose the location of a leak, as that will dictate management. This can often be accomplished by upper endoscopy with administration of contrast under fluoroscopic imaging.

Contained leaks in clinically stable patients can be managed through non-operative strategies including bowel rest, parenteral nutrition, acid suppression, nasogastric drainage, antibiotics, and endoscopic intervention. Depending on the chronicity of the leak, endoscopic strategies include stent placement, cap-mounted clips (including the over-the-scope clip system [OTSC, Ovesco Endoscopy AG, Tübingen, Germany] and the Padlock system [(US Endoscopy, Mentor, OH)]), endoscopic suturing, endoscopic vacuum therapy (EVT), or the administration of tissue sealants. Success varies based on the chronicity and location of the leak.

Esophageal Leaks

Placement of an endoscopic stent is warranted when esophageal dehiscence is between 30 and 70% of the esophageal circumference [19]. Covered and partially covered self-expanding metal stents (SEMS) are well-established therapies for esophageal leaks with recent studies demonstrating success rates of 84–86.2% [20,21]. Stent migration is the most common complication of stent placement, although ineffective defect closure, stricture development, and difficulty of removal due to stent ingrowth have all been reported. Small case series investigating the use of fibrin glue or OTSCs for closure of periesophageal leaks have demonstrated success rates of 72–91% [22–25]. Clips are limited by the need for viable tissue in order to attain successful placement. Novel endoscopic management strategies include the use of novel sealants, Vicryl mesh, biodegradable stents, and EVT. Surgical management is reserved for clinically unstable patients or when tissue necrosis is present.

Duodenal Stump Leak

A duodenal stump leak is a severe complication that can occur following a total or subtotal gastrectomy with an incidence of 3–5% [26, 27]. Risk factors include hematoma formation, inflammation, inadequate closure of the stump, and ischemia. Patients typically present with signs and symptoms of peritonitis. An upright abdominal X-ray may reveal air underneath the diaphragm, and computed tomography (CT) often confirms the diagnosis. Management requires reoperation.

Pancreatic Duct Leak

A pancreatic leak occurs following a pancreaticoduodenectomy, distal pancreatectomy, or total pancreatectomy. The incidence ranges from 3% to 62% [28–31] and can double the risk of death. Clinical presentation includes abdominal complaints, malnutrition, dehydration, pancreatic ascites, infection, or rarely GI bleeding from a pseudoaneurysm. Diagnosis relies on clinical suspicion, although elevation of pancreatic enzymes in the fluid, CT imaging, and/or secretin-stimulated magnetic resonance cholangiopancreatography (MRCP) may be useful. Endoscopic retrograde cholangiopancreatography (ERCP) with pancreatic stent placement is both diagnostic and therapeutic. Other management strategies include endoscopic ultrasound (EUS)-guided drainage, nasopancreatic drain placement, or use of sealants. Perioperative use of somatostatin analogues to decrease the rate of this complication is controversial.

Leak Following Sleeve Gastrectomy (SG)

Leaks following SG occur in the superior aspect of the staple line just below the gastroesophageal junction (Fig. 16.4) [32]. Endoscopic management is dictated by the chronicity and location of the leak. Stent placement is commonly performed for diversion of gastrointestinal contents in early leaks (<6 weeks), whereas techniques focusing on internal drainage such as placement of plastic pigtail stents or endoscopic septotomy are reserved for chronic leaks (>6 weeks). Closure of leaks with OTSCs, endoscopic suturing, EVT, fibrin glue, and other sealants has also been described with variable success. It is always important to treat downstream obstruction with endoscopic balloon dilation to promote healing.

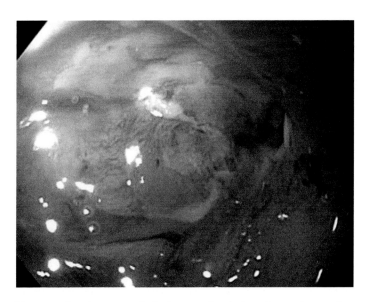

FIGURE 16.4 Anastomotic leak occurring below the gastroesophageal junction after sleeve gastrectomy

Leaks Following RYGB

Leaks after RYGB can occur at any location along a staple line (Fig. 16.5) with the location dictating management strategy. The most common site of occurrence is the gastrojejunal anastomosis.

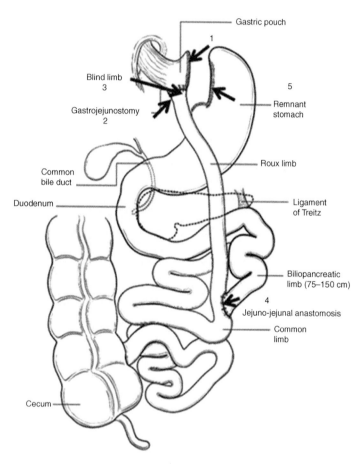

FIGURE 16.5 Multiple points of gastric leak following RYGB. (Adapted from Schulman et al. [32])

Postsurgical Strictures

The etiology of stricture formation is not entirely clear; ischemia and tension at the site of the anastomosis may play a role.

Anastomotic Stricture After Esophagectomy

Anastomotic strictures can occur in 9.1–65.8% of patients after esophagectomy [33, 34]. Resection of the lower esophageal sphincter allows for exposure to gastric acid, thereby resulting in collagen deposition, fibrin production, and ultimately deep ulceration and stricture formation. Risk factors for stricture formation include tumors in the upper esophagus, cardiovascular disease, anastomotic leakage, obesity, and prior chemoradiation. Patients present with dysphagia, odynophagia, decreased intake, and unexplained weight loss. Diagnosis is aided by UGI series and upper endoscopy. Medical therapy is limited to acid suppression, but its role may be more beneficial in a prophylactic setting.

Endoscopic dilation using TTS balloon dilation or Savary dilation is a well-described management strategy with similar efficacy. The role of intralesional steroid injection at the time of dilation is controversial. Patients often require multiple dilations prior to resolution, and recurrence rates can be high as 43% [34]. Major risk factors for stricture recurrence include shorter time of dysphagia onset following surgery, decreased luminal diameter at index dilation, and the presence of an anastomotic leak. Topical mitomycin C and stent placement are emerging methods to treat refractory anastomotic esophageal strictures; however, additional data is needed.

Anastomotic Stricture After Distal Gastrectomy and Pancreaticoduodenectomy

Luminal anastomotic strictures occur with an incidence of 1.1–8.0% following Billroth I reconstruction [35, 36] and up to 1.8% following Billroth II reconstruction [27, 37]. The incidence at the gastroenteral anastomosis is not well reported following pancreaticoduodenectomy. Stricture formation can occur weeks to months following the initial surgery and is often due to the recurrence of malignancy. Diagnosis is made by UGI series, CT scan, or upper endoscopy. Management involves decompression via nasogastric tube, endoscopic balloon dilation, and/or stent placement. Ultimately, patients may require palliative gastrojejunostomy to bypass malignant strictures.

Anastomotic Stricture After RYGB

Gastrojejunal anastomotic stenosis is reported in 2–23% of patients (Fig. 16.6) [38–45]. Surgical techniques using a circular stapler and a retrocolic approach are implicated risk factors for stricture formation. Patients can present weeks to

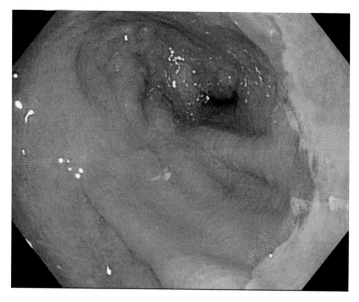

FIGURE 16.6 Stenosis of the gastrojejunal anastomosis after Roux-en-Y gastric bypass

months postoperatively, with patients undergoing open procedures presenting significantly later than those undergoing laparoscopic procedures. Clinical symptoms include progressive dysphagia, postprandial complaints, and inability to tolerate oral intake. Some patients may paradoxically have weight gain as they convert to higher-calorie full liquid diets. Upper endoscopy is the preferred diagnostic modality for direct visualization, as UGI series has a low sensitivity for detection. Endoscopic balloon dilation is the most common modality for treatment and is considered to be effective and safe. The majority of patients will respond in one to four dilation sessions. The most concerning complication of balloon dilation is perforation, with reported rates of up to 2% [46]. Surgical revision is rarely required.

Stenosis Following Sleeve Gastrectomy

The incidence of stenosis following SG is reported between 0.1% and 3.9% [47–52]. It most commonly occurs at the incisura angularis (Fig. 16.7a) and can result in symptoms of gastric outlet obstruction including reflux, dysphagia, nausea, vomiting, early satiety, and rapid weight loss. Diagnosis is typically made by UGI series or upper endoscopy. An algorithmic approach to endoscopic management

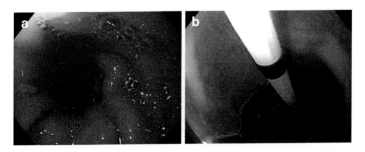

FIGURE 16.7 (**a**) Stenosis of the incisura with reflux of bilious fluid following sleeve gastrectomy (**b**) with subsequent pneumatic balloon dilation

includes TTS radial expansion balloon dilation to 20 mm followed by sequential pneumatic balloon dilation until symptomatic relief has been achieved (Fig. 16.7b). Surgical conversion to RYGB for refractory strictures may be required.

Motility Considerations

Afferent Loop Syndrome

Afferent loop syndrome (ALS) is a rare complication following upper GI surgery and is the result of duodenal or jejunal obstruction at or near an anastomosis. It typically involves the Roux limb created after Billroth II, pancreaticoduodenectomy, or RYGB. It has a reported an incidence of 0.2–1.8% [53–58]. Etiologies of afferent loop syndrome are shown in Table 16.3. Acute ALS occurs within 1 week of surgery and presents with bile leak, fever, leukocytosis, and/or abdominal complaints. Chronic ALS can present months to years following surgery with abdominal pain and distention, obstructive jaundice, cholangitis, and/or pancreatitis. Diagnosis is aided

TABLE 16.3 Etiologies of afferent loop syndrome

Internal hernia
Kinking at the anastomotic site
Recurrent malignancy
Enteroliths
Volvulus
Adhesions
Stricture
Intussusception
Scarring due to inflammation
Surgical technique

by cross-sectional imaging which can reveal a dilated afferent limb, dilated biliary tree, or pancreatitis. The management strategy is dictated by etiology.

Postoperative Ileus

Ileus is characterized by the transient cessation of bowel function, accumulation of gastrointestinal gas and fluid, abdominal complaints, and delayed passage of flatus and stool. The majority of patients will develop postoperative ileus after gastrointestinal surgery. Etiologies of ileus are multifactorial but include iatrogenic, neurologic, metabolic, inflammatory, and hormonal (Table 16.4). Early ambulation, nasogastric tube decompression, and/or early oral intake are key strategies for prevention and management of this condition.

Alkaline Reflux Gastritis

Alkaline, or bile, reflux gastritis is caused by excessive reflux of alkaline duodenal contents into the gastric lumen. This complication is common following surgical procedures that remove or bypass the pylorus. Symptoms commonly include epigastric burning or pain and chronic nausea. Anemia may develop as a result of gastritis. In RYGB, hepatobiliary imino-diacetic acid (HIDA) scan may reveal pooling of the bile in the gastric remnant. Endoscopic evaluation often confirms the presence of bilious fluid in the stomach and gastritis. Ursodeoxycholic acid is a promising agent used to treat abdominal pain related to bile reflux in RYGB patients. Baclofen, a $GABA_B$ agonist, may also have a role.

Delayed Gastric Emptying

Delayed gastric emptying is a complication of pancreatico-duodenectomy and distal gastrectomy, occurring in 18–57%

TABLE 16.4 Etiologies of ileus

Iatrogenic	Surgical	Metabolic	Medical conditions	Hormonal	Neurologic
Opioids	Open technique	Hypokalemia	Pancreatitis	Elevated nitric oxide	Spinal cord injury
Selective serotonin reuptake inhibitor antidepressants (SSRI)	Hematoma	Hyponatremia	Gastroenteritis	Elevated vasoactive intestinal peptide	Diabetes mellitus
Tricyclic antidepressants	Ischemia	Metabolic acidosis	Stroke		
Antipsychotics	Duration of surgical procedure	Hypomagnesemia	Parkinson's disease	Elevated substance P	
Anticholinergics	Handling of bowel during surgery		Botulism		
First-generation H$_1$ antihistamine blockers			Severe burns	Decreased motilin	
Muscle relaxants			Myocardial infarction		
Atropine					
Antineoplastic agents					
Selective antihypertensive agents					
Anesthesia					

TABLE 16.5 Risk factors for the development of postoperative delayed gastric emptying

Diabetes mellitus
Malnutrition
Vagal nerve disruption
Duodenal ischemia
Decreased motilin
Pancreatic fistula
Intra-abdominal abscess
Reconstruction method

[59–63] and 5–30% of patients, respectively [64–66]. The mechanism is not well delineated; however, surgery may disrupt the slow-wave network necessary for mediating gastric motility. Risk factors for the development of this complication are shown in Table 16.5. Symptoms are consistent with gastroparesis. Diagnosis is directed by gastric emptying study, UGI series, and upper endoscopy. Methods for treating primary gastroparesis including diet modification, promotility agents, gastric pacing, and gastric peroral endoscopic pyloromyotomy (G-POEM) may play a role in the management of this disorder, but they have not been well studied in the postoperative setting. Frequently, surgical revision including subtotal gastrectomy and additional reconstruction techniques may be required.

Roux Stasis Syndrome

The incidence of Roux stasis syndrome is not well reported. Pacesetter potentials in the small intestine modulate motility, with those in the duodenum potentiating the fastest action potentials toward the distal ileum, thereby inducing peristalsis. When the jejunum is partially resected in patients with Roux-en-Y reconstruction, the frequency of pacemaker potentials in the distal bowel decreases. Simultaneously, the appearance of ectopic pacemakers drives action potentials retrograde toward the stomach. This disruption in the motility of the Roux limb leads to postprandial abdominal symptoms and weight loss. An UGI series or upper endoscopy often reveals a dilated Roux limb, and promotility agents such as metoclopramide and erythromycin may be trialed. Additional data is needed on the impact of endoscopic gastrointestinal electric stimulation. Ultimately, surgical reconstruction of the Roux limb may be required to remediate ongoing symptoms.

Candy Cane Syndrome

Candy cane syndrome is rare and is characterized by the preferential passage of food and digestive enzymes through an excessively lengthy blind limb following RYGB. Food can become lodged in the blind limb leading to complaints of postprandial nausea, emesis, and pain that resolves after vomiting. The pathophysiology has not been elucidated but may involve surgical technique, dysmotility, or progressive dilation of the blind limb. Diagnosis includes UGI series and upper endoscopy. The classic finding in UGI series includes filling of the blind limb before spillage into the Roux limb. Surgical resection of the redundant limb provided 94–100% success rate in case series studies [67, 68].

Other Complications

Dumping Syndrome

Dumping syndrome is a common complication of upper GI surgery. The pathophysiology is driven by the delivery of hyperosmolar chyme to the small intestine which results in intravascular fluid shifts into the intestinal lumen and release of vasoactive hormones. Early dumping syndrome is characterized by a rapid onset (usually within 15 min) of hypotension and stimulation of the sympathetic nervous system. Late gastric emptying occurs 1–3 h after a meal and follows the

TABLE 16.6 Symptoms of dumping syndrome

Early dumping (within 15 min)

Gastrointestinal symptoms
Abdominal pain
Diarrhea
Nausea
Bloating
Borborygmus

Vasomotor symptoms
Flushing
Palpitations
Tachycardia
Hypotension
Syncope
Diaphoresis

Late dumping (1–3 h)

Hypoglycemic symptoms
Diaphoresis
Palpitations
Hunger
Weakness
Confusion
Tremor
Seizure
Syncope

postprandial insulin peak resulting in symptoms related to hypoglycemia (Table 16.6). Diagnosis is mainly based on clinical suspicion, but provocative testing can be performed by ingestion of glucose after an overnight fast. Medical management is common and includes dietary and lifestyle modifications, in addition to acarbose and/or somatostatin analogues.

Short Bowel Syndrome

Short bowel syndrome is defined as a massive small bowel resection resulting in intestinal failure due to malabsorption leading to inability of maintaining the homeostasis. Management is directed toward balancing nutrients, electrolytes, and fluids.

Small Intestinal Bacterial Overgrowth

Upper GI surgery is a risk factor for the development of small intestinal bacterial overgrowth (SIBO) due to resulting bacterial stasis. This can lead to chronic abdominal pain, bloating, distention, or change in bowel habits. Protein and fat malabsorption is common and can result in vitamin deficiencies and anemia. Small bowel aspirate is the gold standard for diagnosis of SIBO, as breath testing may be less interpretable in altered anatomy. Antibiotic regimens for the treatment of SIBO are listed in Table 16.7.

Gastrogastric Fistulae

Gastrogastric fistula is an abnormal connection between the excluded gastric remnant and the gastric pouch and most commonly occurs following open RYGB (Fig. 16.8). Common symptoms include abdominal pain, nausea, reflux, and weight regain. Diagnosis is confirmed by upper endoscopy or UGI series. Gastrogastric fistula may be managed conservatively with PPI therapy and dietary counseling; closure is indicated in the setting of persistent symptoms that are attributable to the fistula. Endoscopic methods for closure including

TABLE 16.7 Antibiotic choices for treatment of SIBO

Amoxicillin-clavulanate
Trimethoprim-sulfamethoxazole (co-trimoxazole)
Rifaximin
Metronidazole with a cephalosporin
Metronidazole with trimethoprim-sulfamethoxazole (co-trimoxazole)

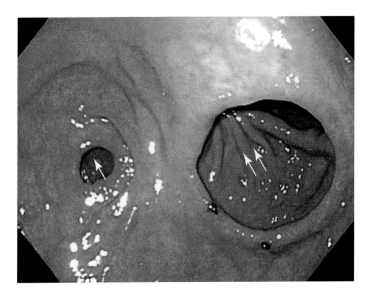

FIGURE 16.8 Gastrogastric fistula following Roux-en-Y gastric bypass. Single arrow is gastrojejunal anastomosis; double arrow is gastrogastric fistula

endoscopic suturing and OTSC placement are most effective in gastrogastric fistula that is less than 1 cm in size; reopening rates can be as high as 65% in larger fistulae [69]. Recently, endoscopic sleeve gastroplasty of the remnant pouch has been proposed as an alternative method to combat weight gain in the setting of a gastrogastric fistula. Surgical management provides definitive treatment.

Conclusion

Postoperative complications following GI surgery are common and can lead to significant morbidity and mortality. Complications vary based on patient characteristics, comorbidities, and the type of surgery performed. Specific knowledge of these unique complications is critical for proper management. Novel minimally invasive endoscopic techniques are emerging and will continue to play a major role in the treatment of these conditions moving forward.

Case Study Follow-Up

The patient was placed on 8 weeks of high-dose proton pump inhibitor therapy with no evidence of active or ongoing bleeding. Follow-up endoscopy 2 months later revealed complete resolution of the anastomotic ulcer.

Clinical Pearls

- Complications are common following gastrointestinal surgery and often occur at the anastomosis given increased tension, relative ischemia, and the presence of foreign material.
- Endoscopic management is often a first-line therapy for the management of anastomotic complications including ulcerations, strictures, leaks, and fistulae.
- Motility-related complications following gastrointestinal surgery should be in the differential for patients with ongoing symptoms and no obvious anatomic complication.
- There are a number of unique complications that arise in the postsurgical patient population and require specific knowledge for proper management.

Self-Test

Question 1. The gastroenterology service is consulted on a 50-year-old man. He is status post Whipple procedure 12 days ago for pancreatic adenocarcinoma and has had inadequate oral intake since surgery. The patient has not passed flatus or had a bowel movement and is thought to have postoperative ileus. He appears malnourished. The team determines that he requires nutritional support. What is the appropriate way to initiate nutritional support at this time?

    A. Total parenteral nutrition.
    B. Nasogastric tube and initiation of feedings with enteral formula.
    C. Placement of gastrostomy tube and initiation of tube feeds.
    D. Continue to delay nutritional support.

Question 2. A 65-year-old female with a history of short bowel syndrome presents to the gastroenterology clinic with complaints of alopecia and a scaly red rash on her hands, face, and groins. What is the most likely etiology?

    A. Vitamin B_{12} deficiency
    B. Zinc deficiency
    C. Vitamin D deficiency
    D. Copper deficiency
    E. Vitamin E deficiency

Question 3. A 55-year-old female with atrial fibrillation on anticoagulation underwent a Roux-en-Y gastric bypass (RYGB) 12 years ago and presents with epigastric pain, nausea, and vomiting. She subsequently undergoes an upper endoscopy, which demonstrates a 1 cm ulcer that is oozing blood. Endoscopic homeostasis is achieved with injection of epinephrine and placement of two hemostatic clips. Which of the following factors *most* likely increased her risk of developing an anastomotic ulcer?

    A. Smoking
    B. Age < 50
    C. Anticoagulation therapy
    D. Current proton pump inhibitor use
    E. Consumption of spicy foods

Question 4. A 70-year-old female complains of watery diarrhea, crampy abdominal pain, bloating, and distention for the past 6 months. She underwent a vagotomy and antrectomy with Billroth II reconstruction 5 years ago. Laboratory studies reveal mild normocytic anemia, vitamin B_{12} deficiency, and positive qualitative test for stool fat. Folate levels are found to be elevated. Endoscopy and colonoscopy with biopsies are normal. All other stool studies, including infectious studies, are negative. What is the most likely diagnosis?

A. Bile salt diarrhea
B. Celiac disease
C. Small intestinal bacterial overgrowth
D. Microscopic colitis
E. Crohn's disease

References

1. Wu JM, Tsai MK, Hu RH, Chang KJ, Lee PH, Tien YW. Reflux esophagitis and marginal ulcer after pancreaticoduodenectomy. J Gastrointest Surg. 2011;15(5):824–8.
2. Azagury DE, Abu Dayyeh BK, Greenwalt IT, Thompson CC. Marginal ulceration after Roux-en-Y gastric bypass surgery: characteristics, risk factors, treatment, and outcomes. Endoscopy. 2011;43(11):950–4.
3. Schulman AR, Abougergi MS, Thompson CC. H. Pylori as a predictor of marginal ulceration: a nationwide analysis. Obesity (Silver Spring, Md). 2017;25(3):522–6.
4. Schulman AR, Chan WW, Devery A, Ryan MB, Thompson CC. Opened proton pump inhibitor capsules reduce time to healing compared with intact capsules for marginal ulceration following Roux-en-Y gastric bypass. Clin Gastroenterol Hepatol. 2017;15(4):494–500.e1.
5. Rawlins L, Rawlins MP, Brown CC, Schumacher DL. Effect of Helicobacter pylori on marginal ulcer and stomal stenosis after Roux-en-Y gastric bypass. Surg Obes Relat Dis. 2013;9(5):760–4.
6. Avgerinos DV, Llaguna OH, Seigerman M, Lefkowitz AJ, Leitman IM. Incidence and risk factors for the development of anemia following gastric bypass surgery. World J Gastroenterol. 2010;16(15):1867–70.

7. D'Hondt MA, Pottel H, Devriendt D, Van Rooy F, Vansteenkiste F. Can a short course of prophylactic low-dose proton pump inhibitor therapy prevent stomal ulceration after laparoscopic Roux-en-Y gastric bypass? Obes Surg. 2010;20(5):595–9.

8. Plaeke P, Ruppert M, Hubens G. Benefits of prophylactic proton pump inhibitors after Roux-en-Y gastric bypass surgery: a retrospective study. Acta Chir Belg. 2015;115(4):273–8.

9. Tanizawa Y, Bando E, Kawamura T, Tokunaga M, Ono H, Terashima M. Early postoperative anastomotic hemorrhage after gastrectomy for gastric cancer. Gastric Cancer. 2010;13(1):50–7.

10. Roulin D, Cerantola Y, Demartines N, Schafer M. Systematic review of delayed postoperative hemorrhage after pancreatic resection. J Gastrointest Surg. 2011;15(6):1055–62.

11. Abell TL, Minocha A. Gastrointestinal complications of bariatric surgery: diagnosis and therapy. Am J Med Sci. 2006;331(4):214–8.

12. Kassis ES, Kosinski AS, Ross P Jr, Koppes KE, Donahue JM, Daniel VC. Predictors of anastomotic leak after esophagectomy: an analysis of the society of thoracic surgeons general thoracic database. Ann Thorac Surg. 2013;96(6):1919–26.

13. Jiang L, Yang K-H, Guan Q-L, Cao N, Chen Y, Zhao P, et al. Laparoscopy-assisted gastrectomy versus open gastrectomy for resectable gastric cancer: an update meta-analysis based on randomized controlled trials. Surg Endosc. 2013;27(7):2466–80.

14. Kumar M, Yang SB, Jaiswal VK, Shah JN, Shreshtha M, Gongal R. Is prophylactic placement of drains necessary after subtotal gastrectomy? World J Gastroenterol. 2007;13(27):3738–41.

15. Alizadeh RF, Li S, Inaba C, Penalosa P, Hinojosa MW, Smith BR, et al. Risk factors for gastrointestinal leak after bariatric surgery: MBSAQIP analysis. J Am Coll Surg. 2018;227:135.

16. Aurora AR, Khaitan L, Saber AA. Sleeve gastrectomy and the risk of leak: a systematic analysis of 4,888 patients. Surg Endosc. 2012;26(6):1509–15.

17. Kim J, Azagury D, Eisenberg D, DeMaria E, Campos GM. ASMBS position statement on prevention, detection, and treatment of gastrointestinal leak after gastric bypass and sleeve gastrectomy, including the roles of imaging, surgical exploration, and nonoperative management. Surg Obes Relat Dis. 2015;11(4):739–48.

18. Morales MP, Miedema BW, Scott JS, de la Torre RA. Management of postsurgical leaks in the bariatric patient. Gastrointest Endosc Clin N Am. 2011;21(2):295–304.

19. Kumar N, Thompson CC. Endoscopic therapy for postoperative leaks and fistulae. Gastrointest Endosc Clin N Am. 2013;23(1):123–36.

20. Dasari BV, Neely D, Kennedy A, Spence G, Rice P, Mackle E, et al. The role of esophageal stents in the management of esophageal anastomotic leaks and benign esophageal perforations. Ann Surg. 2014;259(5):852–60.

21. van Boeckel PG, Sijbring A, Vleggaar FP, Siersema PD. Systematic review: temporary stent placement for benign rupture or anastomotic leak of the oesophagus. Aliment Pharmacol Ther. 2011;33(12):1292–301.

22. Parodi A, Repici A, Pedroni A, Blanchi S, Conio M. Endoscopic management of GI perforations with a new over-the-scope clip device (with videos). Gastrointest Endosc. 2010;72(4):881–6.

23. Pohl J, Borgulya M, Lorenz D, Ell C. Endoscopic closure of postoperative esophageal leaks with a novel over-the-scope clip system. Endoscopy. 2010;42(9):757–9.

24. Surace M, Mercky P, Demarquay JF, Gonzalez JM, Dumas R, Ah-Soune P, et al. Endoscopic management of GI fistulae with the over-the-scope clip system (with video). Gastrointest Endosc. 2011;74(6):1416–9.

25. von Renteln D, Denzer UW, Schachschal G, Anders M, Groth S, Rosch T. Endoscopic closure of GI fistulae by using an over-the-scope clip (with videos). Gastrointest Endosc. 2010;72(6):1289–96.

26. Cozzaglio L, Coladonato M, Biffi R, Coniglio A, Corso V, Dionigi P, et al. Duodenal fistula after elective gastrectomy for malignant disease: an Italian retrospective multicenter study. J Gastrointest Surg. 2010;14(5):805–11.

27. Pedrazzani C, Marrelli D, Rampone B, De Stefano A, Corso G, Fotia G, et al. Postoperative complications and functional results after subtotal gastrectomy with Billroth II reconstruction for primary gastric cancer. Dig Dis Sci. 2007;52(8):1757–63.

28. Bassi C, Buchler MW, Fingerhut A, Sarr M. Predictive factors for postoperative pancreatic fistula. Ann Surg. 2015;261(4):e99.

29. Bassi C, Butturini G, Molinari E, Mascetta G, Salvia R, Falconi M, et al. Pancreatic fistula rate after pancreatic resection. The importance of definitions. Dig Surg. 2004;21(1):54–9.

30. Bassi C, Marchegiani G, Dervenis C, Sarr M, Abu Hilal M, Adham M, et al. The 2016 update of the International Study Group (ISGPS) definition and grading of postoperative pancreatic fistula: 11 years after. Surgery. 2017;161(3):584–91.

31. Peng L, Lin S, Li Y, Xiao W. Systematic review and meta-analysis of robotic versus open pancreaticoduodenectomy. Surg Endosc. 2017;31(8):3085–97.
32. Schulman AR, Thompson CC. Complications of bariatric surgery: what you can expect to see in your GI practice. Am J Gastroenterol. 2017;112:1640.
33. Briel JW, Tamhankar AP, Hagen JA, DeMeester SR, Johansson J, Choustoulakis E, et al. Prevalence and risk factors for ischemia, leak, and stricture of esophageal anastomosis: gastric pull-up versus colon interposition. J Am Coll Surg. 2004;198(4):536–41; discussion 41-2.
34. Mendelson AH, Small AJ, Agarwalla A, Scott FI, Kochman ML. Esophageal anastomotic strictures: outcomes of endoscopic dilation, risk of recurrence and refractory stenosis, and effect of foreign body removal. Clin Gastroenterol Hepatol. 2015;13(2):263–71.e1.
35. Hori S, Ochiai T, Gunji Y, Hayashi H, Suzuki T. A prospective randomized trial of hand-sutured versus mechanically stapled anastomoses for gastroduodenostomy after distal gastrectomy. Gastric Cancer. 2004;7(1):24–30.
36. Mimatsu K, Oida T, Kawasaki A, Kano H, Kuboi Y, Amano S. Anastomotic stricture of Billroth-I gastroduodenostomy using a hemi-double stapling technique. Hepato-Gastroenterology. 2009;56(90):381–4.
37. Shinohara T, Kawano S, Tanaka Y, Fujisaki M, Watanabe A, Yamamoto K, et al. Comparison of the cost and outcomes following totally laparoscopic and laparoscopy-assisted distal gastrectomies for gastric cancer: a single-institution comparison. Surg Endosc. 2016;30(8):3573–81.
38. Khalayleh H, Pines G, Imam A, Sapojnikov S, Buyeviz V, Mavor E. Anastomotic stricture rates following Roux-en-Y gastric bypass for morbid obesity: a comparison between linear and circular-stapled anastomosis. J Laparoendosc Adv Surg Tech. 2018;28(6):631–6.
39. Chang J, Sharma G, Boules M, Brethauer S, Rodriguez J, Kroh MD. Endoscopic stents in the management of anastomotic complications after foregut surgery: new applications and techniques. Surg Obes Relat Diseases. 2016;12(7):1373–81.
40. Kwong WT, Fehmi SM, Lowy AM, Savides TJ. Enteral stenting for gastric outlet obstruction and afferent limb syndrome following pancreaticoduodenectomy. Ann Gastroenterol. 2014;27(4): 413–7.

41. Mathew A, Veliuona MA, DePalma FJ, Cooney RN. Gastrojejunal stricture after gastric bypass and efficacy of endoscopic intervention. Dig Dis Sci. 2009;54(9):1971–8.

42. Ribeiro-Parenti L, Arapis K, Chosidow D, Dumont JL, Demetriou M, Marmuse JP. Gastrojejunostomy stricture rate: comparison between antecolic and retrocolic laparoscopic Roux-en-Y gastric bypass. Surg Obes Relat Dis. 2015;11(5):1076–84.

43. McCarty TM, Arnold DT, Lamont JP, Fisher TL, Kuhn JA. Optimizing outcomes in bariatric surgery: outpatient laparoscopic gastric bypass. Ann Surg. 2005;242(4):494–8; discussion 8-501.

44. Baccaro LM, Vunnamadala K, Sakharpe A, Wilhelm BJ, Aksade A. Stricture rate after laparoscopic Roux-en-Y gastric bypass with a 21-mm circular stapler versus a 25-mm linear stapler. Bariatric Surg Pract Patient Care. 2015;10(1):33–7.

45. Alasfar F, Sabnis AA, Liu RC, Chand B. Stricture rate after laparoscopic Roux-en-Y gastric bypass with a 21-mm circular stapler: the Cleveland Clinic experience. Med Princ Pract. 2009;18(5):364–7.

46. Campos JM, Mello FS, Ferraz AA, Brito JN, Nassif PA, Galvao-Neto Mdos P. Endoscopic dilation of gastrojejunal anastomosis after gastric bypass. Arquivos brasileiros de cirurgia digestiva: ABCD = Brazilian archives of digestive surgery. 2012;25(4):283–9.

47. Burgos AM, Csendes A, Braghetto I. Gastric stenosis after laparoscopic sleeve gastrectomy in morbidly obese patients. Obes Surg. 2013;23(9):1481–6.

48. Boza C, Salinas J, Salgado N, Perez G, Raddatz A, Funke R, et al. Laparoscopic sleeve gastrectomy as a stand-alone procedure for morbid obesity: report of 1,000 cases and 3-year follow-up. Obes Surg. 2012;22(6):866–71.

49. Cottam D, Qureshi FG, Mattar SG, Sharma S, Holover S, Bonanomi G, et al. Laparoscopic sleeve gastrectomy as an initial weight-loss procedure for high-risk patients with morbid obesity. Surg Endosc. 2006;20(6):859–63.

50. Gagner M, Deitel M, Kalberer TL, Erickson AL, Crosby RD. The second international consensus summit for sleeve gastrectomy, March 19–21, 2009. Surg Obes Relat Dis. 2009;5(4): 476–85.

51. Helmiö M, Victorzon M, Ovaska J, Leivonen M, Juuti A, Jaser N, et al. SLEEVEPASS: a randomized prospective multicenter study comparing laparoscopic sleeve gastrectomy and gastric

bypass in the treatment of morbid obesity: preliminary results. Surg Endosc. 2012;26(9):2521–6.

52. Gagner M, Deitel M, Erickson AL, Crosby RD. Survey on laparoscopic sleeve gastrectomy (LSG) at the fourth international consensus summit on sleeve gastrectomy. Obes Surg. 2013;23(12):2013–7.

53. Nageswaran H, Belgaumkar A, Kumar R, Riga A, Menezes N, Worthington T, et al. Acute afferent loop syndrome in the early postoperative period following pancreaticoduodenectomy. Ann R Coll Surg Engl. 2015;97(5):349–53.

54. Fleser PS, Villalba M. Afferent limb volvulus and perforation of the bypassed stomach as a complication of Roux-en-Y gastric bypass. Obes Surg. 2003;13(3):453–6.

55. Aoki M, Saka M, Morita S, Fukagawa T, Katai H. Afferent loop obstruction after distal gastrectomy with Roux-en-Y reconstruction. World J Surg. 2010;34(10):2389–92.

56. Kim HC, Han JK, Kim KW, Kim YH, Yang HK, Kim SH, et al. Afferent loop obstruction after gastric cancer surgery: helical CT findings. Abdom Imaging. 2003;28(5):624–30.

57. Han K, Song HY, Kim JH, Park JH, Nam DH, Ryu MH, et al. Afferent loop syndrome: treatment by means of the placement of dual stents. AJR Am J Roentgenol. 2012;199(6):W761–6.

58. Cho YS, Lee TH, Hwang SO, Lee S, Jung Y, Chung IK, et al. Electrohydraulic lithotripsy of an impacted enterolith causing acute afferent loop syndrome. Clin Endosc. 2014;47(4):367–70.

59. Miedema BW, Sarr MG, van Heerden JA, Nagorney DM, McIlrath DC, Ilstrup D. Complications following pancreaticoduodenectomy. Current management. Arch Surg. 1992;127(8):945–9; discussion 9-50.

60. Wente MN, Bassi C, Dervenis C, Fingerhut A, Gouma DJ, Izbicki JR, et al. Delayed gastric emptying (DGE) after pancreatic surgery: a suggested definition by the International Study Group of Pancreatic Surgery (ISGPS). Surgery. 2007;142(5):761–8.

61. Hanna MM, Gadde R, Allen CJ, Meizoso JP, Sleeman D, Livingstone AS, et al. Delayed gastric emptying after pancreaticoduodenectomy. J Surg Res. 2016;202(2):380–8.

62. Yamaguchi K, Tanaka M, Chijiiwa K, Nagakawa T, Imamura M, Takada T. Early and late complications of pylorus-preserving pancreatoduodenectomy in Japan 1998. J Hepato-Biliary-Pancreat Surg. 1999;6(3):303–11.

63. Richter A, Niedergethmann M, Sturm JW, Lorenz D, Post S, Trede M. Long-term results of partial pancreaticoduodenectomy

for ductal adenocarcinoma of the pancreatic head: 25-year experience. World J Surg. 2003;27(3):324–9.

64. Bar-Natan M, Larson GM, Stephens G, Massey T. Delayed gastric emptying after gastric surgery. Am J Surg. 1996;172(1):24–8.

65. Cohen AM, Ottinger LW. Delayed gastric emptying following gastrectomy. Ann Surg. 1976;184(6):689–96.

66. Jordon GL Jr, Walker LL. Severe problems with gastric emptying after gastric surgery. Ann Surg. 1973;177(6):660–8.

67. Aryaie AH, Fayezizadeh M, Wen Y, Alshehri M, Abbas M, Khaitan L. "Candy cane syndrome:" an underappreciated cause of abdominal pain and nausea after Roux-en-Y gastric bypass surgery. Surg Obes Relat Dis. 2017;13(9):1501–5.

68. Dallal RM, Cottam D. "Candy cane" Roux syndrome--a possible complication after gastric bypass surgery. Surg Obes Relat Dis. 2007;3(3):408–10.

69. Fernandez-Esparrach G, Lautz DB, Thompson CC. Endoscopic repair of gastrogastric fistula after Roux-en-Y gastric bypass: a less-invasive approach. Surg Obes Relat Dis. 2010;6(3):282–8.

Essential Reading

Davis JL, Ripley RT. Postgastrectomy syndromes and nutritional considerations following gastric surgery. Surg Clin North Am. 2017;97(2):277–93. This article provides an overview of postgastrectomy complications.

Kumar N, Thompson CC. Endoscopic therapy for postoperative leaks and fistulae. Gastrointest Endosc Clin N Am. 2013;23(1):123–3. This article provides an overview of endoscopic management of postoperative leaks and fistulae.

Mendelson AH, Small AJ, Agarwalla A, Scott FI, Kochman ML. Esophageal anastomotic strictures: outcomes of endoscopic dilation, risk of recurrence and refractory stenosis, and effect of foreign body removal. Clin Gastroenterol Hepatol. 2015;13(2):263–71.e1.6. This article provides management outcomes of esophageal anastomotic strictures.

Schulman AR, Thompson CC. Complications of bariatric surgery: what you can expect to see in your GI practice. Am J Gastroenterol. 2017;112:1640. This article provides an overview provides an overview of complications associated with bariatric surgery.

Part V

Small Bowel Disorders

Chapter 17
Celiac Disease and Non-celiac Gluten Sensitivity

Amanda K. Cartee and Joseph A. Murray

Case Study

A 33-year-old woman on a gluten-free diet for 5 years is referred for possible celiac disease. She describes postprandial abdominal cramping and loose stools starting in college. Her weight has been stable, and she denies any bone fractures. During that time, a cousin was diagnosed with celiac disease. Our patient started a strict gluten-free diet soon after her cousin's diagnosis and had resolution of her symptoms within several months. She describes nausea, vomiting, abdominal pain, and diarrhea within hours of inadvertent gluten exposure which occurs three to four times per year. She recently met with her primary care provider who checked celiac disease serologies. Serum IgA was within normal limits, and tissue transglutaminase IgA was negative. Besides the family history of celiac disease noted, there are several members with similar postprandial symptoms, some of whom have undergone celiac disease serologies and were negative. In addition, several second-degree relatives have Hashimoto's thyroiditis and systemic lupus erythematosus. Vital signs and physical examination

A. K. Cartee · J. A. Murray (✉)
Mayo Clinic, Rochester, MN, USA
e-mail: cartee.amanda@mayo.edu; murray.joseph@mayo.edu

© Springer Nature Switzerland AG 2019
B. E. Lacy et al. (eds.), *Essential Medical Disorders of the Stomach and Small Intestine*,
https://doi.org/10.1007/978-3-030-01117-8_17

are unremarkable. Recent complete blood count and complete metabolic panel were within normal limits. She wonders if she has celiac disease and if further evaluation is needed.

Objectives

- Describe the pathophysiology of celiac disease.
- List five gastrointestinal and extraintestinal symptoms that celiac disease and non-celiac gluten sensitivity share.
- Diagnose celiac disease in a patient who already adheres to a strict gluten-free diet.
- Develop a treatment and management plan for a patient newly diagnosed with celiac disease.

Epidemiology

Celiac Disease

Celiac disease was once thought to be a rare condition presenting in childhood, affecting mainly people of Northern European ancestry. Over the past decade, epidemiologic studies have shown that celiac disease is actually common, can present at virtually any age, and affects people of various ancestral backgrounds [1]. About 1% of the US population has celiac disease, which is about three million people [2]. Several factors have contributed to the increased incidence and prevalence including improved testing, greater recognition by providers, addition of gluten in processed foods, and increased gluten consumption. Improved serologic testing and greater recognition of subclinical disease, however, cannot fully explain this increase. More people have celiac disease than they did in the past. In addition, celiac disease can present at all ages [1, 3]. Celiac disease incidence is also increasing in countries not traditionally thought to be affected, including Mexico and Asia [5, 6].

These points are best illustrated by a study on Warren Air Force Base recruits. New male military recruits provided blood samples at recruitment during 1948–1954, which were then stored. Years later, the stored samples were tested for tissue transglutaminase IgA (tTG) and, if positive, endomysial antibody (EMA). For comparison, samples were taken from two groups of male residents of Olmsted County, Minnesota, USA. The first group had similar birth years, and the second group was similar in age at sample collection when compared with the historical cohort. More samples tested positive for celiac disease in these groups than the military recruits [4].

This led to several important conclusions: (1) the incidence has increased, and (2) the environmental trigger(s) have affected multiple generations at any age.

Some people are at increased risk of celiac disease. Family history of celiac disease is an important risk factor. When a patient has celiac disease, the chance that a first-degree relative also has celiac disease can be as high as one in seven [7]. There are multiple autoimmune conditions associated with celiac disease including autoimmune thyroid disease and type 1 diabetes, primarily due to shared genetic risk [8]. The genetic predisposition between celiac disease and type 1 diabetes is significant enough that screening for celiac disease in patients with type 1 diabetes is recommended [9]. In addition, a family history of autoimmunity also increases the risk of developing celiac disease [10].

Non-celiac Gluten Sensitivity

In addition to use in people with celiac disease, the popularity of the gluten-free diet is rising [2]. Gluten sensitivity was first described in the 1980s as a cause of diarrhea in a patient who did not have celiac disease or wheat allergy [11]. The number of people sensitive to gluten seems to be increasing, but the lack of a diagnostic test makes it difficult to characterize and study [12].

Etiology and Pathophysiology

Celiac Disease

Like most other autoimmune conditions, celiac disease requires a combination of genetic and environmental triggers. Celiac disease is unique in that the environmental trigger, gluten, is known [1]. The genetic predisposition and environmental factors that contribute to the development of celiac disease are listed in Table 17.1.

An individual must have at least one copy of the genes that encode HLA-DQ2 or HLA-DQ8 to develop celiac disease with extremely rare exceptions [13]. DQ2 is encoded by the carriage of the alleles DQA1:05 with DQB1:02 and DQ8 by DQA1:03 with DQB1:0302. About 30% of the general population carries one of these genes, but only 1% of the population has celiac disease [3]. Thus, genetic susceptibility is not enough to develop celiac disease.

TABLE 17.1 Etiologies of celiac disease and non-celiac gluten sensitivity

Celiac disease	Non-celiac gluten sensitivity
Genetic	Intestinal permeability
HLA-DQ2.5+	Intestinal microbiota dysbiosis
HLA-DQ8+	Alpha-amylase trypsin inhibitors (ATIs)
Environmental triggers	
Gluten exposure (required)	
Amount of gluten	
Timing of gluten	
introduction	
Infections	
Antibiotics	
Medications	
Smoking	

The etiologies of non-celiac gluten sensitivity are mostly proposed, whereas the listed etiologies of celiac disease are more established

There are several proposed environmental triggers that lead to the development of celiac disease in genetically predisposed individuals. The most widely recognized and required environmental trigger is gluten, a peptide found in wheat, barley, and rye. The autoimmune response is dependent on the presence of gluten [1]. Compared to other proteins, gluten is relatively resistant to enzymatic degradation. Gluten is cleaved into three gliadin peptides by peptidases in the stomach. Of the three peptides that result, one is a 33-amino acid sequence rich in glutamine. This peptide enters the small intestine where tissue transglutaminase converts certain glutamine residues to glutamic acid residues. The negative charge on the glutamic acid residues increases their binding affinity to HLA-DQ2 and DQ8 molecules. In people with celiac disease, these gliadin epitopes are recognized by gluten-specific T cells in the lamina propria, which trigger cytokine release and B cell activation. This, in turn, ultimately leads to increased intraepithelial lymphocytosis, villous atrophy, and crypt hyperplasia, the hallmark histologic features of celiac disease. The response to gluten is primarily an adaptive immune response [1, 14]; however, a better understanding of the role of the innate immune system is emerging [14].

Since many people are genetically susceptible but only a minority has celiac disease, there must be other factors that contribute to the development of the disease. The fact that gluten is the known trigger has led researchers to wonder if timing of gluten introduction and amount of gluten alter an individual's risk of developing celiac disease. To date, several groups have studied the age at which infants are first introduced to gluten and subsequent celiac disease diagnosis [15]. Taken together, these studies provide conflicting data. The amount of gluten exposure is also a possible risk factor. Increased gluten intake increases exposure and may lead to an earlier, more symptomatic presentation. The difficulty with studying the amount of gluten exposure is determining the amount itself [16]. There are different amounts of gluten depending on the grain used, and commercially produced products may have added gluten. Other non-dietary triggers are also under study, including childhood infections and antibiotic exposure [1].

Non-celiac Gluten Sensitivity

The etiology and pathophysiology of non-celiac gluten sensitivity remain more elusive [12]. Genetics may have a role in susceptibility; HLA-DQ status may play a role as well. For example, in one study, subjects with diarrhea-predominant irritable bowel syndrome were more likely to respond to a gluten-free diet if they were HLA-DQ2 positive [17]. Some even question if gluten is the true trigger, or if another substrate such as fructans or alpha-amylase trypsin inhibitors are to blame. Intestinal dysbiosis and alterations in intestinal permeability may also contribute [18].

Symptoms

The clinical presentation of celiac disease has also changed over time. Previously, celiac disease was thought to present in childhood with malabsorptive symptoms such as weight loss, diarrhea, and steatorrhea. Now, it is recognized that people with a variety of symptoms and signs, or those without any whatsoever, can also have celiac disease [1, 19]. The symptoms and signs of celiac disease (Table 17.2) are diverse, multi-organ, and non-specific. Patients often describe fatigue, difficulty concentrating, joint pains, abdominal bloating, and loose stools. Often, patients with non-celiac gluten sensitivity have similar symptoms [12]. Thus, differentiating the two conditions based on symptoms alone is nearly impossible.

That being said, there are several symptoms which are more suggestive of celiac disease. Weight loss is a classic malabsorptive symptom. Patients with weight loss on a gluten-containing diet are more likely to have celiac disease, but it is important to keep in mind that food avoidance to minimize

TABLE 17.2 Gastrointestinal and extraintestinal symptoms and signs of celiac disease and non-celiac gluten sensitivity

Gastrointestinal symptoms	Extraintestinal symptoms
Diarrhea	Iron deficiency
Abdominal pain	Osteopenia or osteoporosis
Constipation	Fatigue
Weight loss[a]	Difficulty concentrating, a.k.a. "brain fog"
Bloating	Headaches
Nausea	Rash, dermatitis herpetiformis[a]
Vomiting	Pruritus
Dyspepsia	Arthralgias
Gastroesophageal reflux	Aphthous ulcers
Mildly elevated AST, ALT[a]	Peripheral neuropathy
Small bowel malignancy[a]	Ataxia

There is considerable overlap between the symptoms of celiac disease and non-celiac gluten sensitivity. Symptoms are listed in descending order of frequency for presentation of celiac disease
[a]Symptoms more likely to be seen in celiac disease

gastrointestinal symptoms in a patient with non-celiac gluten sensitivity can also lead to a mild degree of weight loss. In addition, patients with gluten sensitivity may describe pruritus; however, dermatitis herpetiformis is a condition unique to celiac disease. It consists of intensely pruritic erythematous vesicles, particularly on the extensor surfaces of the arms and legs [3].

This change in clinical presentation of celiac disease and the similarity of symptoms between celiac disease and non-celiac gluten sensitivity create a diagnostic challenge, particularly for those patients who present to the clinic for evaluation and are already on a strict gluten-free diet [18].

Diagnostic Evaluation

Celiac Disease

Before describing the diagnostic approach, a brief review of the available diagnostic tests and their utility will be presented (Table 17.3). There are multiple serum celiac antibodies available; however, tissue transglutaminase IgA is the preferred initial screening test as it has both a high sensitivity and specificity. There are several caveats to this test. First, serum IgA level should also be obtained. If the IgA level is low, then tissue transglutaminase IgG and deamidated gliadin IgG should be checked. If the IgA is absent, then transglutaminase IgG and deamidated gliadin IgG should be obtained and selective IgA deficiency considered as a diagnosis in

TABLE 17.3 Laboratory-based tests for celiac disease

Test	Clinical use
Tissue transglutaminase IgA (tTG)	Screening, monitoring
Tissue transglutaminase IgG (tTG)	IgA deficiency
Deamidated gliadin (DGP)	Used to expand sensitivity in patients on a low-gluten-containing diet or during gluten challenge. Positive results suggest persistent gluten exposure in a patient with treated celiac disease
Endomysial antibody (EMA)	Used to expand sensitivity in patients on a low-gluten-containing diet or during gluten challenge
HLA genotyping	Test to exclude celiac disease

Tissue transglutaminase IgA is the most useful test in diagnosing celiac disease and monitoring celiac disease activity except in patients with IgA deficiency itself. Second, in cases where tissue transglutaminase IgA is weakly positive, endomysial antibody can be helpful as it has a high specificity. HLA genotyping is helpful to exclude celiac disease in a patient already following a gluten-free diet [1, 3]. Small bowel biopsies are obtained to confirm the diagnosis of celiac disease. Multiple biopsies should be taken from both the duodenal bulb and the second portion of the duodenum as villous atrophy can be patchy [1, 3].

In patients already on a gluten-containing diet, the first step in the evaluation is to take a thorough dietary history to confirm that they are eating adequate amounts of gluten. The typical westerner eats between 10 and 20 grams of gluten per day. A slice of bread has about 2 grams of gluten [20]. Some patients endorse eating gluten but in fact follow a low-gluten diet, avoiding breads and pastas altogether. Diagnostic tests are dependent on adequate gluten exposure. Patients on a low-gluten diet may have normal serologies and should be encouraged to increase gluten intake before undergoing diagnostic testing.

Diagnosing celiac disease in a patient already following a strict gluten-free diet requires a different process of evaluation than if the patient were eating gluten (Figs. 17.1 and 17.2). With the rise in popularity of the gluten-free diet, patients often try a gluten-free diet prior to visiting with a healthcare provider. Serum autoantibodies and small bowel biopsies can improve or normalize after only several months of a gluten-free diet, especially in young adults or those with mild intestinal inflammation. If the patient has been on a gluten-free diet for a short time frame (i.e., weeks to months) and still has some symptoms, it is reasonable to obtain celiac disease serologies and an endoscopy with small bowel biopsies. How biopsies are obtained in this scenario is important—multiple biopsies should be obtained since villous atrophy can be patchy. In addition, as the small bowel heals from distal to proximal, obtaining several biopsies from the duodenal bulb may aid in diagnosis [1, 3].

In contrast, for patients who have been on a gluten-free diet for a long time (i.e., months to years), the evaluation

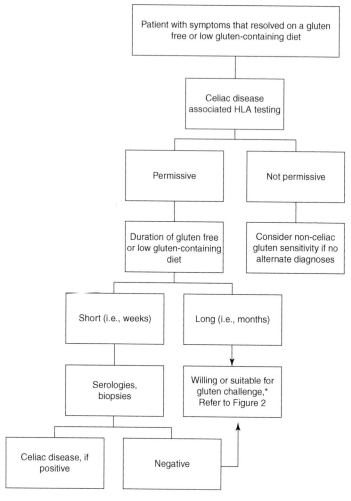

FIGURE 17.1 Approach to diagnose celiac disease in a patient on a gluten-free diet. HLA gene typing and duration of gluten-free diet are important factors that help guide further testing. This algorithm should also be used to diagnose celiac disease when a patient is on a low-gluten-containing diet. *Patients with neurologic symptoms such as dizziness, imbalance, or ataxia should not undergo a gluten challenge

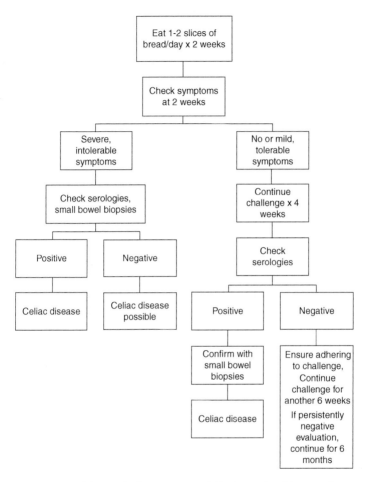

FIGURE 17.2 Gluten challenge protocol. Patients should eat at least one slice of bread per day and increase as able up to three slices of bread per day. Symptoms should be monitored closely to help determine timing of serologies and small bowel biopsies

focuses on exclusion of celiac disease and in those with active symptoms the exclusion of active disease. There are multiple explanations for the patient who continues to have symptoms on a long-standing gluten-free diet. In this scenario, the focus is directed toward excluding celiac disease whether in remission or ongoing active small bowel inflammation and evaluating for other causes. If the patient is on a gluten-free diet and having ongoing symptoms, serologies and biopsies should be ordered to detect active disease. It would also be reasonable to perform celiac disease-associated HLA genotyping as a way to exclude the possibility of celiac disease [3]. If biopsies or serologies are positive, then a careful history should be performed, ideally by an experienced dietitian, to determine possible sources of gluten exposure [20].

Patients may also see a healthcare provider after their symptoms resolve for recommendations about ongoing care. Since differentiating between celiac disease and non-celiac gluten sensitivity based on symptoms and resolution of symptoms is virtually impossible, establishing a diagnosis depends on the patient's willingness to undergo at least a 6-week gluten challenge (Fig. 17.2). For patients unwilling or unable to undergo a gluten challenge, a history and physical should be performed to assess for any evidence of ongoing symptoms, vitamin or mineral deficiencies, or complications of celiac disease such as osteoporosis. Celiac disease-associated HLA genotyping is helpful to exclude celiac disease. A negative result is most helpful since it virtually rules out the possibility of celiac disease. A positive test does not confirm celiac disease but rather makes having celiac disease possible [1, 3, 14, 21]. For willing patients, we recommend starting with a slice of bread per day and, if tolerated, increasing up to three slices of bread per day. At 2 weeks, symptoms should be assessed. If the patient is unable to continue the challenge past 2 weeks because of severe symptoms, serologies and biopsies should be performed at 2 weeks. However, if the patient is able to tolerate the symptoms, we recommend continuing for another 4 weeks to complete a 6-week challenge, at which point serologies should be performed. If serologies are positive, then endoscopy with two biopsies from the duodenal bulb and four biopsies from the second portion of the duodenum should be obtained. In those who remain asymptomatic and seronegative, a further 6 weeks of challenge should be undertaken after ensuring that the patient is adhering to the challenge. If still negative and asymptomatic after 12 weeks, a full 6-month challenge with biopsies at the end should detect disease, if present.

Non-celiac Gluten Sensitivity

Currently, there are no diagnostic tests for non-celiac gluten sensitivity. The main purpose of evaluation is to rule out celiac disease or another cause of the symptoms. HLA typing is particularly useful for excluding celiac disease. Some patients who seek care may not carry permissive genes and/or have persistent symptoms despite a gluten-free diet. For these patients, a thorough history of their symptoms to guide further evaluation is important. Common alternative diagnoses to consider include fructose or fructan intolerance, impaired gastric accommodation, and irritable bowel syndrome.

Treatment

Celiac Disease

There are three main aspects to the management of celiac disease: a gluten-free diet, checking for consequences of malabsorption, and disease monitoring. These are also illustrated in Fig. 17.3.

The only treatment for celiac disease is a strict, lifelong gluten-free diet [3]. Once a patient is diagnosed with celiac disease, they should meet with a dietitian with expertise in celiac disease and begin a gluten-free diet. Gluten is a protein found in wheat, barley, and rye. Since ingestion of even a small amount of gluten activates the immune-mediated response, patients with celiac disease must follow a strict gluten-free diet. This includes avoiding cross-contamination, which is when gluten-free food comes into contact with gluten-containing foods or surfaces. Common

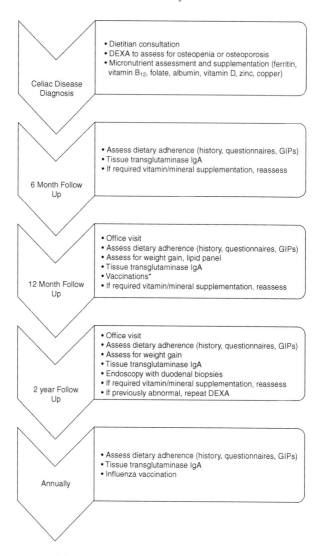

FIGURE 17.3 Management of celiac disease. This flowchart displays the important aspects of caring for a patient with celiac disease in the first 2 years after diagnosis. *Patients who work in a healthcare or high-risk setting for hepatitis B should receive a booster or repeat vaccination if a known non-responder. Older adults (i.e., ≥60 years) should receive pneumonia and shingles vaccinations

sources of cross-contamination in the home include toasters and wooden cutting boards. Medications and cosmetics are also common sources of hidden gluten. Patients should also be given resources about eating out and limiting cross-contamination in this setting [20]. In addition, oats are often become cross-contaminated with gluten while being grown with wheat. Some people with celiac disease react to oats [3, 20].

Once the diagnosis is established, patients should be tested for consequences of malabsorption, including vitamin and mineral deficiencies and osteopenia or osteoporosis [3]. We routinely check ferritin, vitamin B12, folate, vitamin D, zinc, and copper levels at diagnosis. In patients who have a micronutrient deficiency, we replete and recheck levels at 6 and 12 months. Deficiencies should be corrected with supplementation and reversal of the malabsorptive state.

All adult patients with newly diagnosed celiac disease should undergo bone density testing [3]. Patients with osteopenia can often be managed conservatively with calcium and vitamin D supplementation and weight-bearing exercise. Osteoporosis should be managed aggressively, often with bisphosphonate therapy though, anecdotally, oral therapy may not be well tolerated or effective. If the baseline bone density testing is abnormal, it should be repeated in 2 years. Osteomalacia may also be seen in which case treatment of the celiac disease and supplementation with pharmacologic doses of vitamin D (50,000 units weekly) may be needed for a period of time.

Several tests are used to monitor for disease activity and mucosal healing. During the first year, tTG IgA is checked every 6 months. Usually, serologies will have normalized by 1 year if the patient is adhering to the gluten-free diet. Thereafter, tTG IgA is checked annually. Patients without symptoms and with normal serologies at 1 year can try certified gluten-free oats. If symptoms develop, then oats should be avoided altogether. Current guidelines recommend that adults may undergo repeat endoscopy 2 years after diagnosis to assess for small bowel mucosal and histologic healing [3, 20].

Long-term care of a patient with celiac disease focuses on dietary adherence. While following a gluten-free diet has become less cumbersome with increased awareness, greater access to gluten-free products, and FDA gluten-free labeling standards, patients can still be inadvertently exposed to gluten. There are several tools to measure dietary adherence. Monitoring of symptoms and questionnaires are the most basic means of dietary adherence, but assessment by an experienced dietitian remains the gold standard [20]. More recently, tests that detect gluten immunogenic peptides (GIPs) in the urine and stool have been used in clinical trials to assess dietary adherence. These tests are not regulated by the FDA, and their role in clinical practice at this point is unclear [22].

Celiac disease and a gluten-free diet impact several preventive medicine measures. People with celiac disease may have hyposplenism and poor response to vaccinations and be more susceptible to infections with encapsulated bacteria [23]. Patients may not have responded to hepatitis B vaccination, and for those who work in a healthcare correctional or other setting of heightened risk, checking immune status and repeating vaccinations may be worthwhile. Some also advocate for early pneumonia vaccination. The patient may adapt a gluten-free diet that is both calorie dense and has high-fat content. This, coupled with reversal of malabsorption, could lead to hyperlipidemia, excess weight gain, and even metabolic syndrome [20].

Non-celiac Gluten Sensitivity

For non-celiac gluten sensitivity, a gluten-free diet is the only known treatment. There are no known adverse consequences such as micronutrient deficiencies or decreased bone mineral density, and thus, patients with non-celiac gluten sensitivity do not require further evaluation or treatment as long as symptoms resolve on a gluten-free diet. There is likely considerable overlap with fructose intolerance or irritable bowel syndrome [12]. Patients whose symptoms continue despite adherence to a gluten-free diet should be advised to discontinue the diet. The long-term consequences of a gluten-free diet are largely unknown. A gluten-free diet can be associated with weight gain, decreased fiber intake, and increased urine levels of heavy metals [20, 24].

Case Study: Follow-Up

This individual had a long-standing adherence to a gluten-free diet and negative celiac serologies previously which is the reason for obtaining celiac disease-associated HLA typing. She was found to carry HLA-DQ2, making celiac disease a possibility. Since she was asymptomatic and on a strict gluten-free diet for about 5 years, utility of an endoscopy at this point for diagnosis would be low. We discussed a gluten challenge, to which she agreed. She started eating one slice of bread per day and developed abdominal bloating, cramping, and diarrhea but was able to continue the challenge and increase to three slices of bread per day. After 6 weeks, she returned to the clinic. Tissue transglutaminase IgA was positive, and duodenal biopsies revealed partial villous atrophy. She did not have micronutrient deficiencies or decreased bone mineral density. She subsequently met with a dietitian and resumed her gluten-free diet. Tissue transglutaminase will be repeated in 6 months. We counseled her about screening first-degree relatives, particularly her young children. Tissue transglutaminase IgA can be used for celiac disease screening in first-degree relatives starting at age 2, although the frequency of testing remains controversial.

Clinical Pearls

- Levels of serologic tests for celiac disease may decline rapidly while adhering to a gluten-free or low-gluten diet. Broadening the serology panel to include deamidated gliadin and endomysial antibodies maximizes sensitivity in this setting.
- The main purpose of the evaluation in a patient with suspected non-celiac gluten sensitivity is to exclude other etiologies, specifically celiac disease. Sometimes, it may be impossible to rule out celiac disease if the patient who carries the at-risk HLA genotype does not undergo a gluten challenge. In this scenario, the evaluation is limited to assess healing of the intestine and detect alternative diagnoses.
- Patients with newly diagnosed celiac disease should undergo laboratory-based micronutrient and bone mineral density assessments since micronutrient deficiencies and decreased bone mineral density are common complications of celiac disease.
- The main goal of treatment in celiac disease is mucosal healing to reverse and prevent further complications including micronutrient deficiencies, decreased bone mineral density, and malignancy. Patients with celiac disease may benefit from a follow-up endoscopy with duodenal biopsies 2 years after diagnosis to assess for healing.

Self-Test

Question 1. There are both genetic and environmental factors that contribute to celiac disease pathogenesis. Which one of the following is the strongest contributor?

A. Amount of gluten
B. Timing of gluten introduction
C. Childhood infections
D. Presence of HLA-DQ2

Question 2. The clinical presentations of celiac disease and non-celiac gluten sensitivity overlap. Which one of the following differentiates celiac disease from non-celiac gluten sensitivity?

A. Postprandial diarrhea
B. Pruritic, blistering rash
C. HLA-DQ2 positivity
D. Increased intraepithelial lymphocytes (IELs)

Question 3. A patient is referred for possible celiac disease. She has been asymptomatic on a gluten-free diet for several years. Which one of the following test results performed at time of consultation would exclude a diagnosis of celiac disease?

A. Duodenal biopsies
B. Micronutrient testing
C. Tissue transglutaminase
D. HLA genotype

Question 4. A patient was diagnosed with celiac disease 1 year ago. She had no micronutrient or bone density complications at the time of diagnosis. She is following a strict gluten-free diet and denies any symptoms. She works as a nurse. Besides ordering a tissue transglutaminase IgA, which one of the following would you also do?

A. Hepatitis B serologies
B. Bone mineral density scan
C. Dietitian referral
D. Upper endoscopy with biopsies

References

1. Green PH, Cellier C. Celiac disease. N Engl J Med. 2007;357(17):1731–43.
2. Choung RS, Unalp-Arida A, Ruhl CE, Brantner TL, Everhart JE, Murray JA. Less hidden celiac disease but increased gluten avoidance without a diagnosis in the United States: findings from the national health and nutrition examination surveys from 2009 to 2014. Mayo Clin Proc. 2016;92(1):30–8.
3. Kelly CP, Bai JC, Liu E, Leffler DA. Advances in diagnosis and management of celiac disease. Gastroenterology. 2015;148(6):1175–86.
4. Rubio-Tapia A, Kyle RA, Kaplan EL, Johnson DR, Page W, Erdtmann F, et al. Increased prevalence and mortality in undiagnosed celiac disease. Gastroenterology. 2009;137(1):88–93.
5. Remes-Troche JM, Ramirez-Iglesias MT, Rubio-Tapia A, Alonso-Ramos A, Velazquez A, Uscanga LF. Celiac disease could be a frequent disease in Mexico: prevalence of tissue transglutaminase antibody in healthy blood donors. J Clin Gastroenterol. 2006;40(8):697–700.
6. Singh P, Arora S, Singh A, Strand TA, Makharia GK. Prevalence of celiac disease in Asia: a systematic review and meta-analysis. J Gastroenterol Hepatol. 2016;31(6):1095–101.
7. Singh P, Arora S, Lal S, Strand TA, Makharia GK. Risk of celiac disease in the first- and second-degree relatives of patients with celiac disease: a systematic review and meta-analysis. Am J Gastroenterol. 2015;110(11):1539–48.
8. Troncone R, Discepolo V. Celiac disease and autoimmunity. J Pediatr Gastroenterol Nutr. 2014;59(Suppl1):S9–S11.
9. Akirov A, Pinhas-Hamiel O. Co-occurrence of type 1 diabetes mellitus and celiac disease. World J Diabetes. 2015;6(5):707–14.
10. Emilsson L, Wijmenga C, Murray JA, Ludvigsson JF. Autoimmune disease in first-degree relatives and spouses of individuals with celiac disease. Clin Gastroenterol Hepatol. 2015;13(7):1271–7.
11. Cooper BT, Holmes GK, Ferguson R, Thompson RA, Allan RN, Cooke WT. Gluten-sensitive diarrhea without evidence of celiac disease. Gastroenterology. 1981;81(1):192–4.
12. Igbinedion SO, Ansari J, Vasikaran A, Gavins FN, Jordan P, Boktor M, et al. Non-celiac gluten sensitivity: all wheat attack is not celiac. World J Gastroenterol. 2017;23(40):7201–10.

13. Karell K, Louka AS, Moodie SJ, Ascher H, Clot F, Greco L, et al. HLA types in celiac disease patients not carrying the DQQ1*05-DQB1*02 (DQ2) heterodimer: results from the European Genetics Cluster on Celiac Disease. Hum Immunol. 2003;64(4):469–77.

14. Kupfer SS, Jabri B. Pathophysiology of celiac disease. Gastrointest Endosc Clin N Am. 2012;22(4):639–60.

15. Mearin ML. The prevention of coeliac disease. Best Pract Res Clin Gastroenterol. 2015;29(3):493–501.

16. Aronsson CA, Lee H-S, Koletzko S, Uusitalo U, Yang J, Virtanen SM, et al. Effects of gluten intake on risk of celiac disease: a case-control study on a Swedish birth cohort. Clin Gastroenterol Hepatol. 2016;14(3):403–9.

17. Vazquez-Roque MI, Camilleri M, Smyrk T, Murray JA, Marietta E, O'Neill J, et al. A controlled trial of gluten-free diet in patients with irritable bowel syndrome-diarrhea: effects on bowel frequency and intestinal junction. Gastroenterology. 2013;144(5):903–11.

18. Leonard MM, Sapone A, Catassi C, Fasano A. Celiac disease and nonceliac gluten sensitivity: a review. JAMA. 2017;318(7):647–56.

19. Rampertab SD, Pooran N, Brar P, Singh P, Green PH. Trends in the presentation of celiac disease. Am J Med. 2006;119(4):355. e9–355.e14.

20. See JA, Kaukinen K, Makharia GK, Gibson PR, Murray JA. Practical insights into gluten-free diets. Nat Rev Gastroenterol Hepatol. 2015;12:580–91.

21. Coburn JA, Vande Coort JL, Lahr BD, Van Dyke CT, Kroning CM, Wu TT, et al. Human leukocyte antigen genetics and clinical features of self-treated patients on a glute-free diet. J Clin Gastroenterol. 2013;47(10):828–33.

22. Comino I, Fernández-Bañares F, Esteve M, Ortigosa L, Castillejo G, Fambuena B, et al. Fecal gluten peptides reveal limitations of serological tests and food questionnaires for monitoring gluten-free diet in celiac disease patients. Am J Gastroenterol. 2016;111:1456.

23. Noh KW, Poland GA, Murray JA. Hepatitis B vaccine nonresponse and celiac disease. Am J Gastroenterol. 2003;98(10):2289–92.

24. Raehsler SL, Choung RS, Marietta EV, Murray JA. Accumulation of heavy metals in people on a gluten-free diet. Clin Gastroenterol Hepatol. 2018;16(2):244–51.

Essential Reading

Choung RS, Unalp-Arida A, Ruhl CE, et al. Less hidden celiac disease but increased gluten avoidance without a diagnosis in the United States: findings from the national health and nutrition examination surveys from 2009 to 2014. Mayo Clin Proc. 2016;92(1):30–8. This article describes the most up-to-date prevalence of celiac disease in the United States and the rate of people avoiding gluten without celiac disease diagnosis.

Green PH, Cellier C. Celiac disease. N Engl J Med. 2007;357(17):1731–43. This article provides an overview of epidemiology, pathophysiology, diagnosis, and management of celiac disease.

Igbinedion SO, Ansari J, Vasikaran A, et al. Non-celiac gluten sensitivity: all wheat attack is not celiac. World J Gastroenterol. 2017;23(40):7201–10. This review provides an overview of non-celiac gluten sensitivity.

See JA, Kaukinen K, Makharia GK, et al. Practical insights into gluten-free diets. Nat Rev Gastroenterol Hepatol. 2015;12:580–91. This article provides a thorough overview of what it means to be gluten-free for a patient and recommendations on determining adherence.

Chapter 18
Non-celiac Small Bowel Enteropathies

Isabel A. Hujoel and Alberto Rubio-Tapia

Case Study

A 77-year-old woman presents to her primary care physician for fatigue, watery diarrhea, and intermittent lower abdominal pain for the last 6 months. She has had iron-deficiency anemia in the past without response to oral iron. She has hypertension treated with losartan 25 mg daily for the past 5 years and major depressive disorder in remission treated with sertraline 75 mg daily for the past 3 years. Laboratory studies showed iron-deficiency anemia (hemoglobin of 8.6 g/dL, a mean corpuscular volume of 77.9 FL, and a ferritin of 5 ng/mL). A referral to gastroenterology was placed.

I. A. Hujoel · A. Rubio-Tapia (✉)
Division of Gastroenterology and Hepatology,
Mayo Clinic, Rochester, MN, USA
e-mail: hujoel.isabel@mayo.edu; rubiotapia.alberto@mayo.edu

© Springer Nature Switzerland AG 2019   375
B. E. Lacy et al. (eds.), *Essential Medical Disorders
of the Stomach and Small Intestine*,
https://doi.org/10.1007/978-3-030-01117-8_18

Objectives

1. Appreciate the epidemiology of non-celiac enteropathies.
2. Recognize the clinical presentation of non-celiac enteropathies.
3. Formulate a practical differential for non-celiac enteropathies.
4. Review the treatment for non-celiac enteropathies.

Autoimmune Enteropathy

Epidemiology

Autoimmune enteropathy (AIE) is a rare condition. AIE most commonly affects infants (incidence of 1 in 100,000 infants per year) although it is being increasingly recognized in adults [1, 2]. Adults with AIE are typically middle-aged with a delay in diagnosis of 1.5 years [1, 2]. Adult AIE may be a collection of different conditions that share an underlying dysregulation of the immune system [3]. Association with other autoimmune diseases (e.g., hypothyroidism, vitiligo) is common.

Etiology/Pathophysiology

The pathophysiology of AIE in adults appears to stem from dysregulation of the intestinal immune system (Table 18.1). The major histocompatibility complex (MHC) class II molecules are overexpressed in enterocytes. This, along with enterocyte expression of costimulatory markers, may induce CD4+ T cell overactivity with resultant epithelial injury. Antibiotic-induced dysbiosis may lead to loss of tolerance. Anti-enterocyte and anti-goblet cell antibodies are frequently found but are likely not pathogenic [3].

TABLE 18.1 The etiologies of five non-celiac enteropathies

Condition	Etiology

Autoimmune enteropathy	Proposed etiologies
	  Dysregulation of the intestinal immune syndrome
	  Alteration of intestinal microbiome related to antibiotic use
	  In children, it is related to a germline mutation that leads to a reduction in self-tolerance

Common variable immunodeficiency-associated enteropathy	Proposed etiologies
	  Absence of plasma cells leads to a defect in secretory antibodies that in turn causes chronic or repetitive infections
	  Overgrowth of anaerobic bacteria due to deficiency of IgA
	  Decreased CD4+/CD8+ ratio

Whipple's disease	*Tropheryma whipplei* infection

Tropical sprue	Proposed etiologies
	  Infectious factor
	  Bacterial overgrowth (aerobic, gram-negative)
	  Abnormal small bowel permeability
	  Reduced intestinal immune system
	  Hormonal dysregulation
	  Exaggerated ileal brake

Medication-induced enteropathy	Olmesartan → immune-based Nonsteroidal anti-inflammatory drugs → mucosal damage, reduction in prostaglandin levels, intestinal dysbiosis, enterohepatic recycling Mycophenolate mofetil → direct toxic effect, inhibited cell proliferation

In children, AIE is most commonly related to a germ-line mutation causing defects in the regulatory T cells that are required for self-tolerance. The two systemic forms of AIE, immune dysregulation, polyendocrinopathy, enteropathy, X-linked (IPEX) syndrome and autoimmune polyendocrinopathy-candidiasis-ectodermal dystrophy (APECED) syndrome, stem from loss of function mutations in FOXP3 and an autoimmune regulator gene, respectively. These in turn lead to hyperactivation of the immune system and recognition of self-antigens.

Symptoms

Infants less than 6 months old present with severe diarrhea. Children typically present with severe weight loss and failure to thrive. AIE can include systemic manifestations, and in children this includes IPEX and APECED syndromes. IPEX commonly presents with severe diarrhea and an endocrinopathy such as insulin-dependent diabetes. Most children with IPEX die before the age of 3 unless they receive a hematopoietic stem cell transplant. Children with APECED can survive until adolescence and typically present with diarrhea, malabsorption, adrenal gland insufficiency, and hypoparathyroidism.

The typical presentation in adults involves severe weight loss, chronic diarrhea (>90%), and malabsorption [1, 2] (Table 18.2).

Diagnostic Evaluation

Mayo Clinic criteria specify the presence of (1) chronic diarrhea (>6 weeks), (2) malabsorption, (3) specific small bowel histology (partial/complete villous blunting, deep crypt lymphocytosis, increased crypt apoptotic bodies, and minimal intraepithelial lymphocytosis), and (4) exclusion of other causes of villous atrophy [1]. The presence of anti-enterocyte

TABLE 18.2 Common symptoms of five non-celiac enteropathies

Condition	Common symptoms
Autoimmune enteropathy	Infants/children → severe diarrhea, weight loss, failure to thrive; may have systemic manifestations: Endocrinopathies, adrenal gland insufficiencies, hypoparathyroidism Adults → chronic diarrhea (>90%), severe weight loss
Common variable immunodeficiency-associated enteropathy	Chronic diarrhea (>92%) Abdominal pain and dyspepsia are less common but can be seen in over 50% Diminished response to vaccines and infections Recurrent infections (often involving respiratory tract)
Whipple's disease	Early phase: fever, arthralgias/arthritis Middle phase: diarrhea, weight loss, adenopathy Late phase: systemic symptoms (i.e., neurologic symptoms, endocarditis)
Tropical sprue	Acute bouts of diarrhea that progress to chronic diarrhea, abdominal pain, weight loss Symptoms suggestive of underlying nutritional deficiency
Medication-induced enteropathy	Olmesartan → severe diarrhea and weight loss; may require hospitalization Nonsteroidal anti-inflammatory drugs → asymptomatic or symptoms consistent with iron-deficiency anemia Mycophenolate mofetil → chronic persistent diarrhea

or anti-goblet cells is supportive but not required for diagnosis. Anti-enterocyte antibodies have been found in 50–80% of cases and anti-goblet cells in 30%. These antibodies are not specific (Fig. 18.1).

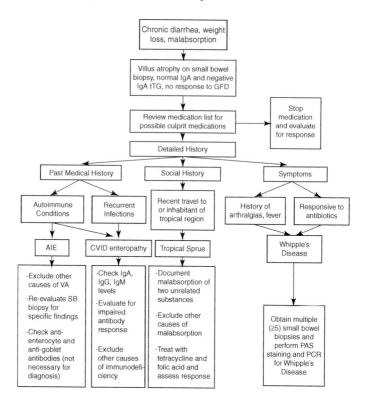

FIGURE 18.1 Diagnostic algorithm to work up the cause of villus atrophy on small bowel biopsy with negative celiac serologies and no response to a gluten-free diet. Evaluation and testing should be guided by a careful history and review of medications

The endoscopic appearance may involve nonspecific duodenal scalloping and fissuring. The histopathologic changes of AIE are highly variable; however, four broad categories have been proposed. These include, in order of prevalence, (1) active chronic enteritis (52%), (2) celiac-like (20%), (3) graft-versus-host disease-like, and (4) mixed pattern. The absence of Paneth or goblet cells may also be seen.

Treatment

One of the key characteristics of AIE is that it does not respond to dietary intervention, such as gluten elimination [2]. In up to roughly 50% of cases, individuals require total parenteral nutrition. The most common medical therapy is with corticosteroids such as prednisone (30–60 mg daily), methylprednisolone (40–50 mg IV daily), or budesonide (3 mg three times daily). Immunomodulators have been used in cases that are refractory to steroids or as steroid-sparing agents. These include azathioprine (2–2.5 mg/kg daily), mycophenolate mofetil (30 mg/kg daily), 6-mercaptopurine (1–1.5 mg/kg daily), cyclosporine (100 mg twice daily), tacrolimus (4 mg twice daily), and infliximab. Unfortunately, only 50–60% of individuals will have a complete response, and relapses are common. Roughly 20% will have no response. In children with IPEX, hematopoietic stem cell transplant can be considered.

Common Variable Immunodeficiency-Associated Enteropathy

Epidemiology

Common variable immunodeficiency (CVID) is the most common symptomatic primary immunodeficiency (prevalence of 1/100,000 to 1/50,000). Most cases are sporadic, but approximately 20% are familial. Up to one-half suffer from chronic diarrhea and malabsorption [4]. The typical age of diagnosis is the mid-30s, and in nearly 40% of cases, the digestive symptoms lead to the diagnosis [4]. Gastrointestinal symptoms can be due to recurrent or chronic intestinal infections. The most common pathogens, in order of frequency, are *Giardia lamblia* (Herman's syndrome), *Campylobacter jejuni*, and *Salmonella* [4]. Noninfectious causes of the gastrointestinal symptoms can include enteropathies that resemble either inflammatory bowel disease or celiac disease [4].

Etiology/Pathophysiology

Common variable immunodeficiency results from different underlying mutations that affect B-cell function and differentiation. While the pathogenesis of enteropathy in CVID is unknown, some hypotheses center on the absence of intestinal plasma cells. There may be a defect in secretory antibodies in the intestine that leads to chronic or repetitive infections that cannot be fully cleared. This, in turn, is thought to lead to chronic inflammation, villous atrophy, and increased intraepithelial lymphocytes. Another hypothesis is that local deficiency in secretory IgA leads to anaerobic bacteria overgrowth (dysbiosis) which in turn stimulates follicular lymphoid hyperplasia (a notable histologic finding in CVID). Abnormalities in T-cells, and specifically a decreased CD4+/CD8+ ratio, have also been implicated (Table 18.1).

Symptoms

Chronic diarrhea is present in 92% of those CVID patients with gastrointestinal symptoms. Dyspepsia and abdominal pain are less common, occurring in 66% and 52%, respectively [4]. Individuals may also have symptoms secondary to concomitant autoimmune conditions found in 46% of cases. CVID is characterized by diminished response to vaccines and recurrent infections (Table 18.2).

Diagnostic Evaluation

CVID is diagnosed when two of the three major immunoglobulin classes (IgA, IgG, or IgM) are two standard deviations below normal, there are impaired antibody responses to vaccinations or infections, and other causes of immunodeficiency have been excluded (Fig. 18.1). In the setting of gastrointestinal symptoms, blood work is often significant for malnutrition (54%) and anemia (56%) [4]. The presence of autoantibodies and peripheral lymphocytic abnormalities is common [4].

In the presence of chronic diarrhea in a CVID patient, upper endoscopy and colonoscopy with biopsies should be performed. Endoscopic and histologic findings in those with CVID and gastrointestinal symptoms are varied. In the stomach, macroscopic abnormalities are common and can include, in order of prevalence, erythema, atrophic mucosa, follicular changes, and ulceration. Stomach histology most frequently demonstrates chronic gastritis. In the small intestine, nearly 70% will have macroscopic findings, specifically nodular lymphoid hyperplasia (44%), loss of folds and mosaic pattern (22%), and ulcerative duodenitis (2%). Small bowel histology is notable for the absence of plasma cells (83%). The most common histologic feature is increased intraepithelial lymphocytes (76%), which is associated with villous atrophy in 51%. Other small bowel findings include follicular lymphoid hyperplasia (49%) and graft-versus-host-like changes (12%). CVID is the most common etiology for duodenal nodular lymphoid hyperplasia in adults [5]. Macroscopic changes in the colon (seen in 70%) include nodular lymphoid hyperplasia, inflammation, and ulcers. The most common histologic finding is microscopic colitis, although lesions mimicking inflammatory bowel disease can also be seen [4].

Treatment

Intravenous immunoglobulin (IVIG; e.g., 300–600 mg/kg IV every 3–4 weeks) is the recommended treatment for CVID, as it reduces the frequency of respiratory infections by 50%, likely by raising circulating immune globulin levels. IgG trough levels should be monitored every 6 months. Treatment goals are to increase IgG levels into the normal range and to significantly reduce major infection rates. Unfortunately, IVIG is not generally effective in reducing gastrointestinal symptoms.

CVID-associated enteropathy frequently requires parenteral nutrition support. Prior to initiation of medical therapy, there needs to be an aggressive investigation for and treatment of infections. While *Salmonella* responds well to quinolone antibiotics, roughly 64% of individuals with *Giardia* developed recurrent infections and require repeated courses of antibiotics. Oral steroids, such as prednisone (10 mg per day) and budesonide (3 mg three times daily), have significant beneficial impact on symptoms and lead to partial mucosal recovery. The ideal length of therapy is unclear.

Whipple's Disease

Epidemiology

Whipple's disease is a rare infectious disease with an estimated prevalence of 3 in 1,000,000 people [6]. Interestingly, *Tropheryma whipplei*, the bacteria responsible, is widespread and found in sewage water (believed to be an environmental source). After exposure, individuals can develop acute or chronic infection or more commonly can become carriers. Asymptomatic carriers are a significant reservoir, and transmission is believed to be oral-oral, fecal-oral, and even possibly respiratory. There is no known nonhuman reservoir [6]. The estimated prevalence of *Tropheryma whipplei* in the stool of the general European population is 4%; however, specific populations, such as sewage workers, cirrhotics, and the homeless, have a prevalence ranging from 12% to 24% [7–9]. Relatives of individuals with Whipple's disease and of carriers have rates reported at 31% and 80%, respectively [10].

Whipple's disease classically affects middle-aged males. Whipple's disease may be rare or underrecognized, in Asia and Africa; however, carriage in these populations is common.

Etiology Pathophysiology

Tropheryma whipplei is a Gram-positive, rod-shaped, periodic acid-Schiff (PAS)-positive bacteria in the actinomycetes family. The prevalence of asymptomatic carriers of *Tropheryma whipplei* together with the rarity of chronic infection suggests that there are likely host, pathogen, and environmental factors that determine susceptibility. Several studies suggest a genetic predisposition that appears to be unique to this bacterium.

The underlying mechanism of infection is *Tropheryma whipplei*'s ability to create an anti-inflammatory environment and to harness the immune system for its own replication and propagation. After macrophages internalize *Tropheryma whipplei* into vacuoles, they then migrate to the deeper mucosa. The bacteria incite a series of changes in the macrophage that lead to an inability of the macrophage to kill the bacteria and inappropriate antigen presentation which prevents differentiation of Th1 cells. The macrophages are induced to both apoptosis, which releases the replicated bacteria into the tissue, and IL-16 secretion, which recruits more macrophages to the area. These recruited macrophages phagocytize the released bacteria leading to further replication and dissemination. It is believed that *Tropheryma whipplei* ultimately reaches the lymphatics before traveling to the circulation and then spreading systemically.

Symptoms

Tropheryma whipplei infection can present as classic Whipple's disease (chronic systemic infection), as a localized infection, and as an acute infection, specifically pneumonia, bacteremia, and gastroenteritis. Localized infection is characterized by involvement of extraintestinal tissues and an absence of gut and systemic involvement [11].

The classic presentation of Whipple's disease is a middle-aged male with fever, diarrhea, abdominal pain, and arthralgias. In reality, the presence of all four symptoms is rare [11]. Classic Whipple's disease has three phases: early, middle, and late [6]. The early phase is characterized by fever and arthralgias that present in a palindromic rheumatic pattern (acute inflammatory attacks). The middle phase is marked by diarrhea and weight loss and the late phase by systemic involvement, commonly seen in the central nervous system, heart, and eyes. Common symptoms, in decreasing prevalence, are weight loss, diarrhea, adenopathy, fever, neurologic symptoms, and arthritis [11]. Neurologic symptoms include memory impairment, abnormal movements including the pathognomonic oculomasticatory myorhythmia, and coma. Other rare symptoms include melanoderma and pseudotumor formation (Table 18.2).

Over half of cases are initially misdiagnosed, commonly as inflammatory arthropathies. Nearly three-fourths of these individuals are placed on immunosuppressant medications [11]. A lack of response to immunosuppressives or an improvement in chronic symptoms when treated with prednisone or antibiotics for an unrelated infection should trigger consideration of Whipple's disease.

Diagnostic Evaluation

The result of blood work is nonspecific. Anemia, particularly microcytic, is a common finding, and leukocytosis is seen in less than one-third of cases. Inflammatory markers, such as C-reactive protein or erythrocyte sedimentation rate, are elevated in up to 82% of cases.

Histopathology and polymerase chain reaction (PCR) are the most common methods used for diagnosis. Endoscopic appearance is rarely remarkable; however, ectatic lymph vessels, dilated villi, and a pale-yellow color may be seen. *Tropheryma whipplei* has a patchy distribution, and several samples should be taken from the duodenum, as well as the gastric antrum, jejunum, and ileum [12]. Histopathology typically uses a PAS stain and identifies PAS-positive foamy macrophages in the lamina propria. This finding is not specific and can be found in other bacterial infections. The Ziehl-Neelsen stain can be used to distinguish Whipple's from mycobacterial infections, as *Tropheryma whipplei* will stain negative while mycobacterium stains positive [13].

Saliva and stool PCR testing have been found to be useful noninvasive screening methods, although they are not yet widely used in the United States. Alternative testing that is infrequently used includes immunohistochemistry, which is highly specific and sensitive, serology, fluorescence in situ hybridization, and electron microscopy [6].

To make the diagnosis, clinicians should perform saliva and stool PCR if available or alternatively proceed with an upper endoscopy with several (>5) small bowel biopsies. The biopsy samples should undergo PAS staining, PCR, and/or immunohistochemistry if available. If PAS-positive and either PCR or immunohistochemistry positive, or PAS-negative but both PCR and immunohistochemistry positive, Whipple's disease is confirmed. If PAS-positive and PCR and immunohistochemistry negative or PAS-negative and either PCR or immunohistochemistry positive, this is a possible diagnosis of Whipple's disease, and further testing needs to be considered [12] (Fig. 18.1).

Treatment

If left untreated, Whipple's disease can be fatal. With treatment, although symptoms typically resolve quickly, relapses are common [13]. Central nervous system involvement has been found in 90% of cases even in the absence of neurologic symptoms, and relapses that involve the central nervous system carry a particularly poor prognosis [6]. Therefore, although there is not currently a consensus on treatment, it is crucial that the regimen chosen has good central nervous system penetrance and sufficient duration to prevent relapse.

There are no clear guidelines on specific drug choices. One currently accepted regimen involves ceftriaxone (2 grams/day) for 14 days followed by oral trimethoprim-sulfamethoxazole (TMP-SMX, 160 mg/800 mg per day) for 1 year. This regimen has a reported response rate of nearly 75%. However, there is increasing evidence that *Tropheryma whipplei* is resistant to TMP-SMX, and a new treatment regimen has been proposed that involves doxycycline (200 mg/day) and hydroxychloroquine (600 mg/day) for 12 months and then maintenance on doxycycline (200 mg/day) daily for life.

Tropical Sprue

Epidemiology

Tropical sprue is a disease of the tropics (India, Southeast Asia, the Caribbean, Mexico, Central America, Central Africa, Venezuela, and Colombia). Tropical sprue is rarely seen in Europe, the Middle East, and North America but has been described in returning travelers, expatriates, and military personnel deployed to affected regions. Several recent studies found that tropical sprue remains the most common cause of malabsorption in certain regions of India, and some hypothesize that cases may be underrecognized [14]. The exact prevalence of tropical sprue is not known, though one estimate of incidence is 0.24 per 100,000 person-years. Women and men appear to be affected equally, and the typical age at presentation is the mid-30s [14]. Prior infectious gastroenteritis is a significant risk factor for tropical sprue (odds ratio of 34.6, 95% confidence intervals 4.8–282.4) [15].

Etiology/Pathophysiology

The exact cause has not yet been determined; however, there are several proposed theories (Fig. 18.2). An underlying infectious component is supported by (1) the reported epidemics, (2) the often-preceding infectious enteritis, (3) the

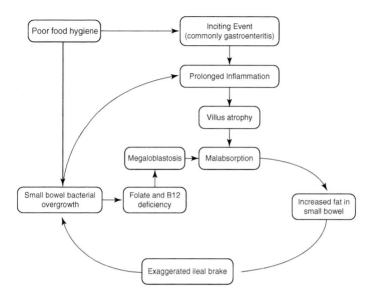

FIGURE 18.2 Current hypothesized pathogenesis of tropical sprue. An inciting event, commonly gastroenteritis, is thought to lead to bacterial overgrowth (commonly aerobic and Gram-negative). These bacteria in turn lead to decreased enterohepatic circulation and fatty acid malabsorption. Other postulated causes not depicted in the figure include reduced gut defense, abnormal small intestinal permeability, hormonal dysregulation, and altered motility

association with small intestinal bacterial overgrowth, (4) a positive response to antibiotic therapy, and (5) the risk of developing tropical sprue after travel to endemic areas.

Symptoms

Tropical sprue typically presents with acute bouts of diarrhea and malaise that progress to chronic diarrhea, abdominal bloating and pain, extreme fatigue, severe weight loss, and steatorrhea [16]. Fever may also be present and is more common in India than the Caribbean [17]. While some cases can undergo spontaneous remission, others can cause severe nutritional deficiencies, with the mortality being as high as 20% in southern India. Nutritional deficiencies can manifest with symptoms related to anemia, glossitis, and dermatitis and may take years to develop. Vitamin B12 and folate deficiencies are classic findings (Table 18.2).

One study comparing celiac disease and tropical sprue found that these two conditions could not be distinguished based on clinical presentation or biopsy, although individuals with tropical sprue were more likely to report recent travel [16].

Diagnostic Evaluation

For diagnosis, there needs to be (1) an appropriate clinical presentation, (2) malabsorption of two unrelated substances, (3) abnormal small intestinal mucosal histology, (4) exclusion of other causes of malabsorption (not including small bowel intestinal overgrowth), and (5) response to treatment with the appropriate antibiotics and folic acid (Fig. 18.1). The criteria to have a compatible clinical presentation are important, as there is a more common entity termed environmental enteropathy that affects low-resource countries with poor sanitation and hygiene and involves abnormal small bowel histology, chronic immune system activation, and impaired response to infections and vaccines [18]. Environmental enteropathy may be the most common cause of villous atrophy worldwide and is potentially a leading etiology for pediatric growth stunting.

Laboratory investigation in tropical sprue is nonspecific. Malabsorption can be demonstrated with tests such as a D-xylose absorption test (carbohydrate malabsorption), stool fat (fat malabsorption), and serum vitamin levels. Low folate levels are characteristic and may help differentiate the condition from small intestinal bacterial overgrowth, where elevated folate levels can be found.

Upper endoscopy typically reveals duodenal scalloping (68%), and the small bowel histology is similar to that found in celiac disease [14, 16]. Megaloblastic changes related to underlying folate and vitamin B12 deficiency may also be present. Tropical sprue may affect the entire small bowel and generally involves the terminal ileum.

Other causes of malabsorption need to be excluded. This includes celiac disease, infection, scleroderma, lymphoma, and severe malnutrition. Anti-endomysial antibodies and anti-tissue transglutaminase antibodies were absent in all tropical sprue patients in one case series; however, antigliadin antibodies are common [16].

Treatment

The treatment of choice is folic acid (5 mg daily) in combination with tetracycline (250 mg four times daily) for 3–6 months. Doxycycline is an alternative (100 mg twice daily). In those populations where tetracycline is contraindicated, poorly absorbed sulfa drugs such as succinylsulfathiazole for 6 months have been used with success. The improvement in anemia and weight loss with initiation of folic acid supplementation is characteristically dramatic. Relapses can be seen in up to 20%.

Individuals with tropical sprue will not respond to a gluten-free diet. A follow-up biopsy may be considered after the course of antibiotics is completed, although this is controversial due to the lack of randomized studies addressing this practice. Secondary pancreatic insufficiency due to loss of enterocyte mass should be suspected as a cause of persistent diarrhea after treatment, and a trial of pancreatic enzymes may be reasonable.

Medication-Induced Enteropathy

Epidemiology

Medications are frequently implicated in self-limited diarrhea. Some drugs may cause inflammation or enteropathy with chronic diarrhea. Several drugs can cause enteropathy, and in one case series, it was the second leading cause of sero-negative villous atrophy, with the majority due to olmesartan [19]. Olmesartan-associated enteropathy has an estimated incidence of 1.3 cases per 1000 individuals per year. Another common medication-induced enteropathy is that secondary to nonsteroidal anti-inflammatory drugs (NSAIDs), which is becoming increasingly recognized due to the use of video capsule endoscopy [20]. Up to 70% of individuals on chronic NSAIDs have been found to have evidence of small intestinal mucosal injury [21]. Finally, pertinent to the solid organ trans-plant population, mycophenolate mofetil is the most common cause of villous atrophy [22]. Case reports have also identi-fied other angiotensin receptor blockers, methotrexate, cyclo-sporine, tacrolimus, idelalisib, and azathioprine as causes of villous atrophy [22, 23].

Etiology/Pathophysiology

The pathophysiology of medication-induced enteropathy is unique to each drug. Olmesartan is believed to have an immune-based pathophysiology and may trigger similar changes in the intestinal epithelial cells as gluten does in celiac disease. This is supported by the identification of simi-lar cytokines, increase in certain cell lines such as CD8+, and IL15 overexpression on biopsy [24]. The enteropathy seen with NSAIDs is postulated to have a multifactorial patho-genesis. This includes direct damage to the mucosa, a reduc-tion in prostaglandin level causing increased intestinal motility and a compromised mucus barrier, and intestinal dysbiosis in the ileum [20]. Enterohepatic recycling of NSAIDs leads to enteropathy even in the setting of non-oral formulations. The use of proton pump inhibitors, in addition to both selective and nonselective NSAIDs, appears to exacerbate enteropathy, possibly through intestinal dys-biosis. Mycophenolate mofetil is postulated to damage the small intestine epithelial cells through a direct toxic effect as well as through inhibition of purine synthesis leading to inhibited cell proliferation (Table 18.1).

Symptoms

The presentation of medication-induced enteropathy is varied and can range in severity. Olmesartan-induced enteropathy typically presents years after initiation of the medication [25]. Typically, individuals suffer from severe diarrhea and significant weight loss and may require hospitalization for dehydration and parenteral nutrition support. They are also more likely to suffer from coexistent autoimmune conditions. In contrast, NSAID-associated enteropathy typically has a subclinical presentation, most commonly involving iron-deficiency anemia that is secondary to occult bleeding (estimated at 1–10 mL of blood loss/day) [20]. Weight loss, abdominal pain, obstructive symptoms, perforation, and overt bleeding are much less frequently seen. Enteropathy can develop within weeks of initiation of a NSAID. Individuals who develop the enteropathy due to mycophenolate mofetil commonly are posttransplant and have been on the medication for a median time of 1 year. The presentation is typically one of chronic and persistent diarrhea [22] (Table 18.2).

Diagnostic Evaluation

The diagnosis of medication-induced enteropathy relies on (1) a history of taking the drug, (2) the presence of enteropathy either clinically or on endoscopy, (3) resolution of symptoms with medication cessation or dose reduction, and (4) exclusion of alternative causes [26]. In approaching a patient with enteropathy, a review of the medication list and a trial off of possible culprit mediations, if possible, is cost-effective and should be done early in the evaluation (Fig. 18.1). Mucosal healing is expected after medication cessation and usually occurs within 6 months.

In the setting of olmesartan and mycophenolate mofetil use, blood work may show signs of malabsorption, hypoalbuminemia, and electrolyte abnormalities [22]. Iron-deficiency anemia may be seen, particularly in the case of NSAID enteropathy [20]. In olmesartan enteropathy, celiac serology is negative, although up to 90% will have either an HLA-DQ2 or DQ8 haplotype. HLA-DQ2 and DQ8 appear to be less prevalent in those affected by mycophenolate mofetil-associated enteropathy, with a prevalence of 45% for the former and 0% for the latter [22].

Pathologic findings are varied. In olmesartan-associated enteropathy, duodenal villous atrophy, intraepithelial lymphocytosis, and a thickened subepithelial collagen layer (collagenous sprue) may be seen. With NSAID enteropathy, mucosal changes are common and include erythema, epithelial breaks, subepithelial hemorrhages, erosions, and ulcerations. The degree of damage has poor correlation with the clinical symptoms. The pathognomonic finding, although rarely seen, is the presence of diaphragm strictures that typically involve numerous concentric fibrinous projections in the small intestine [20]. This can lead to obstructive symptoms. Mycophenolate mofetil-associated enteropathy can similarly present with mucosal erythema, erosions, and ulcerations. Pathologic examination typically shows crypt dilatation, apoptosis, and an edematous lamina propria with little inflammatory infiltrate. Unlike celiac disease, there generally is no hyperplasia of the crypts [22].

Treatment

The mainstay of treatment is withdrawal of the medication if possible. In some cases, such as immunosuppression with mycophenolate mofetil or NSAID therapy in chronic pain, stopping the medication may be difficult. In these cases, reduction of the dose can be trialed and, in the case of mycophenolate mofetil, has been found to lead to symptom resolution [22]. Several additional pharmacologic therapies may help in NSAID enteropathy, such as prostaglandin repletion with misoprostol or rebamipide, the latter of which stimulates prostaglandin production and modulation of dysbiosis with antibiotics or probiotics [20]. Additionally, a selective COX-2 inhibitor without a proton pump inhibitor may minimize risk of enteropathy. In olmesartan-induced enteropathy, steroid therapy (e.g., budesonide 3 mg three times daily with taper) may be reasonable for patients with severe clinical presentation, multiple hospital admissions, or slow clinical response after drug withdrawal.

Case Study: Follow-Up

Following her visit to the gastroenterology clinic, a colonoscopy with random biopsies was performed and was normal. An esophagogastroduodenoscopy was also completed and was normal; however, random duodenal biopsies showed partial villous atrophy (villous-crypt ratio 2:1) with intraepithelial lymphocytosis (80 lymphocytes per 100 epithelial cells). Given these findings, further blood work was obtained. Total IgA, IgA deamidated gliadin, IgA tissue transglutaminase, and IgA endomysial antibodies were all normal. Human leukocyte antigen DQ2 was present. A diagnosis of seronegative villous atrophy was made with a presumed diagnosis of sprue-like enteropathy associated with losartan. Losartan was stopped with close monitoring of blood pressure by her primary care physician; hydrochlorothiazide 12.5 mg daily was initiated to maintain normotension. Iron sucrose IV was given weekly for 5 weeks. A gluten-free diet was not recommended, but the differential diagnosis of seronegative celiac disease was discussed with the patient. The patient reported resolution of her symptoms during a follow-up visit 6 weeks after withdrawal of losartan, and laboratories confirmed resolution of her anemia and iron deficiency (hemoglobin 12.3 g/dL, MCV 84.0 FL, ferritin 188 ng/mL). A follow-up esophagogastroduodenoscopy with duodenal biopsies was performed 6 months after drug withdrawal and showed normal mucosa, confirming the diagnosis of losartan induced enteropathy.

Clinical Pearls

- Not all that "flattens" villi is celiac disease.
- Asymptomatic carriers of *Tropheryma whipplei* represent an important reservoir for the spread of Whipple's disease, and the prevalence of carriage is higher in certain populations including sewage workers, the homeless, and cirrhotics.
- Tropical sprue likely remains a prevalent cause of malabsorption in the tropics and should be considered in returning travelers, expatriates, or deployed military personnel who present with symptoms consistent with enteropathy.
- Medication-induced enteropathy is an emerging cause of chronic unexplained diarrhea.

Self-Test

Question 1. In common variable immunodeficiency-associated enteropathy, what cell line is absent in most small bowel histologic specimens?

    A. Goblet cells
    B. Plasma cells
    C. Paneth's cells
    D. Lymphocytes

Question 2. Rebamipide has been proposed as a pharmacologic therapy to prevent nonsteroidal anti-inflammatory drug-associated enteropathy. What is the mechanism of action of rebamipide?

    A. Prostaglandin analogue
    B. Irreversible blockade of the gastric proton pump
    C. Selective inhibition of cyclooxygenase-2 (COX-2)
    D. Stimulates prostaglandin production

Question 3. Which of the following is the most sensitive and specific diagnostic test for *Tropheryma whipplei* infection?

    A. Polymerase chain reaction (PCR)
    B. Ziehl-Neelsen stain
    C. Periodic acid-Schiff stain (PAS)
    D. Endoscopic appearance

References

1. Akram S, Murray J, Pardi D, Alexander G, Schaffner J, Russo P, et al. Adult autoimmune enteropathy: Mayo Clinic Rochester experience. Clin Gastroenterol Hepatol. 2007;5(11): 1282–90.
2. Sharma A, Choung R, Wang X, Russo P, Wu T, Nehra V, et al. Features of adult autoimmune enteropathy compared with refractory celiac disease. Clin Gastroenterol Hepatol. 2018;16(6):877–83. Available from: https://www.ncbi.nlm.nih.gov/pubmed/?term=Features+of+adult+autoimmune+enteropathy+compared+with+refractory+celiac+disease.
3. Umetsu S, Brown I, Langner C, Lauwers G. Autoimmune enteropathies. Virchows Arch. 2018;472(1):55–66.
4. Malamut G, Verkarre V, Suarez F, Viallard J, Lascaux A-S, Cosnes J, et al. The enteropathy associated with common variable immunodeficiency: the delineated frontiers with celiac disease. Am J Gastroenterol. 2010;105(10):2262–75.
5. Rubio-Tapia A, Hernandez-Calleros J, Trinidad-Hernandex S, Uscanga L. Clinical characteristics of a group of adults with nodular lymphoid hyperplasia: a single center experience. World J Gastroenterol. 2006;12(12):1945–8.
6. Dolmans R, Boel C, Lacle M, Kusters J. Clinical manifestations, treatment, and diagnosis of Tropheryma whipplei infections. Clin Microbiol Rev. 2017;30(2):529–55.
7. Fenollar F, Trani M, Davoust B, Salle B, Birg M, Rolain J, et al. Prevalence of asymptomatic Tropheryma whipplei carriage among humans and nonhuman primates. J Infect Dis. 2008;197(6): 880–7.

8. Schoniger-Hekele M, Petermann D, Weber B, Muller C. Tropheryma whipplei in the environment: survey of sewage plant influxes and sewage plant workers. Appl Environ Microbiol. 2007;73(6):2033–5.

9. Keita A, Brouqui P, Badiaga S, Benkouiten S, Ratmanov P, Raoult D, et al. *Tropheryma whipplei* prevalence strongly suggests human transmission in homeless shelters. Int J Infect Dis. 2013;17(1):e67–8.

10. Fenollar F, Keita A, Buffet S, Raoult D. Intrafamilial circulation of Tropheryma whipplei, France. Emerg Infect Dis. 2012;18(6):949–55.

11. Hujoel I, Johnson D, Lebwohl B, Leffler D, Kupfer S, Tsung-Teh W, et al. *Tropheryma whipplei* infection (Whipple disease) in the United States. Dig Dis Sci. 2018. Available from: https://www.ncbi.nlm.nih.gov/pubmed/29572616.

12. Schneider T, Moos V, Loddenkemper C, Marth T, Fenollar F, Raoult D. Whipple's disease: new aspects of pathogenesis and treatment. Lancet Infect Dis. 2008;8(3):179–90.

13. Fenollar F, Puechal X, Raoult D. Whipple's disease. N Engl J Med. 2007;356(1):55–66.

14. Pipaliya N, Ingle M, Rathi C, Poddar P, Pandav N, Sawant P. Spectrum of chronic small bowel diarrhea with malabsorption in Indian subcontinent: is the trend really changing? Intest Res. 2016;14(1):75–82.

15. McCarroll M, Riddle M, Gutierrez R, Porter C. Infectious gastroenteritis as a risk factor for tropical sprue and malabsorption: a case-control study. Dig Dis Sci. 2015;60(11):3379–85.

16. Langenberg M, Wismans P, van Genderen P. Distinguishing tropical sprue from celiac disease in returning travellers with chronic diarrhoea: a diagnostic challenge? Travel Med Infect Dis. 2014;12(4):401–5.

17. Nath S. Tropical sprue. Curr Gastroenterol Rep. 2005;7:343–9.

18. Rogawski E, Guerrant R. The burden of enteropathy and "subclinical" infections. Pediatr Clin N Am. 2017;64(4):815–36.

19. DeGaetani M, Tennyson C, Lebwohl B, Lewis S, Abu Daya H, Arguelles-Grande C, et al. Villous atrophy and negative celiac serology: a diagnostic and therapeutic dilemma. Am J Gastroenterol. 2013;108(5):647–53.

20. Tai F, McAlindon M. NSAIDs and the small bowel. Curr Opin Gastroenterol. 2018;34(3):175–82.

21. Shin S, Noh C, Lim S, Lee K, Lee K. Non-steroidal anti-inflammatory drug-induced enteropathy. Intest Res. 2017;15(4):446–55.

22. Weclawiak H, Ould-Mohamed A, Bournet B, Guilbeau-Frugier C, Fortenfant F, Muscari F, et al. Duodenal villous atrophy: a cause of chronic diarrhea after solid-organ transplantation. Am J Transplant. 2011;11(3):575–82.
23. Louie C, DiMaio M, Matsukuma K, Coutre S, Berry G, Longacre T. Idelalisib-associated enterocolitis: clinicopathologic features and distinction from other enterocolitides. Am J Surg Pathol. 2015;39(12):1653–60.
24. Marietta E, Nadeau A, Cartee A, Singh I, Rishi A, Choung R, et al. Immunopathogenesis of olmesartan-associated enteropathy. Aliment Pharmacol Ther. 2015;42(11):1303–14.
25. Rubio-Tapia A, Herman M, Ludvigsson J, Kelly D, Mangan T, Wu T, et al. Severe spruelike enteropathy associated with olmesartan. Mayo Clin Proc. 2012;87(8):732–8.
26. Hujoel I, Rubio-Tapia A. Sprue-like enteropathy associated with olmesartan: a new kid on the enteropathy block. GE Port J Gastroenterol. 2016;23(2):61–5.

Essential Reading

Dolmans R, Boel C, Lacle M, Kusters J. Clinical manifestations, treatment, and diagnosis of Tropheryma whipplei infections. Clin Microbiol Rev. 2017;30(2):529–55. This article provides an extensive and updated review on the manifestations, treatment, and diagnosis of Tropheryma whipplei infections.

Malamut G, Verkarre V, Suarez F, Viallard J, Lascaux A-S, Cosnes J, et al. The enteropathy associated with common variable immunodeficiency: the delineated frontiers with celiac disease. Am J Gastroenterol. 2010;105(10):2262–75. This article describes a large case series of common variable immunodeficiency and provides extensive data on the clinical presentation, endoscopic, histologic, and laboratory findings, as well as treatment response.

Rubio-Tapia A, Herman M, Ludvigsson J, et al. Severe sprue-like enteropathy associated with olmesartan. Mayo Clin Proc. 2012;87(8):732–8. This article is the first report of enteropathy associated with olmesartan, and describes a series of 22 cases.

Tai F, McAlindon M. NSAIDs and the small bowel. Curr Opin Gastroenterol. 2018;34(3):175–82. This article provides an updated review on the topic of nonsteroidal anti-inflammatory enteropathy and details theories on the underlying pathophysiology.

Chapter 19
Protein-Losing Enteropathy

Brooke Corning and Andrew P. Copland

Case Study

A 49-year-old man with hypertension, diabetes, depression, and anxiety presented with a history of intermittent epigastric abdominal pain and non-pitting edema in the bilateral lower extremities. For 10 years, his abdominal pain occurred two to three times a day. He denied nausea or vomiting, and there was no association with eating. He also denied melena, hematochezia, or steatorrhea and reported well-formed stools. He experienced weight gain associated with his fluid retention and was unable to work due to the abdominal pain and lower extremity edema. Diuretic therapy failed to improve the edema and resulted in a prerenal azotemia. Due to recurrent transudative pleural effusions, a chest tube had been placed so that he could drain pleural fluid daily at home.

He was evaluated on multiple occasions by the emergency department where computed tomography scans reported dilated small bowel loops with associated enteri-

B. Corning · A. P. Copland (✉)
Division of Gastroenterology and Hepatology, University of Virginia Health System, Charlottesville, VA, USA
e-mail: apc8d@virginia.edu

© Springer Nature Switzerland AG 2019
B. E. Lacy et al. (eds.), *Essential Medical Disorders of the Stomach and Small Intestine*,
https://doi.org/10.1007/978-3-030-01117-8_19

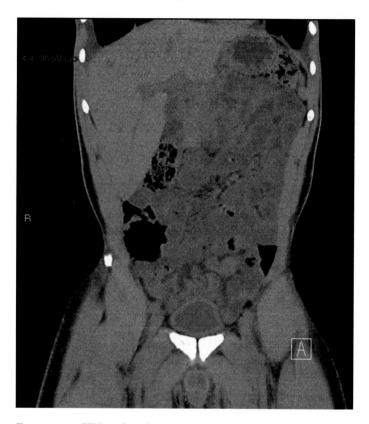

FIGURE 19.1 CT imaging showing dilated and thickened loops of the bowel

tis as well as small bilateral pleural effusions (Fig. 19.1). Labs were notable for low levels of serum total protein (4.8 g/dL) and albumin (2.9 g/dL). Blood counts and metabolic panels were otherwise unremarkable. An upper endoscopy was done that showed normal-appearing duodenal mucosa; however, biopsies of the duodenum showed dilated lymphatics (Fig. 19.2). Nutritional labs revealed low iron (iron 59 mcg/dL, transferrin 163 mg/dL) and low vitamin E (4.6 mg/dL).

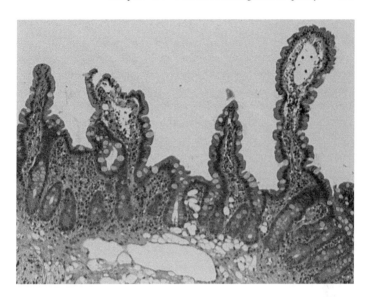

FIGURE 19.2 Mucosal biopsy of the duodenum showing dilated lacteals in the mucosa and submucosa

Objectives

- Recognize the clinical presentation of protein-losing enteropathy (PLE).
- Appreciate the diverse possible etiologies of PLE.
- Understand the appropriate diagnostic evaluation for PLE.
- Review treatment options for PLE, including management of the underlying disorder and nutritional optimization.

Epidemiology

Protein-losing enteropathy (PLE) is an uncommon syndrome leading to hypoproteinemia. Symptomatic hypoalbuminemia resulting from enteric losses is the defining characteristic of PLE. However, it is often underappreciated as low serum albumin more frequently occurs as a result of hemodilution, under-production due to malnutrition or hepatic dysfunction, and renal losses (e.g., nephrotic syndrome) or as a negative acute phase reactant. Epidemiologic studies are complicated by the numerous potential causes of PLE which can include erosive and nonerosive gastrointestinal conditions and non-gastrointestinal conditions that affect the gut (Table 19.1). Because of this, the exact epidemiology of PLE is unclear.

TABLE 19.1 Etiologies of PLE

Nonerosive gastrointestinal disease	Erosive gastrointestinal disease
Collagenous colitis	Inflammatory bowel disease
Amyloidosis	
Menetrier's	NSAID enteropathy
Gastric polyposis	Gut malignancies
Celiac sprue	Graft-versus-host disease
Tropical sprue	
Eosinophilic gastroenteritis	Sarcoidosis
Lymphocytic gastritis	Ulcerative jejunoileitis
Bacterial infections (small intestinal bacterial overgrowth, strongyloides, tuberculosis, *Helicobacter pylori*, Whipple's disease)	
CMV with hypertrophic gastropathy	
Systemic lupus erythematosus	
ANCA (+) vasculitis	
Connective tissue disorders (e.g., Sjögren's syndrome)	
Congenital metabolic abnormalities (e.g., Gaucher's disease)	
Lymphatic congestion/obstruction	**Cardiac disease**
Primary lymphangiectasia	Congenital heart disease
Secondary lymphangiectasia (heart failure, mesenteric panniculitis, retroperitoneal fibrosis, tuberculous infiltration, lymphoma, neoplastic lymphoid invasion)	Fontan operation for univentricular heart
Thoracic duct obstruction	Congestive heart failure (particularly right heart failure)
Portal hypertension	
Congenital malformation of the lymphatics	Constrictive pericarditis

The preponderance of epidemiologic data comes from congenital heart disease patients having undergone the Fontan procedure, a surgery employed in the treatment of single-ventricle cardiac malformations that are associated with PLE in at least 5–8% of patients [1, 2]. In addition to post-Fontan patients, PLE has been described in patients with chronic systemic inflammatory conditions ranging from rheumatologic disorders such as systemic lupus erythematosus [3, 4] to infectious diseases (e.g., tuberculosis). Gastrointestinal (GI) mucosal inflammatory states such as inflammatory bowel disease, celiac sprue, Whipple's disease, eosinophilic gastroenteritis, and microscopic colitis are among the many diagnoses implicated in causing PLE (Table 19.1). Twenty cases of PLE induced by Menetrier's disease, a rare form of hypertrophic gastropathy, were identified over a 10-year period at a referral center [5]. Finally, causes of impaired lymphatic outflow such as GI tract lymphoma and primary lymphangiectasia have also been reported as potential underlying causes of PLE. Regardless of the cause, the key to identifying PLE involves the recognition that hypoalbuminemia may result from GI tract protein loss, even in the absence of diarrhea.

Etiology and Pathophysiology

Normal physiologic protein losses account for no more than 1–2% of the body's daily albumin loss [6]. In PLE, the pathologic loss of protein from the GI tract may approach 60% of the total serum albumin per day. Serum protein loss, of which albumin makes up a significant component, results in third spacing of fluids due to loss of intravascular oncotic pressure. The body's ability to increase albumin and immunoglobulin synthesis is limited, as compared to other serum proteins resulting in a net loss of albumin daily [7]. Despite the loss of other proteins, including immunoglobulins and clotting factors, clinically related sequelae such as an increase in opportunistic infections, thrombosis, or bleeding are rarely seen in patients with PLE.

The etiologies of PLE may be broadly grouped into those that cause GI mucosal injury and those that cause obstruction of the intestinal lymphatic system which may involve intestinal or extraintestinal disease processes [8] (Table 19.1). Among these etiologies, the underlying pathophysiology of enteric protein loss likely differs.

Inflammatory processes resulting in epithelial ulceration and protein loss include inflammatory bowel disease (IBD), Behcet's disease, NSAID enteropathy, peptic ulcer disease, and certain malignancies such as lymphoma. These processes result in leakage of protein-rich fluid into the lumen of the GI tract, the degree to which is related to the extent and severity of mucosal involvement. In fact, the degree of protein loss (measured by alpha-1-antitrypsin loss) has been suggested to be useful in assessing disease activity in inflammatory bowel disease [8].

Mucosal damage without overt ulceration may lead to enteric protein loss through permeability changes in the mucosal surface. This is hypothesized to occur when intercellular tight junctions are compromised or vascular permeability is altered. This mechanism has been implicated in PLE caused by Menetrier's disease (giant hypertrophic gastropathy) and small bowel enteropathies such as celiac, amyloid, Whipple's disease, eosinophilic enteritis, and collagenous colitis as well as AIDS-associated gastroenteropathy, systemic lupus erythematosus, and graft-versus-host disease.

Lymphatic obstruction may contribute to PLE in several clinical settings. Increased lymphatic pressure results in lymphatic rupture and spillage of lymph into the intestine with loss of both albumin and other proteins. Secondary lymphangiectasia can result from damage to the lymphatic system (malignancy, chemotherapy, radiation, or infection) or venous hypertension from cirrhosis, Budd-Chiari syndrome, constrictive pericarditis, or heart failure. Primary intestinal lymphangiectasia is typically diagnosed in childhood as a congenital malformation or obstruction of intestinal lymphatic drainage; however, some groups have used direct lymphangiography to show that 90% of these patients may have thoracic duct outlet obstruction [9].

The exact pathophysiology related to PLE associated with the Fontan procedure for univentricular congenital heart disease remains somewhat unclear; however, prevailing thought suggests that Fontan physiology results in increased central venous pressure and decreased capacity for reabsorption of interstitial fluid, with compensatory dependence on the lymphatic system as well as increased lymph production from the liver and portal circulation [10].

It is possible for a disease process to cause PLE through a combination of the above mechanisms. Systemic lupus erythematosus, for example, may cause enteric protein loss via vasculitis causing mucosal injury, from related dysmotility causing small intestinal bacterial overgrowth which impairs the GI mucosa, and also from increased hydrostatic forces due to pericarditis or pericardial effusion [11]. Patients with Crohn's disease may display features of both ulcerative mucosal disease and lymphatic obstruction with submucosal edema, dilation of lacteals, and granulomatous involvement of blood vessels and mesenteric lymph nodes [12, 8].

Signs and Symptoms

The overarching driver of symptoms in PLE relates to decreased oncotic pressure from hypoalbuminemia which is typically <3.0 g/dL. This results in the third spacing of fluid into interstitial spaces and leads to edema, pleural effusions, pericardial effusion, bowel wall edema, and ascites which in turn contributes to shortness of breath, fatigue, abdominal pain, and weeping of fluid from the legs. Edema may not be limited to the lower extremities and can also be noted in the face, upper extremities, and sacrum. Patients are often unable to maintain their weight except for weight related to fluid retention [13]. Symptoms related to fat-soluble vitamin deficiencies are less common though certainly symptomatic vitamin and essential fatty acid deficiencies have been described and typically manifest with characteristics of the particular vitamin deficiency (e.g., night blindness in vitamin A deficiency). Some patients with PLE will present with a diarrhea that has secretory characteristics; however, it is important to recognize that diarrhea is neither uniformly present nor necessary to make a diagnosis of PLE. Most patients experience other symptoms directly related to the underlying cause of the PLE. This is particularly true for the gastroenterologist managing inflammatory bowel disease where fistulas, abscesses, and bloody diarrhea can be prominent features of the disease.

Diagnostic Evaluation

PLE is an uncommon cause of hypoalbuminemia. A key step in the diagnostic process is to perform a thorough history and physical to evaluate a potential PLE patient for acute illness, malnutrition, impaired protein synthetic function related to malnutrition or chronic liver disease, and renal losses due to a nephrotic syndrome prior to assessing for a potential GI tract source of protein loss (Table 19.2).

The preferred test for diagnosis of PLE is a measurement of alpha-1-antitrypsin (A1AT) clearance. A1AT is made in the liver and does not undergo degradation in the bowel. Clearance in

TABLE 19.2 Core testing in PLE assessment

1. Assess for alternate causes of hypoalbuminemia

    (a) Renal losses – 24-hr urine collection for urine protein
    (b) Hepatic synthetic impairment – biochemical and imaging-guided assessment of liver function
    (c) Malnutrition causing impaired synthesis – global clinical assessment
    (d) Consider acute inflammatory response in acute settings

2. Assess stool loss of alpha-1-antitrypsin (A1AT)

    (a) Test of choice = 24-hr A1AT clearance
    (b) Spot stool A1AT level has lower sensitivity

3. Assess and evaluate potential causes of PLE (gastrointestinal, cardiac, vascular/lymphatic, systemic inflammatory)

TABLE 19.3 Stool alpha-1-antitrypsin (A1AT) clearance

A1AT clearance = (24-hr stool volume × stool A1AT)/serum A1AT

In the absence of diarrhea, normal <27 mL/24-hr

In the presence of diarrhea, normal <56 mL/24-hr

the stool is calculated using a plasma A1AT level and a quantitative measurement of A1AT from a 24-hr stool collection (Table 19.3). Normal A1AT clearance levels are <27 mL/24-hr. A higher cutoff value of 56 mL/24-hr is used in the presence of diarrhea, as this will increase the apparent A1AT clearance leading to false-positive values [7]. In a suspected gastric hypersecretory state (such as Menetrier's), measurement of A1AT should be performed on acid suppressive therapy as A1AT is susceptible to acid degradation.

An A1AT level from a spot stool sample is less sensitive than A1AT clearance for the diagnosis of PLE, although it may be useful to track the disease following its diagnosis. A nuclear study utilizing radiolabeled albumin may be available at specialized centers; however, this is not routinely available at most institutions and does incur the risk of radiation exposure.

Once PLE is confirmed, additional evaluation should be directed toward identifying the underlying etiology. Endoscopy, while not strictly necessary for the diagnosis of PLE, is often useful to evaluate for GI mucosal disease. Further testing to evaluate potential causes of PLE may be quite extensive and includes a thorough evaluation of the GI tract, cardiovascular system, and lymphatic system.

Endoscopic appearance of the mucosa may provide a clue in many cases where GI disease is the primary cause of PLE. Menetrier's disease will appear as thickened gastric folds on examination of the stomach. The presence of mucosal ulceration, while nonspecific, may signify a number of diseases. Both celiac and non-celiac small bowel enteropathies may appear grossly as atrophic small bowel mucosa and histologically as blunted villi. Lymphangiectatic mucosa, either primary or secondary, is characterized by white-tipped villi due to dilated lacteals. Small bowel biopsies for histologic examination are often helpful as some mucosal findings may be subtle.

Treatment

The cornerstones of PLE treatment are threefold: (1) management of the underlying disease process, (2) nutritional optimization, and (3) supportive care. It is important to consider that no controlled studies exist for the management of PLE with which to base treatment decisions. Infection, cardiac disease, primary GI mucosal disease, and other potential underlying causes should be approached with routine therapy as dictated by the disease process. Generally, a high-protein diet (2.0–3.0 mg/kg/day) administered enterally, if possible, is recommended. If oral intake is inadequate, enteral feedings should be considered, reserving the use of parenteral nutrition to those patients who fail the enteral approach. It is also important to recognize that there is often a substantial delay in clinical response to treatment of PLE with response being measured in weeks or months.

For primary intestinal lymphangiectasia, a high-protein, low-fat diet with added medium-chain triglycerides results in resolution of symptoms in up to two-thirds of patients [14]. Medium-chain fatty acids are absorbed directly into the portal circulation rather than through lymphatics, reducing lymphatic pressure and rupture with protein leakage. In some diseases causing PLE, such as primary intestinal lymphangiectasia and Crohn's disease, surgical resection may be curative if the disease is limited to a short segment of the bowel [15]. In a small study of patients with congestive heart disease and PLE, liver lymphangiography with embolization of hepatic lymphatic ducts resulted in sustained albumin increase in 3/8 of patients [16]. Menetrier's disease has been associated with *Helicobacter pylori* in up to 90% of cases and may result in improvement with *H. pylori* therapy [17], although in refractory cases gastrectomy may be necessary. There are numerous case reports and case series in the literature describing the use of a variety of therapeutic agents ranging from budesonide, subcutaneous heparin, octreotide, everolimus, and cetuximab as treatment of PLE. Given the limited data available, however, these agents should be used cautiously and only in clinical scenarios similar to the published reports.

Management of edema is generally supportive and similar to the management of lymphedema with compression stockings and skin care. Diuretic therapy, unless being used to manage underlying cardiac issues, is typically unsuccessful at shifting fluid from the tissue to the intravascular space because of the low oncotic pressure and may result in kidney injury. Wrapping the lower extremities may provide some relief of chronic otherwise refractory edema. While intravenous albumin infusions may help patients suffering from severe third spacing of fluid in the acute setting, albumin administration is not a practical long-term therapy due to both cost and very rapid excretion of the infused albumin.

Case Study: Follow-Up

An evaluation for underlying liver and renal disease was pursued; liver synthetic function appeared intact, and proteinuria was absent. Due to high suspicion for PLE, an A1AT clearance was obtained, which returned at 191 mL/24-hr (normal <27 mL/24-hr). The patient was diagnosed with primary lymphangiectasia based on prior imaging and small bowel biopsy results. He received nutritional counseling for a high-protein, low-fat diet. Physical therapy and high-quality compression stockings helped managed peripheral edema and improve ambulation. His pleural effusion subsequently improved, and his chest tube was able to be removed. In addition, his weight stabilized with improvement in prior micronutrient deficiencies.

Clinical Pearls

- Consider PLE in patients with unexplained moderate-severe hypoalbuminemia (<3.0 g/dL), even in the absence of overt GI symptoms, after ruling out hepatic synthetic dysfunction and renal protein losses.
- The diagnostic test for PLE with the highest sensitivity is the stool A1AT clearance rather than spot stool A1AT level. This is calculated using both serum A1AT and 24-hr stool A1AT as follows:
- A1AT clearance = (24-hr stool volume × stool AIAT)/serum A1AT
- The threshold of normal A1AT clearance differs based on the presence or absence of diarrhea.
- In the absence of diarrhea, normal clearance level is <27 mL/24-hr.
- In the presence of diarrhea of any cause, normal is <56 mL/24-hr.
- Treatment of PLE is based on the underlying disease process responsible.

Self-Test

Question 1: PLE is most commonly described in the literature in what patient population?

    A. Post-Fontan procedure for congenital heart disease
    B. Inflammatory bowel disease
    C. Systemic rheumatologic disorders (e.g., lupus)
    D. Menetrier's disease

Question 2: A patient is referred for evaluation of symptomatic hypoalbuminemia (albumin 1.9 g/dL) and has an exam notable for peripheral edema and small pleural effusions. They have a history of Crohn's disease and experience ongoing nonbloody diarrhea. You suspect a diagnosis of protein-losing enteropathy. Which of the following would best confirm this diagnosis?

   A. A spot stool A1AT of 25 mg/dL
   B. Stool A1AT clearance of 30 mL/24-hr
   C. Stool A1AT clearance of 80 mL/24-hr
   D. Echocardiogram to rule out heart failure and urinalysis to rule out proteinuria.

Question 3: Which medical therapy would most benefit the patient with Crohn's disease described in the previous question after confirmation of PLE?

   A. Oral furosemide daily
   B. Initiation of a biologic therapy
   C. Daily intravenous albumin infusion
   D. Low-protein diet

References

1. Atz AM, Zak V, Mahony L, Uzark K, D'Agincourt N, Goldberg DJ, et al. Longitudinal outcomes of patients with single ventricle after the Fontan procedure. J Am Coll Cardiol. 2017;69(22):2735–44. https://doi.org/10.1016/j.jacc.2017.03.582.
2. Wilson TG, Shi WY, Iyengar AJ, Winlaw DS, Cordina RL, Wheaton GR, et al. Twenty-five year outcomes of the lateral tunnel Fontan procedure. Semin Thorac Cardiovasc Surg. 2017;29(3):347–53. https://doi.org/10.1053/j.semtcvs.2017.06.002.
3. Perednia DA, Curosh NA. Lupus-associated protein-losing enteropathy. Arch Intern Med. 1990;150(9):1806–10.
4. Zheng WJ, Tian XP, Li L, Jing HL, Li F, Zeng XF, et al. Protein-losing enteropathy in systemic lupus erythematosus: analysis of the clinical features of fifteen patients. J Clin Rheumatol. 2007;13(6):313–6. https://doi.org/10.1097/RHU.0b013e31815bf9c6.
5. Rich A, Toro TZ, Tanksley J, Fiske WH, Lind CD, Ayers GD, et al. Distinguishing Menetrier's disease from its mimics. Gut. 2010;59(12):1617–24. https://doi.org/10.1136/gut.2010.220061.
6. Schmidt PN, Blirup-Jensen S, Svendsen PJ, Wandall JH. Characterization and quantification of plasma proteins excreted in faeces from healthy humans. Scand J Clin Lab Invest. 1995;55(1):35–45.
7. Umar SB, DiBaise JK. Protein-losing enteropathy: case illustrations and clinical review. Am J Gastroenterol. 2010;105(1):43–9; quiz 50. https://doi.org/10.1038/ajg.2009.561.

8. Levitt DG, Levitt MD. Protein losing enteropathy: comprehensive review of the mechanistic association with clinical and subclinical disease states. Clin Exp Gastroenterol. 2017;10:147–68. https://doi.org/10.2147/CEG.S136803.

9. Sun X, Shen W, Chen X, Wen T, Duan Y, Wang R. Primary intestinal lymphangiectasia: multiple detector computed tomography findings after direct lymphangiography. J Med Imaging Radiat Oncol. 2017;61(5):607–13. https://doi.org/10.1111/1754-9485.12606.

10. Menon S, Chennapragada M, Ugaki S, Sholler GF, Ayer J, Winlaw DS. The lymphatic circulation in adaptations to the Fontan circulation. Pediatr Cardiol. 2017;38(5):886–92. https://doi.org/10.1007/s00246-017-1576-y.

11. Ebert EC, Hagspiel KD. Gastrointestinal and hepatic manifestations of systemic lupus erythematosus. J Clin Gastroenterol. 2011;45(5):436–41. https://doi.org/10.1097/MCG.0b013e31820f81b8.

12. Ferrante M, Penninckx F, De Hertogh G, Geboes K, D'Hoore A, Noman M, et al. Protein-losing enteropathy in Crohn's disease. Acta Gastro-Enterol Belg. 2006;69(4):384–9.

13. Vignes S, Bellanger J. Primary intestinal lymphangiectasia (Waldmann's disease). Orphanet J Rare Dis. 2008;3:5. https://doi.org/10.1186/1750-1172-3-5.

14. Desai AP, Guvenc BH, Carachi R. Evidence for medium chain triglycerides in the treatment of primary intestinal lymphangiectasia. Eur J Pediatr Surg. 2009;19(4):241–5. https://doi.org/10.1055/s-0029-1216389.

15. Kim NR, Lee SK, Suh YL. Primary intestinal lymphangiectasia successfully treated by segmental resections of small bowel. J Pediatr Surg. 2009;44(10):e13–7. https://doi.org/10.1016/j.jpedsurg.2009.06.034.

16. Itkin M, Piccoli DA, Nadolski G, Rychik J, DeWitt A, Pinto E, et al. Protein-losing enteropathy in patients with congenital heart disease. J Am Coll Cardiol. 2017;69(24):2929–37. https://doi.org/10.1016/j.jacc.2017.04.023.

17. Bayerdorffer E, Ritter MM, Hatz R, Brooks W, Ruckdeschel G, Stolte M. Healing of protein losing hypertrophic gastropathy by eradication of Helicobacter pylori--is Helicobacter pylori a pathogenic factor in Menetrier's disease? Gut. 1994;35(5):701–4.

Essential Reading

1. Levitt DG, Levitt MD. Protein losing enteropathy: comprehensive review of the mechanistic association with clinical and subclinical disease states. Clin Exp Gastroenterol. 2017;10:147–68. https://doi.org/10.2147/CEG.S136803. In-depth review of the pathophysiologic mechanism and diagnosis of PLE.
2. Umar SB, DiBaise JK. Protein-losing enteropathy: case illustrations and clinical review. Am J Gastroenterol. 2010;105(1):43–9; quiz 50. https://doi.org/10.1038/ajg.2009.561. Additional case illustrations of causes of PLE with accompanying high yield clinical features.

Chapter 20
Small Intestinal Bacterial Overgrowth

Eamonn M. M. Quigley

Case Study

A 72-year-old retired male initially presented with a long history of abdominal bloating and watery diarrhea with urgency. He had experienced a number of episodes of fecal incontinence which had been most distressing and made him virtually housebound. His only other medical problem was atrial fibrillation. He was under significant stress and at that time was caring for his wife who was terminally ill with myeloma. He himself had a history of depression and had expressed suicidal ideation in the past. Investigations included celiac serology, esophagogastroduodenoscopy with duodenal biopsies, colonoscopy with random biopsies, and radiographic imaging. The only positive findings were colonic diverticula and a stable aneurysm of the ascending aorta. A diagnosis of diarrhea-predominant irritable bowel syndrome had been made and loperamide and an antispasmodic prescribed.

When seen in our clinic 2 years later, he continued to report several loose bowel movements daily despite loperamide in a dose of 2 mg twice daily, and there had been two

E. M. Quigley (✉)
Division of Gastroenterology, Houston Methodist Hospital, Houston, TX, USA
e-mail: equigley@houstonmethodist.org

© Springer Nature Switzerland AG 2019
B. E. Lacy et al. (eds.), *Essential Medical Disorders of the Stomach and Small Intestine*,
https://doi.org/10.1007/978-3-030-01117-8_20

417

recent episodes of fecal incontinence. Bloating also persisted. On reviewing his medical record, it was noted that he had received a course of vitamin B_{12} injections in the past for documented B_{12} deficiency. Apart from being rather thin and having well-controlled atrial fibrillation, his physical examination was unremarkable.

Objectives

- Provide a clinical definition of SIBO.
- Name common causes and the principal clinical consequences of SIBO.
- List the advantages and limitations of breath hydrogen testing and jejunal aspiration.
- Develop a management plan for SIBO.

Epidemiology

The very term bacterial overgrowth succinctly conveys what those who coined this term sought to transmit: a situation where an increase in the numbers and/or change in the type of bacteria in the small intestine results in clinical consequences. The idea that an alteration in the bacterial contents of the small intestine and, specifically, the presence of bacterial species normally confined to the colon could lead to problems may date as far back as the late nineteenth century. The impact of such overgrowth, or "contamination," on a variety of intestinal functions and human nutrition was elegantly demonstrated in a series of classical studies in the 1950s, 1960s, and 1970s [1, 2]. Until recently, the clinical context most typically linked with small intestinal bacterial overgrowth (SIBO) was malabsorption/maldigestion. Latterly, SIBO has been incriminated in a host of other intestinal and extraintestinal disorders often on the basis of imprecise methodology and/or limited data. Such studies have generated considerable controversy and thrown the definition of SIBO into sharp relief.

The patient described above illustrates what I regard to be the classical presentation of SIBO and that which fulfills the original definition of this clinical entity – a clinical syndrome featuring clinical and/or laboratory evidence of maldigestion/malabsorption related to qualitative and/or quantitative alterations in the small intestinal microbiota [1]. However, in more recent years, a much more liberal definition of SIBO as "a condition in which the small bowel is colonized by excessive numbers of aerobic and anaerobic microbes that are normally found in the small intestine" has been advanced [2, 3] and seems to have been widely adopted in clinical practice. Consequently, SIBO has come to be recognized in association with a wide range of symptoms and clinical entities in the absence of evidence of maldigestion/malabsorption. The association of SIBO with irritable bowel syndrome (IBS) is a prime example of this expanded concept which moves SIBO from a well-circumscribed clinical context (maldigestion and malabsorption) into deeper and murkier waters where the focus is shifted to how we test for SIBO. As we will see later, this has led to considerable debate and controversy such that the very concept of SIBO has been questioned [4].

There are few if any large population studies on the incidence or prevalence of SIBO in the community. In two of the few such studies, Khin-Maung U and colleagues described SIBO among 21% of village children in rural Myanmar [5], and Lewis and colleagues identified SIBO in 14.5% of 62 residents of elderly people's homes [6]. Others have suggested that the latter is a reflection of frailty and not of aging *per se* [7]. Another insight into the background prevalence of SIBO can be gained (with all its limitations) from reports of positive tests for SIBO among control subjects in studies examining the prevalence of SIBO in disease groups. Grace and colleagues, in their excellent summary of the literature, reported a prevalence which ranged from 0% to 20% among such apparently healthy subjects [8]. All other studies are in symptomatic individuals where SIBO has been described as a common cause of diarrhea in children [9] and the elderly [10]. SIBO also appears to be common among the morbidly obese [11].

Etiology and Pathophysiology

Disorders Associated with SIBO

Many disease states have been linked with SIBO. Many of these can be predicted from our understanding of the factors that prevent small intestinal contamination in health and, in particular, gastric acid and intestinal motor activity. Other protective factors include the integrity of the intestinal mucosa, including its protective mucus layer and intrinsic antibacterial mechanisms, such as defensins and immuno-globulins; the enzymatic activities and bacteriostatic proper-ties of intestinal, pancreatic, and biliary secretions; the protective effects of the commensal microbiota; and the mechanical and physiological properties of the ileocecal valve [1]. Disorders commonly associated with SIBO are listed in Table 20.1 [1, 8].

TABLE 20.1 Diseases and disorders linked to SIBO

Abnormal small intestinal motility:

Diabetic autonomic neuropathy

Systemic sclerosis/scleroderma

Amyloidosis

Hypothyroidism

Idiopathic intestinal pseudo-obstruction

Acromegaly

Gastroparesis

Myotonic muscular dystrophy

Chronic opiate use

Long-standing use of motility-suppressing drugs

Anatomic abnormalities:

Small intestinal diverticulosis

Surgically induced alterations in anatomy (Billroth II gastrectomy, end-to-side anastomosis)

TABLE 20.1 (continued)

Strictures (Crohn's disease, radiation, surgery)

Blind loops

Gastrocolic or jejunocolic fistula

Ileocecal valve resection

Hypochlorhydria

Postsurgical

Long-term acid suppression (?)

Immune deficiency

Inherited immune deficiencies

Acquired immune deficiency (e.g., AIDS, severe malnutrition)

Multifactorial

Chronic pancreatitis

Celiac disease

Tropical sprue

Crohn's disease

Cystic fibrosis

Intestinal failure

Radiation enteropathy

Liver disease

End-stage renal disease

It has long been recognized that hypochlorhydria is a risk factor for SIBO. In the past, this association was largely identified in the context of surgical procedures such as vagotomy and gastrectomy. Nowadays, there is concern for the possible development of SIBO among individuals on long-term treatment with proton-pump inhibitors (PPIs). Results have been conflicting, however, with meta-analyses suggesting a small but definite link of uncertain clinical significance with SIBO [12, 13].

SIBO has long been regarded as a potential complication of celiac disease and one of the causes of a failure to respond to gluten withdrawal. Rubio-Tapia and colleagues documented SIBO in 9.3% of their patients with unresponsive disease [14].

An association between SIBO and several other disorders has been proposed but remains controversial including rosacea, interstitial cystitis, restless legs syndrome, Parkinson's disease, erosive esophagitis, and, most notably, IBS [1, 8]. Diverticula in the jejunum occur in 0.07–2% of the population and tend to be large and multiple, whereas those in the ileum are small and single. These features explain the observation that symptoms and complications, such as SIBO, have been reported more frequently in association with jejunal than with ileal diverticula. Jejunal diverticula are twice as frequent in men and are observed predominantly among those over 60 years of age – demographics that accord with our case. Morphological studies suggest that disorders of intestinal motility such as progressive systemic sclerosis and visceral myopathies and neuropathies play an important role in the formation of these small bowel diverticula [15]. Dysmotility may also explain the high prevalence of SIBO among those with diabetes, intestinal pseudo-obstruction, and scleroderma.

Pathogenesis of Symptoms and Clinical Signs in SIBO

The impact of SIBO on gut morphology and physiology has been elegantly demonstrated in a series of classical clinical and laboratory studies performed during the latter half of the last century (reviewed in Ref. [1]). The clue that led to the diagnosis of SIBO in our patient was B_{12} deficiency. This arises, in SIBO, as a consequence of the consumption of cobalamin by anaerobes, as well as from malabsorption of the vitamin as a result of competition for binding at the binding site with bacterially generated metabolites of cobalamin.

In instances of more severe overgrowth, mucosal damage may directly involve and compromise the binding site. While SIBO may also result in thiamine and nicotinamide deficiency, serum folate levels may be high due to bacterial synthesis of folic acid.

Mucosal injury will also contribute to symptomatology via the loss of brush border enzymes. Damage to the epithelial barrier will enhance permeability and, rarely, could lead to a protein-losing enteropathy. Bacterial digestion of luminal protein will contribute to malnutrition and fermentation of carbohydrates to cause such symptoms as bloating and flatulence. Deconjugation of bile acids and consequent depletion of the bile acid pool will lead to maldigestion of fat and fat-soluble vitamins.

Among individuals with short bowel syndrome levels of overgrowth can lead to the generation of large amounts of D-lactic acid and result in an encephalopathic state [16].

Signs and Symptoms

The clinical manifestations of SIBO, even in the classical context of maldigestion/malabsorption, are protean and can range from the detection of laboratory abnormalities (e.g., vitamin B_{12} or iron deficiency) in an asymptomatic individual to florid steatorrhea and a protein-losing enteropathy. SIBO is an important cause of otherwise unexplained diarrhea in the elderly and may also present with weight loss and such relatively non-specific symptoms as bloating, flatulence, and abdominal discomfort – many of the features present in our case. However, for a variety of reasons including earlier diagnosis and the disappearance of those surgical procedures that accounted for many past instances of SIBO, the classical features of SIBO are rarely seen nowadays. SIBO is now primarily recognized as a cause of unexplained diarrhea and occult malabsorption in the elderly and is associated with, at most, a negligible inflammatory response and very little in the way of mucosal injury.

In clinical practice, the big controversy has been the nature of the association between IBS and SIBO, an issue that arose in our case. Initial reports on this association documented SIBO in 84% of patients with IBS with a significant improvement in IBS symptoms linked to a normalization of the lactulose breath test following the use of neomycin [17, 18]. Subsequent studies provided conflicting results leading some to question this association [19–23]. In an important systematic review and meta-analysis of the link between SIBO and IBS, Ford and colleagues drew attention to the impact of test modality on SIBO prevalence, the average prevalence of SIBO on breath tests being 54%, in sharp contrast to a mean prevalence of just 4% for tests based on cultures of jejunal aspirates [24]. These authors also drew attention to the impact of diagnostic criteria, which varied considerably between studies, on study outcome [24]. This controversy will not be resolved until a more accurate test for SIBO emerges. For now, and as exemplified by our case, it is reasonable to conclude that SIBO can certainly present with symptoms that mimic those of IBS.

Diagnostic Evaluation

Jejunal Aspiration

Classically, SIBO was defined as the presence, in an aspirate from the jejunum, of $\geq 10^5$ colony-forming units (CFU) per mL of bacteria or of $\geq 10^3$ CFU/mL of bacterial species that normally colonize the large bowel, such as *Enterobacteriaceae*, enterococci, *Pseudomonas* spp., and *Bacteroides* spp.

It is vital to appreciate that a variety of techniques have been used to obtain bowel contents for culture, including the classic technique of jejunal intubation under fluoroscopic guidance, a variety of endoscopically guided aspiration methods, mucosal brushings using a cytology brush, and mucosal biopsies. It is particularly important not to extrapolate diagnostic criteria from one technique to another, as is commonly done in the case of endoscopically derived aspirates, where samples are often derived from the second part of the duodenum and not the jejunum, locations where the microbiota may differ both quantitatively and qualitatively. Though widely quoted and applied, it must be emphasized that, while the so-called gold standard for the definition of SIBO based on aspirate and culture (i.e., $\geq 10^5$ CFU/mL of bacteria in the proximal small bowel) correlates well with clinical features in "classical" SIBO, its application to the diagnosis of SIBO outside of this context has not been validated [25].

Aspiration-based approaches also suffer from being invasive, time-consuming, and costly. Moreover, this approach is vulnerable to contamination of the aspirate by oropharyngeal microbes, and the culture technique itself is also beset with potential problems ranging from challenges inherent to maintaining anaerobic conditions during the collection, transport, and evaluation of samples to the enthusiasm and skill of the microbiologist. It should come as no wonder that the reproducibility of this approach has been reported to be low. Novel approaches to optimize jejunal aspiration are in development [26]; such approaches coupled with culture-independent techniques for the evaluation of the small intestinal microbiota may, hopefully, provide a true gold standard.

Breath Tests

For patient convenience, as well as simplicity in their execution, breath tests have become the most widely employed modalities for the diagnosis of SIBO in clinical practice. While a number of breath tests have been evaluated over the years, the hydrogen breath test has become by far the most popular. These breath tests are based on the premise that carbohydrate fermentation by bacteria within the gut and, most notably, anaerobic bacteria in the colon is the only source of H_2 production in the body. When "colonic" bacteria colonize the small intestine in SIBO, exposure of carbohydrate to these bacteria in the small intestine produces a large and premature amount of H_2 gas which diffuses into the systemic circulation and is excreted via the lung in the expired air.

Hydrogen breath tests employ either simple sugars, such as glucose, which should normally be absorbed in the small intestine, or nonabsorbable compounds, such as lactulose, which are fermented by intestinal bacteria. Following a 12-h overnight fast and a low fiber diet for 1 day, subjects are asked to exhale into a tube connected to a bag and syringe to obtain baseline H_2 values before intake of the sugar substrate. Then the substrate is administered orally and sequential end-expiratory breath samples collected at timed intervals for 2–3 h. These tests are not without their own problems. Firstly, in individuals who harbor methanogenic and/or sulfide-reducing bacteria, H_2 produced by fermentation will be utilized by these bacteria and converted into methane and hydrogen sulfide, respectively, leading to a false-negative test if only H_2 is assayed. Secondly, and an important cause of a false-positive lactulose breath hydrogen test, any condition that leads to accelerated intestinal transit will lead to an early rise in breath H_2 due to the premature arrival of lactulose into the colon. Thirdly, the oral microbiota may contribute a confusing early peak, as will the ingestion of a high fiber diet on the day before the test. Fourthly, recent food ingestion may lead to an exaggeration and smoking and exercise a suppression of the breath H_2 response. The impact of these potential confounders can be minimized by attention to patient preparation, the inclusion of assays for methane and hydrogen sulfide, and the addition of a test for intestinal transit [3, 27, 28].

The criteria for the diagnosis of SIBO, particularly when using lactulose as the sugar substrate, have generated controversy ever since its inception, and this test, despite being the most widely employed test in the diagnosis of SIBO, has yielded the most conflicting data. The principal criteria proposed include:

1. A high basal level of H_2 is related, it is thought, to the action of the bacterial on a previous meal or unabsorbed carbohydrate in the gut. Some consider this finding, in of itself, as diagnostic.

2. A double peak on the breath H_2 expiration graph has become an established criterion for the diagnosis of SIBO by the lactulose breath test: the first peak due to production of the gas by the effect of bacterial overgrowth in the small bowel and the second resulting from the action of cecal microbes on lactulose. However, it may be difficult to distinguish a double peak in many cases.

3. A rise in H_2 of ≥ 20 ppm above baseline within 90 min [3]. This definition of a positive test must be mindful of the fact that the average orocecal transit time is only slightly longer; it should come as no surprise, therefore, that so many apparently healthy subjects will appear to have SIBO. Rapid transit, as may occur in conditions such as IBS, will compound interpretation further, especially, given the propensity of lactulose itself to accelerate transit. It has been proposed that rapid transit, rather than SIBO, may explain positive breath hydrogen tests in diarrhea-predominant IBS. For all these reasons and despite the recommendations of a recent expert panel, this criterion remains controversial [29].

The use of glucose as the sugar substrate is the other commonly performed breath test used to diagnose SIBO. Glucose is normally given in a dose 50–75 g dissolved in water as a 10% solution and the expired breath sampled at baseline and every 15–20 min after glucose ingestion for 2–3 h. A glucose breath test is considered positive if the basal H_2 level is >12 ppm or a rise of >12 (or 20 according to some) ppm above the baseline value occurs within 2 h. In general, the glucose breath test has been demonstrated to be more accurate than the lactulose test, and as a result, this is the preferred test for the diagnosis of SIBO in some centers.

My approach is to interpret breath tests with caution, mindful of the clinical context and of the various pitfalls that surround their interpretation. They should be regarded as corroborative rather than conclusive evidence.

Other Tests

Apart from identifying causative factors such as jejunal diverticulosis or a stricture, imaging studies are of little value in the direct diagnosis of SIBO as small intestinal mucosal changes in SIBO are neither specific nor diagnostic and mucosal injury and villous atrophy are evident only in the most severely affected individuals.

The Therapeutic Trial

Given the problems associated with all of the above-described tests for the diagnosis of SIBO, it should come as no surprise that clinicians have turned to therapeutic trials of antibiotics as an alternative "diagnostic" strategy. However appealing as the therapeutic trial may seem, it currently lacks standardization with respect to choice of antibiotic, dose, duration of therapy, or appropriate outcome measures. It is for now an entirely empirical approach.

Treatment

There are three components to the treatment of SIBO: firstly, treating the underlying disease; secondly, altering small intestinal bacteria; and thirdly, addressing any associated nutritional deficiencies. Clearly, the primary goal should be the treatment or correction of any underlying disease or defect, when possible. Unfortunately, several of the clinical conditions that are associated with SIBO, such as visceral myopathies and multiple jejunal diverticula, are not readily reversible. It stands to reason that medications associated with intestinal stasis such as those drugs known to inhibit intestinal motility or gastric acid secretion should be eliminated or substituted.

When correction of the clinical condition associated with SIBO is not an option, management is based on antibiotic therapy. Its objective should not be to eradicate the bacterial flora but to alter it in a way that leads to symptomatic improvement. Although, ideally, the choice of antimicrobial agents should reflect *in vitro* susceptibility testing, this is usually impractical as many different bacterial species, with different antibiotic sensitivities, typically coexist. Antibiotic treatment remains, therefore, primarily empirical [8]. There have been few randomized controlled trials of antibiotics in SIBO – rifaximin being the notable exception [30]. In theory, an antibiotic regimen for SIBO should cover both aerobic and anaerobic enteric bacteria. In general, a single 7- to 10- day course of antibiotic may improve symptoms for up to several months in

TABLE 20.2 Antibiotic regimens for SIBO

Ciprofloxacin (250 mg BID)
Norfloxacin (800 mg/day)
Metronidazole (250 mg TID)
Trimethoprim-sulfamethoxazole (1 double strength BID)
Doxycycline (100 mg BID)
Amoxicillin-clavulanic acid (500 mg TID)
Tetracycline (250 mg QID)
Neomycin (500 mg BID)
Rifaximin (800–1200 mg/day)

46–90% of patients with SIBO and render breath tests negative in 20–75%. Some antibiotic options are listed on Table 20.2.

In a recent meta-analysis, the overall eradication rate for SIBO with rifaximin was over 70% with symptom improvement noted in over two-thirds of those who were successfully eradicated [30]. Higher doses were associated with higher eradication rates.

Recurrence following one course of therapy remains an issue, and some patients will need either repeated (e.g., the first 5–10 days out of every month) or continuous courses of antibiotic therapy. In this setting, rotating antibiotic regimens are recommended to prevent the development of resistance. Decisions on management should be individualized and consider such risks of long-term antibiotic therapy as diarrhea, *Clostridium difficile* infection, intolerance, bacterial resistance, and cost. Antibiotics with less toxicity, lower systemic absorption, and greater affordability should be preferred. Following antibiotic therapy, it is not necessary to repeat diagnostic tests for SIBO should gastrointestinal symptoms respond.

Finally, the identification and treatment of nutritional disturbances, commonly present in patients with SIBO, are important components of the overall management of SIBO. In particular, correction of micronutrient (e.g., fat-soluble vitamins, vitamin B12) and electrolyte (e.g., calcium, magnesium) deficiencies, when present, is important. As mucosal damage may persist for some time even after complete eradication of bacterial overgrowth, nutritional therapies may be required over a prolonged period of time. The role of dietary modifications (e.g., lactose-free diet, low FODMAP diet) in the management of SIBO remains unclear and requires additional study.

Case Study: Follow-Up

A lactulose breath test was performed (see Fig. 20.1) which demonstrated a rapid rise to 111 parts per million (ppm) in breath hydrogen within 20 min of lactulose ingestion which was sustained throughout the test. There was no significant rise in breath methane level. The patient reported bloating and diarrhea during the test. A barium small bowel examination revealed multiple small intestinal diverticula but no evidence of obstruction or mucosal disease (see Fig. 20.2).

He was commenced on a rotating schedule of ciprofloxacin and metronidazole. At follow-up, his diarrhea had resolved, there were no further episodes of fecal incontinence, and he had gained almost 7 pounds in weight.

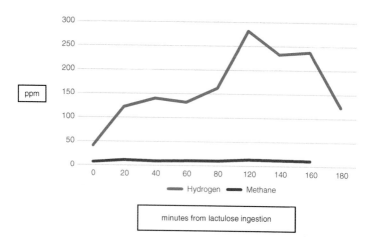

FIGURE 20.1 Lactulose breath test

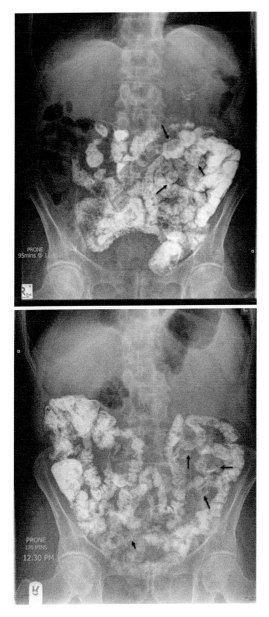

FIGURE 20.2 Two views from a barium small bowel study revealing multiple small intestinal diverticula (arrowed)

Clinical Pearls

- Small intestinal bacterial overgrowth (SIBO) in its classical presentation leads to maldigestion and malabsorption.
- Congenital, acquired, and surgically induced changes in intestinal anatomy may predispose to SIBO.
- Disorders resulting in impaired motility of the small intestine may be complicated by SIBO.
- SIBO has been implicated in the pathogenesis of "functional" symptoms such as bloating and diarrhea in the absence of maldigestion and malabsorption, but here the diagnosis relies on tests that are not well validated or reliable.
- In the absence of high-quality clinical trials of antibiotic treatment for SIBO, treatment remains largely empirical.

Self-Test

Question 1. *SIBO may be complicated by which one of the following?*

A. Vitamin B_{12} deficiency.
B. Folate deficiency.
C. Small intestinal lymphoma.
D. Elevated levels of vitamin B_{12} in serum.

Question 2. *Which one of the following is regarded as diagnostic of SIBO?*

A. $>10^3$ CFU/mL of Gram-positive organisms in a jejunal aspirate.
B. A rise in breath hydrogen of more than 10 ppm within 120 min of lactulose ingestion.
C. The detection of any hydrogen or methane in the basal breath sample, before either lactulose or glucose is administered.
D. $> 10^5$ CFU/mL of bacteria in a jejunal aspirate.

Question 3. *Regarding the use of rifaximin in SIBO, which one of the following is correct?*

A. Systemic side effects are a long-term issue because of the rapid absorption of the drug.
B. It can only be used for one 2-week course as efficacy is lost at that stage.
C. Eradication rates in excess of 60% are to be expected.
D. *Clostridium difficile*-associated disease (CDAD) is a common side effect.

References

1. Quigley EMM. Small intestinal bacterial overgrowth. In: Feldman M, Friedman LS, Brandt LJ, editors. Sleisenger and Fordtran's gastrointestinal and liver disease. 10th ed. New York: Elsevier; 2016. p. 1824–31.
2. Rezaie A, Pimentel M, Rao SS. How to test and treat small intestinal bacterial overgrowth: an evidence-based approach. Curr Gastroenterol Rep. 2016;18:8.
3. Rezaie A, Buresi M, Lembo A, Lin H, McCallum R, Rao S, Schmulson M, Valdovinos M, Zakko S, Pimentel M. Hydrogen and methane-based breath testing in gastrointestinal disorders: the north American consensus. Am J Gastroenterol. 2017;112:775–84.
4. Quigley EM. Small intestinal bacterial overgrowth: what it is and what it is not. Curr Opin Gastroenterol. 2014;30:141–6.
5. Khin-Maung U, Bolin TD, Duncombe VM, Myo-Khin, Nyunt-Nyunt-Wai, Pereira SP, Linklater JM. Epidemiology of small bowel bacterial overgrowth and rice carbohydrate malabsorption in Burmese (Myanmar) village children. Am J Trop Med Hyg. 1992;47:298–304.
6. Lewis SJ, Potts LF, Malhotra R, Mountford R. Small bowel bacterial overgrowth in subjects living in residential care homes. Age Ageing. 1999;28:181–5.
7. Mitsui T, Shimaoka K, Goto Y, Kagami H, Kinomoto H, Ito A, Kondo T. Small bowel bacterial overgrowth is not seen in healthy adults but is in disabled older adults. Hepato-Gastroenterology. 2006;53:82–5.
8. Grace E, Shaw C, Whelan K, Andreyev HJ. Review article: small intestinal bacterial overgrowth--prevalence, clinical features,

current and developing diagnostic tests, and treatment. Aliment Pharmacol Ther. 2013;38:674–88.

9. de Boissieu D, Chaussain M, Badoual J, Raymond J, Dupont C. Small-bowel bacterial overgrowth in children with chronic diarrhea, abdominal pain, or both. J Pediatr. 1996;128:203–7.

10. McEvoy A, Dutton J, James OF. Bacterial contamination of the small intestine is an important cause of occult malabsorption in the elderly. Br Med J. 1983;287:789–93.

11. Sabaté JM, Jouët P, Harnois F, Mechler C, Msika S, Grossin M, Coffin B. High prevalence of small intestinal bacterial over-growth in patients with morbid obesity: a contributor to severe hepatic steatosis. Obes Surg. 2008;18:371–7.

12. Lo WK, Chan WW. Proton pump inhibitor use and the risk of small intestinal bacterial overgrowth: a meta-analysis. Clin Gastroenterol Hepatol. 2013;11:483–90.

13. Su T, Lai S, Lee A, He X, Chen S. Meta-analysis: proton pump inhibitors moderately increase the risk of small intestinal bacte-rial overgrowth. J Gastroenterol. 2018;53:27–36.

14. Rubio-Tapia A, Barton SH, Rosenblatt JE, Murray JA. Prevalence of small intestine bacterial overgrowth diagnosed by quantitative culture of intestinal aspirate in celiac disease. J Clin Gastroenterol. 2009;43:157–61.

15. Krishnamurthy S, Kelly MM, Rohrmann CA, et al. Jejunal diverticulosis: a heterogeneous disorder caused by a vari-ety of abnormalities of smooth muscle or myenteric plexus. Gastroenterology. 1983;85:538–47.

16. Uribarri J, Oh MS, Carroll HJ. D-lactic acidosis. Medicine. 1998;77:73–82.

17. Pimentel M, Chow EJ, Lin HC. Eradication of small intestinal bacterial overgrowth reduces symptoms of irritable bowel syn-drome. Am J Gastroenterol. 2000;95:3503–6.

18. Pimentel M, Chow EJ, Lin HC. Normalization of lactulose breath testing correlates with symptom improvement in irritable bowel syndrome: a double-blind, randomized, placebo-controlled study. Am J Gastroenterol. 2003;98:412–9.

19. Quigley EM. A 51-year-old with irritable bowel syndrome: test or treat for bacterial overgrowth? Clin Gastroenterol Hepatol. 2007;5:1140–3.

20. Vanner S. The lactulose breath test for diagnosing SIBO in IBS patients: another nail in the coffin. Am J Gastroenterol. 2008;103:964–5.

21. Vanner S. The small intestinal bacterial overgrowth. Irritable bowel syndrome hypothesis: implications for treatment. Gut. 2008;57:1315–21.

22. Spiegel BM, Chey WD, Chang L. Bacterial overgrowth and irritable bowel syndrome: unifying hypothesis or a spurious consequence of proton pump inhibitors? Am J Gastroenterol. 2008;103:2972–6.

23. Spiegel BM. Questioning the bacterial overgrowth hypothesis of irritable bowel syndrome: an epidemiologic and evolutionary perspective. Clin Gastroenterol Hepatol. 2011;9:461–9.

24. Ford AC, Spiegel BM, Talley NJ, Moayyedi P. Small intestinal bacterial overgrowth in irritable bowel syndrome: systematic review and meta-analysis. Clin Gastroenterol Hepatol. 2009;7:1279–86.

25. Khoshini R, Dai SC, Lezcano S, Pimentel M. A systematic review of diagnostic tests for small intestinal bacterial overgrowth. Dig Dis Sci. 2008;53:1443–54.

26. Shanahan ER, Zhong L, Talley NJ, Morrison M, Holtmann G. Characterisation of the gastrointestinal mucosa-associated microbiota: a novel technique to prevent cross-contamination during endoscopic procedures. Aliment Pharmacol Ther. 2016;43:1186–96.

27. Gasbarrini A, Corazza GR, Gasbarrini G, Montalto M, et al. Methodology and indications of H_2 breath testing in gastrointestinal diseases: the Rome consensus conference. Aliment Pharmacol Ther. 2009;29(Suppl 1):1–49.

28. Yu D, Cheeseman F, Vanner S. Combined oro-caecal scintigraphy and lactulose hydrogen breath testing demonstrate that breath testing detects oro-caecal transit, not small intestinal bacterial overgrowth in patients with IBS. Gut. 2011;60:334–40.

29. Paterson W, Camilleri M, Simren M, Boeckxstaens G, Vanner SJ. Breath testing consensus guidelines for SIBO: RES IPSA LOCQUITOR. Am J Gastroenterol. 2017;112:1888–9.

30. Gatta L, Scarpignato C. Systematic review with meta-analysis: rifaximin is effective and safe for the treatment of small intestine bacterial overgrowth. Aliment Pharmacol Ther. 2017;45:604–16.

Essential Readings

Rezaie A, Buresi M, Lembo A, Lin H, McCallum R, Rao S, Schmulson M, Valdovinos M, Zakko S, Pimentel M. Hydrogen and methane-based breath testing in gastrointestinal disorders: the North American consensus. Am J Gastroenterol. 2017;112:775–84. *Though its recommendations are not without its critics, this recent consensus document discusses the current status of breath testing in some detail*

Ford AC, Spiegel BM, Talley NJ, Moayyedi P. Small intestinal bacterial overgrowth in irritable bowel syndrome: systematic review and meta-analysis. Clin Gastroenterol Hepatol. 2009;7:1279–86. *The most complete assessment of the role of SIBO in irritable bowel syndrome*

Gatta L, Scarpignato C. Systematic review with meta-analysis: rifaximin is effective and safe for the treatment of small intestine bacterial overgrowth. Aliment Pharmacol Ther. 2017;45:604–16. *A detailed assessment of the impact of rifaximin in SIBO*

Chapter 21
Food Allergies, Food Intolerances, and Carbohydrate Malabsorption

John Leung, Apaar Dadlani, and Sheila Eileen Crowe

Case Study

Caroline is a 24-year-old female who presents with a 2-year history of bloating, abdominal pain, and diarrhea. She has experienced mild generalized abdominal pain, 2–3 days a week, and it is associated with frequent loose stools with a Bristol scale of

J. Leung
Center for Food Related Diseases at Tufts Medical Center, Boston, MA, USA

Food Allergy Center at Floating Hospital of Tufts Medical Center, Boston, MA, USA

Department of Gastroenterology and Department of Pediatric Allergy and Immunology, Tufts Medical Center, Boston, MA, USA

A. Dadlani
Department of Gastroenterology, Tufts Medical Center, Boston, MA, USA

S. E. Crowe (✉)
Division of Gastroenterology, Department of Medicine, University of California in San Diego, La Jolla, CA, USA
e-mail: secrowe@ucsd.edu

© Springer Nature Switzerland AG 2019
B. E. Lacy et al. (eds.), *Essential Medical Disorders of the Stomach and Small Intestine*,
https://doi.org/10.1007/978-3-030-01117-8_21

437

6–7, at least three times a week. Her abdominal pain is often relieved with bowel movements. She also notes postprandial bloating. Because of a family history of celiac disease, Caroline put herself on a gluten-free diet. She finds it helpful, but it does not completely remit her symptoms. She, therefore, obtained a "food intolerance panel" through a commercial laboratory that she found on the internet, and results showed elevations in specific IgG levels for wheat, milk, pork, salmon, shrimp, and 15 other foods. She started avoiding all these food items, and consequently lost over 10 pounds. Because of her extensive dietary restriction, she finds it difficult to eat out with friends, and it has taken a toll on her social life. Despite avoiding all these foods for 2 months, her symptoms have persisted. Otherwise, a review of systems is negative. She is a nonsmoker, denies consuming alcohol, and works as a receptionist in a law firm. She does not take any medications except oral contraceptive pills. She denies any drug allergy. Her brother has peanut allergy, and her mother has celiac disease. Laboratory testing showed normal complete blood count, thyroid stimulating hormone, liver tests, and celiac disease serology (while she was consuming gluten). *Helicobacter pylori* urea breath test was also negative.

Objectives

- Recognize the key pathophysiologic differences between food allergy and food intolerance
- Identify the diagnostic strategies in differentiating food intolerance from food allergy
- Review the therapeutic options in managing food allergy and food intolerance

Epidemiology

It is estimated that up to 20% of the population has experienced adverse reactions to specific foods or food groups [1]. More than one-half of the patients with irritable bowel syndrome (IBS) report symptoms associated with certain foods [2]. The majority of the adverse food reactions are not immunological and are not life-threatening. These are referred to as food intolerances. In contrast, food allergy is an abnormal immunologic response following consumption of a food, which can potentially be life-threatening. It is less common than food intolerance, and the prevalence of IgE-mediated food allergy is estimated to be 1–2% in adults and less than 10% in children [3].

Etiology/Pathogenesis

While food allergy is an abnormal immune response to an ingested food, food intolerance does not arise from immune system dysregulation. Food intolerance is a nonallergic adverse food reaction (AFR) that can be caused by a variety of disease processes including intolerance of foods containing fermentable oligosaccharides, disaccharides, monosaccharides, and polyols (FODMAPs), gastroesophageal reflux disease (GERD), gastrointestinal infections, disorders resulting from structural and functional abnormalities (e.g., gallbladder disease, pancreatic insufficiency), metabolic diseases, and toxin-mediated reactions (Table 21.1) [4].

Food allergy results from a breakdown of immunologic tolerance to a food. It is often categorized based on the immune pathway leading to the breakdown into IgE-mediated, non-IgE-mediated, or mixed IgE/non-IgE-mediated (Fig. 21.1). There has been an apparent increase in the prevalence of food allergy in the recent years which cannot be explained by genetics alone. Several hypotheses have been advanced to explain the role of specific environmental factors, and their respective supporting evidence were summarized in a recent report published by the National Academies of Sciences, Engineering and Medicine (Table 21.2) [6].

Development of an IgE-mediated allergic reaction is a multistep process at the molecular level, with the involve-

TABLE 21.1 Causes of food intolerance

Cause	Examples
Structural gastrointestinal (GI) causes	Hiatal hernia Pyloric stenosis Tracheoesophageal fistula
Enzymatic causes	Disaccharidase deficiency (lactase, sucrase-isomaltase, glucose-galactose) Galactosemia
Other disorders	Malignancy Pancreatic insufficiency (cystic fibrosis, Shwachman-Diamond syndrome) Gallbladder disease Peptic ulcer disease Irritable bowel syndrome

Contaminants and additives	Flavorings and Preservatives
	    Monosodium glutamate
	    Nitrites/nitrates
	Toxins
	    Bacterial: *Clostridium botulinum*, *Staphylococcus aureus*
	    Fungal: Aflatoxins, trichothecenes, ergot
	    Seafood associated:
	        Scombroid poisoning (tuna, mackerel)
	        Ciguatera poisoning (grouper, snapper, barracuda)
	        Saxitoxin (shellfish)
	Infectious Organisms
	    Bacteria: *Salmonella, Shigella, Escherichia coli, Yersinia, Campylobacter*
	    Parasites: *Giardia, Trichinella*
	    Viruses: Hepatitis, rotavirus, enterovirus
	Accidental Contaminants
	    Heavy metals (mercury, copper)
	    Pesticides

TABLE 21.1 (continued)

Cause	Examples
Pharmacologic agents	Caffeine (coffee, tea, soft drinks, cocoa) Histamine (fish, beer, wine, chocolate, sauerkraut) Tyramine (cheeses, pickled herring, avocado, orange, banana, tomato) Serotonin (banana, tomato, plum, avocado, pineapple juice) Alcohol
Psychologic	Food aversion

Adapted with permission from Ref. [4]

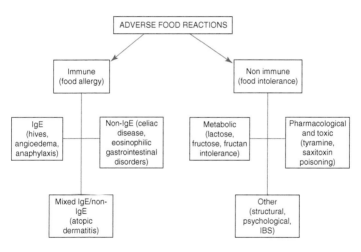

FIGURE 21.1 Classification of adverse food reactions. IgE immunoglobulin E, IBS irritable bowel syndrome. (Adapted with permission from Ref. [5])

ment of multiple cell types. When an allergen is first exposed to a genetically predisposed individual, it activates Th-2 lymphocytes (contrary to the regulatory T-reg subtype in nonpredisposed individuals, which helps in oral tolerance development). These Th-2 cells secrete cytokines (particu-

TABLE 21.2 Hypotheses supporting role of environmental factors in food allergy

Hypothesis	Details
Hygiene hypothesis	Reduced microbial exposure associated with improved hygiene practices may increase our susceptibility to allergic diseases secondary to under-developed immune system.
Microbiome depletion hypothesis	This hypothesis evolves from hygiene hypothesis. It states that reduced diversity of our microbiome leads to aberrant development of our immune systems, leading to increased risk of allergies.
Allergen avoidance hypothesis	It hypothesizes that avoidance of allergen in early years of life prevents normal development of tolerance.
Dual antigen exposure hypothesis	It suggests allergic sensitization to food occurs through low-dose cutaneous exposure, while early oral consumption of food protein induces oral tolerance. This is one of the leading hypotheses and is derived based on data from well-conducted clinical trials.
Nutritional immunomodulation hypothesis	It proposes deficiency or excess of certain nutrients can influence the normal development of oral tolerance. Vitamin D, antioxidants (vitamin C, beta-carotene), omega-3 fatty acids, and dietary fat (e.g., omega-3 fatty acids and n-6 fatty acids) have been shown to have immunomodulatory effects.

TABLE 21.2 (continued)

Hypothesis	Details
Other hypotheses (e.g., short chain fatty acid hypothesis, food processing hypothesis, genetically modified foods)	Specific gut microbiota may lead to production of short chain fatty acids, contributing to diminished sensitization to allergens via complex molecular mechanisms. Food additives may lead to a toxic immune reaction. Genetically modified foods might harbor new allergens, leading to allergy.

Adapted with permission from Ref. [6]

larly IL-4 and IL-13) to drive production of allergen-specific IgE immunoglobulin from B cells. The IgE antibodies bind to the IgE receptors on the surfaces of mast cells and basophils. This process is known as sensitization. Upon reexposure to the same allergen, IgE bound on mast cells and basophils get cross-linked, resulting in the release of preformed and de-novo synthesized inflammatory and vasoactive mediators such as histamine, tryptase, chymase, carboxypeptidase, platelet-activating factor (PAF), and leukotriene. These induce vasodilation, mucus secretion, smooth muscle contraction, and influx of other inflammatory cells [7, 8]. This is known as type-1 hypersensitivity reaction and is responsible for IgE-mediated food allergy. Non-IgE-mediated and mixed IgE/non-IgE-mediated food allergies have distinct pathogenesis, and their discussion is beyond the scope of this chapter.

In contradistinction, food intolerance is non-immune-mediated. Of the multiple causes of food intolerance, we will limit our discussion to IBS and carbohydrate malabsorption. IBS is a common functional gastrointestinal disorder that is characterized by a chronic episodic alteration in bowel habits with associated abdominal discomfort/pain in the absence of an organic cause. The pathophysiology of IBS remains uncertain, but it has been suggested that visceral hypersensitivity, gastrointestinal dysmotility, small intestinal bacterial overgrowth, altered gut microbiota, psychosocial dysfunction, and other factors play a role [9]. Carbohydrate intolerance is another important entity which can be caused by loss of brush border enzymes (lactose, isomaltose), disorder of transport proteins (fructose-sorbitol malabsorption, glucose-galactose malabsorption), or inability of gut enzymes to fully metabolize the sugar (e.g., fructan) [10, 11]. All conditions lead to increased transport of partially metabolized sugar into the colon, where they are fermented, leading to flatulence and bloating.

Symptoms

Patients who suffer from adverse food reactions manifest a spectrum of symptoms ranging from transient and benign symptoms such as bloating, hives, and loose stools to potentially life-threatening reactions such as anaphylaxis (associated with IgE-mediated allergy). Since the patient in our case reported partial improvement of symptoms by avoiding wheat products, we will use adverse reactions to wheat (ARW) as an example to demonstrate the key similarities and differences between food allergy and intolerances. ARW can be seen in disorders such as celiac disease, eosinophilic esophagitis (EoE), IgE-mediated wheat protein allergy, and fructan intolerance (which presents as a subset of IBS). Making a diagnosis based on symptoms alone is not always possible as the individual presentations of different ARW can be quite nonspecific and may overlap to a great extent (Fig. 21.2).

A patient presenting with weight loss, diarrhea, abdominal discomfort, and nutritional deficiency along with extra-intestinal manifestations such as anemia, type 1 diabetes mellitus, or dermatitis herpetiformis should be suspected to have celiac disease rather than other wheat-related disorders [12]. Wheat-induced EoE should be suspected in a patient who presents with dysphagia, heartburn, and episodic esophageal food impactions, with remission of symptoms upon avoidance of wheat [13]. IgE-mediated allergic reactions to wheat are

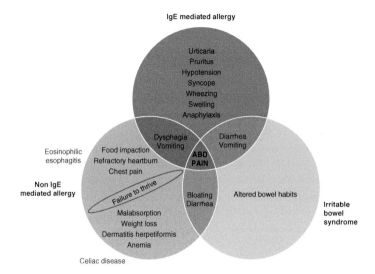

FIGURE 21.2 Overlapping symptoms between various wheat-related disorders. IgE immunoglobulin E, GERD gastroesophageal reflux disease, ABD abdominal

associated with rapid-onset of urticaria, angioedema, vomiting, wheezing, and/or anaphylaxis. Fructan intolerance typically presents with bloating and abdominal distension with consumption of fructan-rich foods such as wheat, cereals, onions, and garlic. Thus, a particular food can cause several different AFR, and their associated symptoms can be quite similar.

Diagnostic Evaluation

From a clinical perspective, it is important to distinguish food intolerance from food allergy because the prognosis, management, and nutritional implications are very different. There is, however, no single reliable diagnostic study or symptom that can differentiate food allergy from intolerance. Instead, a thorough history and physical exam remains the cornerstone of narrowing down the differential diagnoses, and selective tests can then be used to confirm the diagnosis. Table 21.3 shows the key diagnostic tests for the evaluation of different wheat-related disorders.

The diagnostic evaluation of celiac disease includes serology (IgA anti-tTG antibodies, anti-gliadin antibodies), HLA typing, and the gold standard small bowel biopsy [12]. Esophageal biopsies are required to confirm the diagnosis of EoE [13].

Skin testing and specific IgE level of wheat are used for evaluation of IgE-mediated wheat allergy, but the results must be interpreted in the context of the clinical history. Supervised oral food challenge (OFC) is accepted as the gold

TABLE 21.3 Key diagnostic tests for various wheat-related disorders

Wheat-related disease	Key diagnostic tests
Celiac disease	Serology: tTG IgA (preferred), tTG IgG, EMA IgA, DGP IgA, and IgG Small bowel biopsy: required in cases with positive serology and/or high probability of celiac disease Other tests: HLA testing and capsule endoscopy
Eosinophilic esophagitis	Endoscopic esophageal biopsy (>15 eos/hpf)
IgE-mediated allergy	Compatible clinical history is essential Skin prick tests, wheat-specific serum IgE levels (ImmunoCAP) Supervised oral challenge in select cases
Fructan intolerance	Trial elimination

tTG tissue transglutaminase, *IgA* immunoglobulin A; *IgG* immunoglobulin G, *EMA* endomysial antibody, *DGP* deamidated gliadin peptide, *HLA* human leukocyte antigen, *eos/hpf* eosinophils per high power field, *IgE* immunoglobulin E

standard for IgE-mediated wheat allergy [5]. Each test has its own advantages and disadvantages, as listed in Table 21.4.

Patients with fructan intolerance do not require the diagnostic tests mentioned above. However, if performed, they would have negative celiac disease serology, normal duodenal

TABLE 21.4 Standardized diagnostic tests for IgE-mediated food allergy

Test	Advantages	Disadvantages
ImmunoCAP specific IgE test	Noninvasive Easy availability High negative predictive value	Can only be interpreted in the context of clinical history Sensitivity differs for different foods Modest positive predictive value
Skin prick test (SPT)	High sensitivity Result is available within few minutes	Can only be interpreted in the context of clinical history Sensitivity differs for different foods Can only be conducted by allergists Cannot be performed in patients with generalized eczema, or other skin diseases Cannot be performed in patients on antihistamines and/or montelukast
Oral food challenge (OFC)	*Gold standard* for the diagnosis of IgE-mediated food allergy	Resource and time intensive Risk of allergic reaction, including anaphylaxis during challenge Can be performed only in a specialized center with resources to manage reactions, thereby limiting availability

and esophageal biopsy, and usually have negative IgE serology and skin prick test to wheat. In recent years, there have been reports describing a new entity known as non-celiac gluten sensitivity (NCGS). These patients' symptoms improve with elimination of gluten from the diet, but they do not have celiac disease; they do not have duodenal inflammation or positive celiac disease serology. In 2018, a randomized, double-blind, placebo-controlled, crossover study of individuals with self-reported NCGS found that fructans, rather than gluten, seem to be the cause of their symptoms [14]. Gluten is a protein found in grains, including wheat, barley, and rye. Fructans are carbohydrates, which are also found in wheat and barley. A gluten-free diet eliminates over 50% of the major source of fructans (wheat) in a typical American diet [15]. Therefore, it is not surprising that patients suffering from fructan intolerance respond to gluten-free diet. Fructan intolerance is often found in patients with IBS, along with other carbohydrate intolerances such as lactose and fructose intolerance. Hydrogen (and methane) breath tests are often used to evaluate for these carbohydrate intolerances because of availability, low cost, and noninvasive nature. Whereas breath tests for lactose and fructose are commonly used, there is no standardized test for diagnosis of fructan intolerance. However, a fructan breath test (serial measurements of breath hydrogen and methane, with the substrate being fructan) may aid in its diagnosis, if conducted in a specialized center [10]. A recently published guideline strongly recommends performing breath test using either glucose or lactulose to rule out small intestinal bacterial overgrowth prior to diagnosing carbohydrate intolerance [16]. In our practice, we always rule out small intestinal bacterial overgrowth before proceeding with carbohydrate intolerance breath tests, as this decreases the risk of false-positive results for carbohydrate malabsorption.

Many commercial laboratories offer a "food intolerance IgG/IgG4 panel" directly to consumers with the claim that they can pinpoint food trigger(s) causing intolerances. These antibodies have been ascribed to form immune complexes with ingested food [17]; however, they do not cause adverse reactions, unlike IgE-mediated reactions. An expert consensus concluded that the presence of these antibodies does not indicate the presence of food allergy or intolerance, but is rather a physiological response of the body on food exposure, and use of these tests only results in false positive diagnoses [18], which might cause unnecessary food avoidance leading to malnutrition and weight loss. Furthermore, performance of these tests only adds to the cost of treatment, and dietary restriction may hamper one's social life. It has been our experience that IgG and/or IgG4 tests are not helpful in identifying food trigger(s) causing gastrointestinal symptoms. Due to lack of sufficient scientific evidence, tests such as provocation test, kinesiology, cytotoxic tests and electro-dermal testing have also not been proven to be beneficial in the diagnosis of food related diseases [19]. More extensive research is required to understand their diagnostic utility.

Treatment

Although avoidance of wheat products is the cornerstone treatment for various wheat-related adverse reactions, there are few subtle but important differences in the management of each of them.

A "four-E" approach, as highlighted in Fig. 21.3, is useful in the management of IgE-mediated food allergy [20]. It consists of:

1. *Elimination of the food trigger*: This is the key to prevent a food allergic reaction, as there is no cure for food allergy. To eliminate the food trigger, one must be able to correctly identify it.
2. *Early recognition of allergic reaction and anaphylaxis*: Dangerous fatal and near-fatal reactions may occur if the symptoms of the reaction are not recognized quickly and epinephrine administration is delayed [21].
3. *Epinephrine autoinjector use when required*: Patients with IgE-mediated food allergy should always carry self-

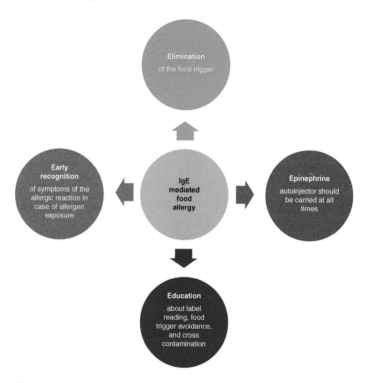

FIGURE 21.3 The four-E approach in the management of IgE-mediated food allergy

injectable intramuscular epinephrine in case of anaphylaxis due to accidental exposure [5]. Indications to use epinephrine may include mild or severe symptoms from various organ systems [22] and are highlighted in Table 21.5. In contrast, patients with non-IgE-mediated food allergic diseases such as celiac disease and EoE do not require self-injectable epinephrine.

4. *Education about food trigger avoidance and cross contamination*: Food trigger avoidance comprises of the avoiding the sources of food harboring the food allergen. This might appear easy in theory, but its practical application may be challenging. For example, wheat is usually present in pasta, bran, bread crumbs etc.; however, hidden sources may

TABLE 21.5 Indications to use epinephrine in food allergic reaction

Indications to use epinephrine in food allergic reaction:
1. If there are severe symptoms from any one organ system
2. If there are combination of symptoms from ≥2 organ systems
3. If mild symptoms from one organ/organ system continue to worsen despite treatment with antihistamines

Organ system	Severe symptoms	Mild symptoms
Skin	Generalized hives	Few hives, mild pruritus
Gastrointestinal	Intractable vomiting, severe diarrhea	Mild nausea or abdominal discomfort
Mouth	Lip/tongue angioedema	Oral pruritus
Throat	Difficulty in breathing, dysphagia, hoarseness, and tightness	
Respiratory	Respiratory distress, wheeze, intractable cough	
Cardiovascular	Circulatory collapse presenting as weak pulse, dizziness, pale or blue skin, fainting	
Other	Anxiety, confusion, sense of impending doom	Nasal symptoms including sneezing, itchy and runny nose

include vegetable gum, soy sauce, and flavoring agents. Hence, one must check the label of the food product to ensure it is free from the allergen.

Patients with IgE-mediated allergy should also be explained about cross-reactivity with other related foods which the patient has never consumed (as their tolerance is not known), which may lead to restriction of more than just the known allergen. Cross reactivity arises when related foods share the same allergenic protein. For example, fish and tree nuts are commonly cross-reactive, and hence allergy testing (skin prick test and oral food challenge) should be considered in case tolerance to other nuts or shellfish, respectively, is not known. Grains including wheat, and fruits & vegetables are less likely to be cross reactive [23]. Patients should also be educated about safe storage and cleaning if there is possibility of cross-contamination with the allergen, (in case other nonallergic members of the family continue to consume the food that the patient is allergic to). Additionally, some medications and vaccines usually harbor common allergens, and it is important to inquire about the relevant food allergies before administering them. Figure 21.4 enlists some useful resources for more information about food allergy.

In patients with food intolerance and carbohydrate intolerance, treatment might involve avoidance of carbohydrates

Useful websites for general information

- https://www.fda.gov/Food/IngredientsPackagingLabeling/FoodAllergens/ucm079311.htm
- https://newsinhealth.nih.gov/2017/03/understanding-food-allergies
- https://www.foodallergies.org/
- https://acaai.org/allergies/types/food-allergy
- https://www.aaaai.org/conditions-and-treatments/allergies/food-allergies
- Food allergy action plan (English): https://www.foodallergy.org/sites/default/files/2018-06/emergency-care-plan.pdf
- Food allergy action plan (Spanish): https://www.foodallergy.org/sites/default/files/2018-06/emergency-care-plan-spanish.pdf

Useful websites for recipes

- https://www.aaaai.org/conditions-and-treatments/allergies/food-allergies/allergy-free-recipes
- https://www.kidswithfoodallergies.org/page/recipes-diet.aspx?cat=17#res

Useful mobile apps

- NIH: Food allergy information
- Belay

FIGURE 21.4 Useful resources for patients with food allergy

in addition to fructans, such as lactose and fructose (FODMAPs). FODMAPs are short-chain carbohydrates and sugar alcohols (lactose, fructose, fructan, galactans and polyols) which are poorly absorbed in the GI tract and are rapidly fermented by bacteria. In a recent randomized, controlled, single-blind, crossover trial of IBS patients, Halmos et al. found significant reduction of symptoms in more than 50% of patients treated with the low FODMAP diet [24].

Case Study Follow-Up

Caroline was initially diagnosed with IBS based on Rome IV criteria (2-year history of chronic abdominal pain, 2–3 days/week, loose stools, no alarm symptoms), after ruling out other potential causes of wheat-related disorders (celiac disease, EoE and IgE-mediated allergy) based on the detailed history, physical examination and selective diagnostic testing. She was treated with a low FODMAP diet for 4 weeks with significant symptomatic improvement; however, at subsequent clinic visits she reported difficulty in adhering to the restrictive diet. In an attempt to liberalize her diet, she was advised by a dietitian to reintroduce different FODMAP group foods one by one, based on results of carbohydrate breath tests. Breath testing for small intestinal bacterial overgrowth and lactose and fructose malabsorption were negative, but positive for fructans. It was concluded that fructan intolerance was responsible for her symptoms, explaining why she experienced partial improvement with gluten-free diet, which eliminated the major source of dietary fructan (wheat). Therefore, lactose and fructose were able to be successfully reintroduced into her diet, while continuing to avoid fructan-containing foods such as wheat, onions, garlic, artichokes, bananas and cereals [25]. Caroline noted a better symptomatic improvement with fructan restriction as compared to gluten-free diet. She also reported that this less restrictive diet involving elimination of only fructan-containing foods was easier to follow than the low FODMAP diet.

Clinical Pearls

- It is important to distinguish food intolerance from food allergy because the prognosis, management and nutritional implications are very different.
- Food allergy can be IgE-mediated (IgE-mediated food protein allergy), non-IgE-mediated (celiac disease, eosinophilic esophagitis) or mixed IgE/non-IgE-mediated (atopic dermatitis).
- One should be aware of the nonvalidated and unproven diagnostic tests for food related diseases, as unnecessary dietary restriction can result in malnutrition and disruption of social life.
- The "four-E" approach, consisting of elimination of dietary allergen, early recognition of anaphylaxis, epinephrine use when indicated, and education about the allergen identification and cross contamination are the key points in in the management of IgE-mediated food allergy.

Self-Test

Question 1. Which one of the following disorders is classified as food allergy?

A. Eosinophilic esophagitis
B. Pancreatitis
C. Irritable bowel syndrome
D. Fructan intolerance

Question 2. A 20-year-old female comes to the office complaining of 3-year history of altered bowel movements, vomiting, and abdominal pain relieved with defecation and often associated with consumption of fruit juices, soda, honey, and maple syrup. Which one of the following will not be helpful in determining the diagnosis?

A. History and physical examination
B. Presence of serum IgG4 antibodies
C. Fructose hydrogen and methane breath test
D. Small intestinal bacterial overgrowth breath test

Question 3. Which one of the following is not a part of the "four-E" approach indicated in the management of IgE-mediated food allergy?

A. Exposure of allergen later in life leads to development of tolerance
B. Elimination of known allergen from all possible dietary sources
C. Education about the allergen, its sources, symptoms caused in case of reaction, and management of the reaction
D. Early recognition of symptoms of allergic reaction
E. Epinephrine administration when indicated

References

1. Lomer MCE. Review article: the aetiology, diagnosis, mechanisms and clinical evidence for food intolerance. Aliment Pharmacol Ther. 2015;41(3):262–75.
2. Böhn L, Störsrud S, Törnblom H, Bengtsson U, Simrén M. Self-reported food-related gastrointestinal symptoms in IBS are common and associated with more severe symptoms and reduced quality of life. Am J Gastroenterol. 2013;108(5):634–41.
3. Turnbull JL, Adams HN, Gorard DA. Review article: the diagnosis and management of food allergy and food intolerances. Aliment Pharmacol Ther. 2015;41(1):3–25.
4. Sampson HA. Differential diagnosis in adverse reactions to foods. J Allergy Clin Immunol. 1986;78(1):212–9.
5. Boyce JA, Assa'ad A, Burks AW, Jones SM, Sampson HA, Wood RA, et al. Guidelines for the diagnosis and management of food allergy in the United States: report of the NIAID-sponsored expert panel. J Allergy Clin Immunol. 2010;126(6 0):S1–58.

6. Sicherer SH, Sampson HA. Food allergy: a review and update on epidemiology, pathogenesis, diagnosis, prevention, and management. J Allergy Clin Immunol. 2018;141(1):41–58.

7. Valenta R, Hochwallner H, Linhart B, Pahr S. Food allergies: the basics. Gastroenterology. 2015;148(6):1120–1131.e4.

8. Leung J, Beukema KR, Shen AH. Allergic mechanisms of eosinophilic oesophagitis. Best Pract Res Clin Gastroenterol. 2015;29(5):709–20.

9. Saha L. Irritable bowel syndrome: pathogenesis, diagnosis, treatment, and evidence-based medicine. World J Gastroenterol: WJG. 2014;20(22):6759–73.

10. Fedewa A, Rao SSC. Dietary fructose intolerance, fructan intolerance and FODMAPs. Curr Gastroenterol Rep. 2014;16(1):370.

11. Raithel M, Weidenhiller M, Hagel AF-K, Hetterich U, Neurath MF, Konturek PC. The malabsorption of commonly occurring mono and disaccharides. Dtsch Ärztebl Int. 2013;110(46):775–82.

12. Parzanese I, Qehajaj D, Patrinicola F, Aralica M, Chiriva-Internati M, Stifter S, et al. Celiac disease: from pathophysiology to treatment. World J Gastrointest Pathophysiol. 2017;8(2):27–38.

13. Dellon ES, Gonsalves N, Hirano I, Furuta GT, Liacouras CA, Katzka DA, et al. ACG clinical guideline: evidenced based approach to the diagnosis and management of esophageal eosinophilia and eosinophilic esophagitis (EoE). Am J Gastroenterol. 2013;108(5):679–92; quiz 693.

14. Skodje GI, Sarna VK, Minelle IH, Rolfsen KL, Muir JG, Gibson PR, et al. Fructan, rather than gluten, induces symptoms in patients with self-reported non-celiac gluten sensitivity. Gastroenterology. 2018;154(3):529–539.e2.

15. Moshfegh AJ, Friday JE, Goldman JP, Ahuja JK. Presence of inulin and oligofructose in the diets of Americans. J Nutr. 1999;129(7 Suppl):1407S–11S.

16. Rezaie A, Buresi M, Lembo A, Lin H, McCallum R, Rao S, et al. Hydrogen and methane-based breath testing in gastrointestinal disorders: the North American consensus. Am J Gastroenterol. 2017;112(5):775–84.

17. Marinkovich V. Specific IgG antibodies as markers of adverse reactions to foods. Monogr Allergy. 1996;32:221–5.

18. Bock SA. AAAAI support of the EAACI position paper on IgG4. J Allergy Clin Immunol. 2010;125(6):1410.

19. Hammond C, Lieberman JA. Unproven diagnostic tests for food allergy. Immunol Allergy Clin North Am. 2018;38(1):153–63.

20. Crowe SE, Leung J. Food allergy and food intolerance. In: Mullin GE, Matarese LE, Palmer M, editors. Gastrointestinal and liver disease nutrition desk reference. Boca Raton: CRC Press; 2011. p. 72–4.
21. Sampson HA, Mendelson L, Rosen JP. Fatal and near-fatal anaphylactic reactions to food in children and adolescents. N Engl J Med. 1992;327(6):380–4.
22. Food Allergy & Anaphylaxis Emergency Care Plan|Food Allergy Research & Education [Internet]. [cited 2018 Jul 19]. Available from: https://www.foodallergy.org/life-with-food-allergies/ food-allergy-anaphylaxis-emergency-care-plan
23. Sicherer SH. Clinical implications of cross-reactive food allergens. J Allergy Clin Immunol. 2001;108(6):881–90.
24. Halmos EP, Power VA, Shepherd SJ, Gibson PR, Muir JG. A diet low in FODMAPs reduces symptoms of irritable bowel syndrome. Gastroenterology. 2014;146(1):67–75.e5.
25. Gibson PR, Shepherd SJ. Evidence-based dietary management of functional gastrointestinal symptoms: the FODMAP approach. J Gastroenterol Hepatol. 2010;25(2):252–8.

Essential Reading

Sicherer SH, Sampson HA. Food allergy: a review and update on epidemiology, pathogenesis, diagnosis, prevention, and management. J Allergy Clin Immunol. 2018;141(1):41–58. This review article comprises of recent updates in the understanding of food allergy.

Skodje GI, Sarna VK, Minelle IH, Rolfsen KL, Muir JG, Gibson PR, et al. Fructan, rather than gluten, induces symptoms in patients with selfreported non-celiac gluten sensitivity. Gastroenterology. 2018;154(3):529–539.e2. This paper shares the details of the first randomized, placebo-controlled trial to demonstrate that patients with NCGS actually appear to be intolerant to fructan, not gluten.

Halmos EP, Power VA, Shepherd SJ, Gibson PR, Muir JG. A diet low in FODMAPs reduces symptoms of irritable bowel syndrome. Gastroenterology. 2014;146(1):67–75. e5. This article reports the results of the first multicenter, randomized, controlled, single-blind trial to show the efficacy of low FODMAP diet in the treatment IBS.

Appendix: Answers to Self-Test Questions

Chapter 1

1. Answer: B. Dorsal lateral reticular formation of the medulla

Explanation

The vomiting center is where many neuroanatomical pathways converge, and stimulation of this area can lead to the development of nausea and vomiting. Afferent signaling pathways from the GI tract, vestibular system, musculoskeletal system, the heart, and the oropharynx converge here, and efferent pathways travel to the GI tract, diaphragm, abdominal wall muscles, and oropharynx to coordinate the complex act of vomiting.

2. Answer: D. Aprepitant

Explanation

Many different medications can cause nausea and vomiting. Chemotherapeutic agents, such as cis-platinum, are a classic example. A number of cardiovascular medications including digoxin, calcium channel blockers, beta blockers, diuretics, and antiarrhythmics are associated with nausea and vomiting. Antibiotics, including tetracycline and erythromycin, and other commonly used medications to treat GI disorders, such

© Springer Nature Switzerland AG 2019
B. E. Lacy et al. (eds.), *Essential Medical Disorders of the Stomach and Small Intestine*,
https://doi.org/10.1007/978-3-030-01117-8

as sulfasalazine, can also cause nausea and vomiting. Aprepitant is a neurokinin-1 receptor antagonist used to treat nausea and vomiting.

3. Answer: A. Remove the offending agent

Explanation

In a patient with nausea and vomiting, after ruling out a life-threatening illness, the most important item to remember is performing a thorough and thoughtful history and physical examination. If an offending agent is identified in the history and physical, this should first be removed to see if there is improvement in the patient's symptoms. If no offending agent is identified or if symptoms don't improve, then the next step would be empiric symptom control and diagnostic testing with an abdominal x-ray (KUB), upper endoscopy (EGD), and possibly a fluoroscopic examination of the small intestine (SBFT). If symptoms persist further testing can be done to see if an underlying etiology can be found. See Fig. 1.1.

Chapter 2

1. Answer: A. Postsurgical

Explanation

Nissen fundoplication, Billroth gastric resection, and heart and lung transplantation are the most common causes of vagal injury, resulting in postsurgical gastroparesis. Although idiopathic gastroparesis is the most common etiology for gastroparesis, it can only be diagnosed after all other possible etiologies have been excluded. The patient did not have complications associated with his diabetes, most notably a lack of retinopathy. Additionally, the patient had type 2 diabetes for only 5 years' duration with good glycemic control (HbA1c). Lastly, the patient did have an upper gastrointestinal viral infection 1 year ago, but that was not complicated by autonomic dysfunction. If he had developed post-viral gastroparesis, the majority of symptoms should have resolved at 1 year, not just started late after the infection. The timing of the surgical intervention 2 weeks ago is much more closely tied to the development of symptoms.

2. Answer: B. Breath test, 4-h, solid meal

Explanation

Gastric scintigraphy and breath test are the gold standard tests to measure gastric emptying. Gastric emptying utilizing solid meals measured over 3 h (not 2 h) has the highest correlation with upper gastrointestinal symptoms. Thus, breath test over 4 h using a solid meal is the correct answer. Ultrasound and MRI only use a liquid meal. The wireless motility capsule usually empties from the stomach with the return of fasting motility (migrating motor complex) and therefore may not assess gastric emptying of digestible food.

3. Answer: D. Metoclopramide

Explanation

Metoclopramide is the only medication that has FDA approval for the indication of gastroparesis. Although erythromycin is FDA approved, it is not approved for the indication of gastroparesis. Currently, erythromycin for gastroparesis is off-label use. Domperidone is used under expanded access use provided by the FDA with a single patient or multi-patient IND (investigational drug) application, if the QTc is <450 ms in men and <470 ms in women. Cisapride was an effective medication to improve gastric emptying and upper gastrointestinal symptoms. However, cardiac side effects resulted in removal of cisapride from the market. Relamorelin is a promising new ghrelin agonist that could improve the amount of food intake and gastric emptying. However, it is still undergoing investigational trials to obtain FDA approval.

Chapter 3

1. Answer: C. Tobacco use

Explanation

Tobacco use is associated with a lower incidence of nausea and vomiting in pregnancy. Tobacco use results in lower levels of both HCG and estradiol, thought to be the mechanism of protection. All other answers listed are known risk factors and increase the incidence of nausea and vomiting of pregnancy.

2. Answer: D. Ondansetron

Explanation

The ACOG recommends that prenatal vitamins be started at least 1 month prior to becoming pregnant. This has been associated with a lower incidence of symptoms. For women that develop symptoms, first-line agents include those that can be obtained over the counter including both ginger and vitamin B6. Both medications have been shown to reduce both nausea and vomiting. While ondansetron is effective for all levels of nausea and vomiting in pregnancy, the ACOG states that there is insufficient evidence to assess safety for the fetus; some studies have suggested an increased incidence of cleft palate in infants of women taking ondansetron. Pregnant women thus should be warned of this risk prior to taking this medication.

3. Answer: A. Female sex

Explanation

Female sex has been shown to be an independent risk factor for development of postoperative nausea and vomiting. The other factors listed are all protective. Non-smoking status is related to increased risk for development of symptoms. Likewise, younger patients have a higher incidence of PONV. The use of local anesthesia, compared to general or volatile anesthetics, is associated with a decreased incidence of PONV.

4. Answer: B. Neurokinin-1 receptor antagonist

Explanation

Aprepitant works through its antagonistic effect on the neurokinin-1 receptor, a receptor found centrally in the emesis center. This results in decreased symptoms of nausea and vomiting. The other options are all mechanisms of action for other drugs commonly used for PONV but are not the mechanism of action for aprepitant. 5-hydroxytryptamine receptor antagonists include ondansetron and granisetron. Dopamine receptor antagonists include droperidol, haloperidol, and metoclopramide. Antihistamines include dimenhydrinate and meclizine. Anticholinergics include scopolamine patches.

Chapter 4

1. Answer: C. Three attacks per year, typically 12–18 h per episode, none of which have led to ED visits or hospital admission

Explanation

The severity of CVS (or CHS) should guide all management decisions, particularly when offering prophylaxis using daily medications, as many of the typical prophylactic medications are associated with some side effects. For example, first-line prophylaxis agents such as TCAs and topiramate may be associated with daytime drowsiness or fatigue. The goal is to reduce the number of days per year that patients suffer from CVS-related symptoms, secondarily reducing the risk of complications, reducing healthcare utilization, and improving quality of life. The general guidance is that patients with *more than three episodes per year* and/or individual episodes *lasting more than 3 days* should be offered prophylactic medication. This is particularly the case if past attempts at abortive treatment at home are unsuccessful and episodes frequently lead to ED visits and hospital admission. Thus, Answer A is clearly incorrect, as the patient has had more than three fairly severe episodes per year that routinely lead to ED visits and hospital admissions. Answer B is incorrect because the episode frequency is high, and although the patient has access to a fairly effective abortive therapy, there are some episodes that fail to abort. Answer D is incorrect because there are more than three episodes a year, all of which end up being treated in the ED setting. Answer E is incorrect because there are more than three episodes per year with some episodes that fail a home-based abortive regimen.

2. Correct Answer: D. Alprazolam

Explanation

All of the other agents lists in Answers A, B, C, and E are used as prophylactic medications in CVS (or CHS). First-line prophylactic medication options include TCAs (i.e., amitriptyline, nortriptyline, or doxepin) or topiramate. Anti-epileptic drugs (AEDs) as a class may be effective prophylactic approaches, with the AEDs topiramate, levetiracetam, and zonisamide having the best evidence for use.

Mitochondrial stabilizers such as coenzyme Q10 and L-carnitine may also be useful agents for CVS (or CHS) prophylaxis. Alprazolam may be useful as an acute abortive treatment, but has no clear role as a prophylactic agent.

3. Answer: D. Migraine

Explanation

CVS (and CHS) are associated with several comorbidities. The most common associations are with migraine, but mood disorders such as generalized anxiety disorder, panic disorder, depression, and bipolar disorder are common as well. A personal or family history of migraine is supportive of the CVS diagnosis using Rome IV criteria. Although some CVS patients also have epilepsy (and AEDs can be useful in CVS treatment), Answer A is incorrect because this is not a defining comorbidity in CVS. Answers B, C, and E are incorrect because these common medical conditions are not known to have an increased prevalence in the CVS (or CHS) population.

Chapter 5

1. Answer: C

Explanation

The patient has chronic intestinal pseudo-obstruction (CIPO). This may be due to a myopathic process affecting smooth muscle of the gastrointestinal tract; measuring ANA is indicated in the evaluation of a possible myopathy (Answer D is correct). CIPO may also be secondary to a neuropathic etiology, thus TSH and fasting glucose should also be performed (Answers A and B are correct). Measuring a fasting gastrin level is not part of the evaluation of CIP (Answer C is incorrect and thus the right choice).

2. Answer: B

Explanation

Explanation: Octreotide 50 mcg s.c. QHS has been shown to improve nausea, bloating, and abdominal pain in patients with CIPO (Answer B is correct). Simethicone and proton pump inhibitors have not been shown to improve bloating, in patients with or without CIPO (Answers A and C are incorrect). PEG-3350 may improve bowel movement frequency, but has not been shown to improve bloating in CIP (Answer D is incorrect).

3. Answer: A

Explanation

Venting gastrostomy tube placement has been demonstrated to reduce hospitalizations in patients with CIPO (Answer A is correct). While prokinetics such as cisapride and metoclopramide may help symptoms, they have not been demonstrated to reduce hospitalizations (Answers B and C are incorrect). Surgical pyloroplasty has not been demonstrated to benefit patients with CIPO (Answer D is incorrect).

Chapter 6

1. Answer: D. Order *H. pylori* stool antigen testing

Explanation

The patient is under age 60 with one alarm feature (family member diagnosed with an upper gastrointestinal malignancy). Thus, she should undergo *H. pylori* "test and treat" as the first step in her diagnostic evaluation. Answer A is incorrect as a trial of PPI therapy is warranted only after investigation for an organic cause is performed and is negative. Answer B is incorrect as EGD is the first step for patients under age 60 years with >1 alarm feature, clinically significant weight loss (typically >5% of body weight), overt gastrointestinal bleeding, or a rapidly progressive alarm feature. Answer C is incorrect as gastric emptying testing should only be considered after organic causes such as *H. pylori* infection are excluded.

2. Answer: B. Perform EGD with gastric biopsies

Explanation

The patient is over age 60 and meets criteria for dyspepsia. Patients with uninvestigated dyspepsia aged 60 years and over should undergo initial evaluation with EGD with gastric biopsies to rule out malignancy and *H. pylori*. Answer A is incorrect as a trial of PPI therapy is warranted only after investigation for an organic cause is performed and negative. Answer C is incorrect as gastric emptying testing should only be considered after organic causes are excluded. Answer D is incorrect as any patient age 60 or older should undergo EGD with gastric biopsies as the first step in evaluation to rule out both malignancy and *H. pylori*.

3. Answer: B. Functional dyspepsia

Explanation

Evaluation for an organic cause of this patient's dyspepsia has been unrevealing, thus a diagnosis of functional dyspepsia can be made. Answer A is incorrect as the patient has not undergone gastric emptying testing. Answer C is incorrect since, although she takes daily aspirin, her EGD with gastric biopsies was grossly and histologically negative for evidence of NSAID-induced gastritis. Answer D is incorrect because she denies heartburn symptoms, her EGD was negative for reflux-associated esophagitis, and she has not responded to PPI treatment.

Chapter 7

1. Answer: D. Treat with a PPI, bismuth, tetracycline, and metronidazole for 14 days

Explanation

Patients with persistent *H. pylori* infection after treatment with a clarithromycin-containing regimen should not be re-treated with clarithromycin. When the infection persists after a clarithromycin-containing regimen, this indicates that the *H. pylori* is clarithromycin-resistant. Therefore, options A and B are incorrect. Option B is also incorrect based on its suggested duration of 28 days of treatment; prolonging treatment with a clarithromycin-containing regimen would not increase the chance of successful cure. The combination suggested by option C is not recommended (see Table 7.2). Option D does not contain clarithromycin and would be the most appropriate next step in this patient's management (see Reference 8 in Chap. 7).

2. Answer: A. Amoxicillin

Explanation

H. pylori readily acquires resistance to clarithromycin and levofloxacin. Such resistance is absolute; prescribing either of these drugs in a higher dose or giving them for a prolonged duration would not be helpful. Therefore, options B and C are incorrect. Metronidazole resistance is common so option D is incorrect. However, this is more of a relative phenomenon, such that metronidazole might still be effective against a "metronidazole-resistant" strain of *H. pylori* assuming that the patient could tolerate it in a sufficiently high dose and within an appropriate combination. For reasons that are unclear, *H. pylori* hardly ever becomes resistant to amoxicillin, so option A is the correct response. This is an important practical point; amoxicillin can be included in a rescue regimen for a patient who was not truly allergic to penicillin, even if it had been part of the initial (failed) regimen (see Table 7.2 and Reference 8).

3. Answer: D. Discontinue omeprazole for 14 days and perform a UBT

Explanation

All patients who are treated for *H. pylori* infection should be re-tested after treatment. However, PPIs should be avoided for at least 2 weeks before the posttreatment test, as they reduce the sensitivity of both the UBT and the fecal antigen test. Therefore, options A and B are incorrect. The PPI (in this case, omeprazole) needs to be stopped in order to perform either the UBT or fecal antigen test optimally. This should be feasible, as the patient is described as having only "mild, intermittent heartburn." However, if the patient was reluctant to stop all treatment for heartburn, it would be appropriate for him to receive a standard dose of an H_2RA, instead of the PPI, for the 2 weeks prior to testing. Option C is incorrect because 5 days off the PPI is inadequate. Option D is the correct response (see Reference 8 in Chap. 7).

Chapter 8

1. Answer: C. Abdominal CT scan

Explanation

Clinicians should entertain a broad differential list when reviewing a patient with epigastric pain. Specific questioning should help narrow the diagnosis and exclude unlikely causes, to avoid unnecessary and potentially harmful investigations. The presence of progressive symptoms and stools that are difficult to flush (suggesting steatorrhea) should lead to the suspicion of chronic pancreatitis. A diagnosis of FD in this setting is unlikely. Celiac disease has likely been excluded by normal duodenal biopsies 2 years ago. Glucose hydrogen breath testing is useful to investigate small bowel bacterial overgrowth, which is less likely based on the information provided. *H. pylori* does not cause diarrhea but should be considered in any patient with epigastric symptoms.

2. Answer: A. Trial of PPI

Explanation

First-line pharmacologic therapy for FD consists of a PPI trial, which should be done in conjunction with reassurance. Answers C and E are usually recommended as the second-line. Dietary changes, including gluten restriction and low FODMAP diet, should be discussed with patients as potential options, although the evidence for these is currently less robust than in patients with IBS. No treatment, based on the symptom severity, would be a suboptimal approach. The subtle duodenal eosinophilia is associated with PDS, but specific treatment for this is not yet standard of care.

3. Answer: C. Frequent postprandial vomiting

Explanation

Vomiting warrants a careful evaluation for alternative disorders. Although impaired gastric motility is seen in a subset of patients, it correlates poorly with symptoms, and vomiting should not be considered a typical symptom of FD. Postprandial vomiting should alert clinicians to the possibility of a gastric outlet obstruction or gastroparesis, with appropriate investigations to follow.

Chapter 9

1. Answer: D. All of the above

Explanation

All of the above is the correct answer, as the gastric pressure has to be higher than LES and UES pressure, in order to allow free flow of gastric contents into the mouth. This is achieved by a concordant increase in gastric pressure and a decrease in both sphincter pressures.

2. Answer: A. A careful history

Explanation

The mainstay of diagnosis for rumination syndrome is by the Rome criteria, which outline typical and supportive symptoms. The other tests are non-specific but could reveal other disorders that cause regurgitation and which are not rumination syndrome.

3. Answer: C. Baclofen

Explanation

Baclofen is the only medication of these four that has been tested in a randomized controlled trial and shown efficacy in rumination syndrome. The mechanism of action is via an increase in LES tone and inhibition of transient lower esophageal sphincter relaxations. The other treatments listed will either not be effective (this is not an issue of acid reflux) or have not been tested.

Chapter 10

1. Answer: D. Helping the patient inhibit intercostal and diaphragmatic muscular activity while contracting the anterior abdominal muscles to reduce distension

Explanation

These biofeedback favored-maneuvers reshape the abdomen and reduce anterior protrusion. Experimental studies employing CT imaging have shown the importance of chest expansion, diaphragmatic contraction, and anterior lower oblique muscle relaxation in the pathogenesis of functional abdominal distension. Biofeedback aims at reversing these pathogenetic factors. Answer A is incorrect because repeated belching tends to increase, rather than decrease, the flow of air penetrating the gastrointestinal tract. Answer B is incorrect because intraluminal gas expansion is not the usual cause of functional bloating and distension. Answer C is incorrect because patient relaxation may not by itself correct abdominal distension. Answer E is incorrect because CT imaging studies do not substantiate such organ reallocation.

2. Answer: C. Prior surgery such as anti-reflux Nissen-type fundoplication

Explanation

Prior Nissen fundoplication is a well-recognized, although relatively uncommon, risk factor for the development of bloating and distension. Answer A is incorrect, because there is no firm evidence that *Helicobacter pylori* infection relates to the development of bloating and abdominal distension. Answer B is incorrect, because high protein diets tend to induce ketosis and weight loss, rather than bloating or distension. Answer D is incorrect, because there is no evidence that gallstones induce such manifestations. Answer E is incorrect, because carcinoid syndrome due to liver metastasis may produce flushing and diarrhea, but it does not cause bloating.

3. Answer: D. Bloating may occur without flatulence and may resolve without apparent expelling of gas by mouth or anus.

Explanation

Bloating and flatulence, defined as evacuation of large volumes of gas per anus, may coexist but are produced by different mechanisms and may respond to different treatments. Answer A is incorrect because bloated patients often indicate that passing flatus does not relieve their bloating and abdominal distension. Answer B is incorrect because psyllium is poorly fermented, yet ingestion of excessive amounts of this fiber may induce bloating on account of its mass effect. Answer C is incorrect because CO_2 is highly diffusible through the small bowel wall and hence unlikely to cause bowel distension. Answer E is incorrect because although activated charcoal may help flatulence, albeit unpredictably, it is not an effective remedy for bloating or abdominal distension.

Chapter 11

1. Answer: B. Functional dyspepsia

Explanation

The most likely etiology for this woman's abdominal pain is functional dyspepsia, given the presence of upper gastrointestinal symptoms and a negative work-up for structural causes. The Rome IV criteria for functional dyspepsia require the presence of one or more of the following symptoms: postprandial fullness, early satiety, epigastric pain, or epigastric burning, symptoms present during the last 3 months with onset at least 6 months prior to diagnosis, and no evidence of structural disease to explain the symptoms (see Reference 4 in Chap. 11). Without any diarrhea or constipation, irritable bowel syndrome is unlikely. Although gastroesophageal reflux disease is a possibility, it is less likely given the absence of heartburn symptoms, negative esophagogastroduodenoscopy (EGD), and lack of improvement in symptoms with acid reduction therapy. Similarly, peptic ulcer disease is unlikely in the setting of a normal EGD. While biliary colic can cause meal-associated abdominal complaints, the normal ultrasound makes this less likely.

2. Answer: C. Chronic mesenteric ischemia

Explanation

The patient has numerous risk factors for atherosclerotic disease, including hypertension, hyperlipidemia, and tobacco use, and his presentation is most consistent with chronic mesenteric ischemia. Patients with chronic mesenteric ischemia classically present with postprandial abdominal pain that starts soon after initiating a meal and often have weight loss due to sitophobia, or fear of eating, due to the pain that will likely ensue [14]. With a normal esophagogastroduodenoscopy within the last 6 months, gastric malignancy is unlikely. While aspirin therapy could cause medication-induced dyspepsia or put the patient at increased risk of peptic ulcer disease, the nature of his symptoms, degree of weight loss, and cardiovascular risk factors make chronic mesenteric ischemia more likely. Without a history of alcohol use and in the absence of diarrhea or hyperglycemia, chronic pancreatitis is less likely.

3. Answer: E. Esophagogastroduodenoscopy

Explanation

The most likely etiology of this man's epigastric pain is peptic ulcer disease (PUD), likely a result of his over-the-counter arthritis medications, which most probably contain nonsteroidal anti-inflammatory drugs (NSAIDs). An esophagogastroduodenoscopy (EGD) is the most direct and accurate method of establishing this diagnosis and assessing its size and location. Given the patient's age, weight loss, and microcytic anemia, an EGD is warranted in the evaluation of his epigastric pain (see Reference 16 in Chap. 11). Neither a computed tomography scan of the abdomen nor an abdominal ultrasound would be recommended next, given that there is a higher pretest probability for PUD. Given that the patient had a normal colonoscopy 1 year prior, it is less likely to be needed in the evaluation of his microcytic anemia, which could be explained from a peptic ulcer. If an ulcer was found on EGD, then testing for *H. pylori* could be pursued, given NSAIDs and *H. pylori* can synergistically increase the risk for PUD. However, a positive *H. pylori* stool antigen would not negate the need for an EGD given the weight loss and anemia.

4. Answer: A. Anorectal manometry with balloon expulsion

Explanation

The patient's constellation of symptoms and examination findings are likely secondary to pelvic floor dysfunction (dyssynergic defecation), and anorectal manometry with balloon expulsion would be the best next step in her evaluation (see Reference 4 in Chap. 11). If the diagnosis is confirmed, then biofeedback therapy would be the treatment of choice for this disorder. Increasing the dose of stimulant laxatives would not help to address the primary disorder and may lead to overflow diarrhea. A defecating proctogram may be helpful if there was concern over prolapse, which is not reported by the patient or noted on examination. Colonic transit may be secondarily delayed in a patient with pelvic floor dysfunction, so colonic transit testing could be done if the constipation does not improve with biofeedback therapy. A subtotal colectomy would not be recommended for patients suspected of having pelvic floor dysfunction, given it would not address the primary abnormality.

Chapter 12

1. Answer: C. The mortality rates of acute mesenteric ischemia due to mesenteric venous thrombosis are more favorable than other forms of acute mesenteric ischemia.

Explanation

Of the causes of acute mesenteric ischemia, mesenteric venous thrombosis is associated with lower mortality rates. Answer A is incorrect as histories of myocardial infarction and atrial fibrillation are risk factors for acute thromboembolic arterial (not venous) ischemia. Option B is incorrect as patients with acute mesenteric thrombosis typically have a history of chronic or subacute symptoms consistent with chronic mesenteric ischemia. Option D is incorrect as upper GI series is actually contraindicated in cases of suspected mesenteric ischemia, as barium will obscure visualization of the mesenteric vessels on CT or MRI scanning.

2. Answer: B. Postprandial abdominal pain, aversion to eating, weight loss

Explanation

The classic triad of symptoms of chronic mesenteric ischemia consists of postprandial abdominal pain, food aversion for fear of provoking pain (sitophobia), and concomitant weight loss. Option A is incorrect and is typical of irritable bowel syndrome. Option C is incorrect and is suggestive of an inflammatory colitis, which could be infectious, idiopathic, or ischemic. These are not symptoms typically reported in patients with small intestinal ischemia. Option D is incorrect and better describes patients with decompensated cirrhosis and portal hypertension, as manifested by ascites, hepatic encephalopathy, and variceal bleeding.

3. Answer: D. Significant weight loss following several courses of chemotherapy

Explanation

Patients with SMA syndrome generally have an antecedent history of significant weight loss, which results in reduction of the aortic-superior mesenteric artery angle from loss of the mesenteric fat pad. Options A, B, and C are incorrect and are risk factors for mesenteric venous thrombosis.

Chapter 13

1. Answer: B. CAPS is associated with chronic constant or near constant abdominal pain with relative independence from gastrointestinal physiological events.

Explanation

The answer is B as per the Rome IV criteria shown in Table 13.1.

2. Answer: C. Norepinephrine, serotonin, acetylcholine, and histamine

Explanation

The answer is C, as illustrated in Table 13.2. Tricyclic antidepressants possess noradrenergic and serotonergic properties, which help toward pain and mood, respectively. However, they can be limited by their antimuscarinic and antihistaminic side effects. In contrast, SNRI lack the antimuscarinic and antihistaminic side effects, but their use is theoretically based given the paucity of randomized controlled trials evaluating their clinical effectiveness in functional gastrointestinal disorders.

3. Answer: A. Selective serotonin reuptake inhibitors (SSRI)

Explanation

The answer is A, as although SSRI possess serotonergic properties (thus improve mood), they lack noradrenergic properties and would therefore be insufficient toward alleviating pain. In contrast, TCA and SNRI increase both serotonin and norepinephrine levels within the neurosynaptic cleft (see Table 13.2)

Chapter 14

1. Answer: B. Is similar to the pain triggered by distension of the esophagus

Explanation

Answer A is incorrect as biliary pain lacks a precise localization as biliary tract is highly innervated by afferent nerves that convey mechanical and noxious stimuli to several dorsal root ganglion and multiple segments of the spinal cord. Such diffuse innervation explains how the viscero-somatic nerve connections may account for the localization of biliary pain in different areas of the abdomen and thorax. Answer C is incorrect as biliary pain radiates to the back in less than half of the cases. Answer D is incorrect as the pain is not always triggered by eating a fatty meal.

2. Answer: D: Complex interaction among altered innervation of the SO.

Explanation

Experimental evidence indicates a complex and nuanced pathophysiology leading to biliary pain in patients who previously had undergone cholecystectomy. Answer A is incorrect as such a mechanism cannot be advocated in the presence of residual or recurrent stones. Answer B is incorrect as SO manometry shows abnormality of SO motor function in a variable percentage of patients according to the different (12–59%) subgroups evaluated. Answer C is incorrect as there are few studies that have systematically looked at change in SO function before and after cholecystectomy in humans.

3. Answer: A. Postcholecystectomy biliary pain and one of the objective findings of bile flow obstruction

Explanation

Answer B is incorrect as it has been shown that patients without increased liver enzymes >2 times normal on at least two occasions during biliary pain and/or increased CBD diameter do not respond to endoscopic sphincterotomy. Answer C is incorrect as it has been shown that the endoscopic sphincterotomy is useful in more than 90% of patients with biliary obstruction indicating a structural defect (e.g., stenosis) of the SO. Answer D is incorrect as it has been shown that even if the abnormal manometry and hepatobiliary scintigraphy correlate with SO dysfunction and predict outcome of sphincterotomy, the results of the different studies are not equivalent.

Chapter 15

1. Answer: C. Prompt operation, with intraoperative endoscopy to confirm location of ulcer, inclusion of anterior duodenal bulb perforated ulcer into pyloroplasty incision, Heineke-Mikulicz closure of pyloroplasty, and truncal vagotomy, for definitive ulcer therapy.

Explanation

In this patient with prior peptic ulcer and no ulcerogenic medications and prior documentation of Helicobacter negativity, definitive ulcer therapy is appropriate. This patient has multiple risk factors for failure of non-operative therapy (e.g., age, tachycardia, and large pneumoperitoneum). Answer A is therefore not correct. Large pyloric channel ulcer is more likely associated with obstruction of the gastric outlet, and intraoperative endoscopy is optimal for ulcers in this location. Answer B therefore is not optimal therapy. Ulcers in an unusual location of the stomach should arouse suspicion for gastric cancer. This perforated ulcer is best resected with wedge gastrectomy technique to allow definitive pathology and ulcer closure. Answer D is therefore not correct. Because patients with uncontrolled spillage into the peritoneum may deteriorate rapidly, indefinite delay in control of peritoneal sepsis is likely to lead to morbidity. Answer E is therefore incorrect.

Chapter 16

1. Answer: B. Nasogastric tube and initiation of feedings with enteral formula

Explanation

Enteral nutritional support should be considered in any patient who is unable to eat orally for 10–14 days unless high-grade bowel obstruction is present. Total parental nutrition should be considered only after enteral nutrition has been attempted. Delaying nutritional support may worsen patient outcomes. Given that postoperative ileus is a transient complication, the placement of a permanent gastrostomy tube would not be required at this time.

2. Answer: B. Zinc deficiency

Explanation

Short gut syndrome can lead to malabsorption and zinc deficiency. It is characterized by loss of taste, poor wound healing, a scaly rash, and alopecia. Vitamin B_{12} deficiency can lead to macrocytic anemia, pancytopenia, hypersegmented neutrophils, and unexplained neurologic or psychiatric symptoms. Prolonged vitamin D deficiency presents with osteomalacia. Copper deficiency leads to anemia and bone abnormalities. Vitamin E deficiency leads to hemolysis and neuromuscular disorders.

3. Answer: A. Smoking

Explanation

Marginal ulcers in RYGB patients can occur any time postoperatively at the gastrojejunal anastomosis. These ulcers are likely to form due to ischemia or anastomotic tension. Smoking and NSAID use are independent predictors of marginal ulcer occurrence. PPI use postoperatively can be protective. While anticoagulation therapy may increase the risk of bleeding from a marginal ulceration, it has not proven to increase the risk of ulcer development.

4. Answer: C. Small intestinal bacterial overgrowth

Explanation

The patient's presentation suggests a malabsorptive process. Of the choices listed, only small intestinal bacterial overgrowth is most likely associated with a previous upper gastrointestinal surgery. Bile salt diarrhea typically occurs in patients who have undergone cholecystectomy or ileal resection less than 100 centimeters. Celiac disease presents with diarrhea and abdominal pain with gluten containing foods as a trigger. Laboratory findings in celiac disease may reveal iron deficiency anemia, vitamin D deficiency, and abnormal liver chemistries. Furthermore, duodenal examination may reveal villous blunting and biopsies would demonstrate increased intraepithelial lymphocytes. Microscopic colitis would demonstrate pathognomonic changes on colonic biopsies. Crohn's disease typically presents with loose stools, abdominal pain, weight loss, and iron deficiency anemia and often demonstrates ulcerations, skip lesions, and/or small bowel disease (specifically terminal ileitis) on endoscopic evaluation.

Chapter 17

1. Answer: D. Presence of HLA-DQ2

Explanation

Individuals with celiac disease must have a genetic predisposition. HLA-DQ2 or HLA-DQ8 molecules bind to and present gliadin peptides to T-cell receptors. Answer A is incorrect because while many agree that increased gluten consumption increases the risk of celiac disease, people must first have a genetic predisposition. Answer B is incorrect as evidence of timing of gluten introduction and subsequent development of celiac disease is controversial. Answer C is incorrect; childhood infections may later increase risk of celiac disease development, but this does not contribute as strongly as permissive HLA genotype and gluten.

2. Answer: B. Pruritic, blistering rash

Explanation

The clinical presentations of celiac disease and non-celiac gluten sensitivity overlap. Answer B gives a classic description of dermatitis herpetiformis, which is pathognomonic for celiac disease. Answer A is incorrect as patients with gluten sensitivity often describe gastrointestinal symptoms, including postprandial diarrhea. Answer C is incorrect because patients with non-celiac gluten sensitivity can have celiac permissive genes. Nearly 30% of the general population has celiac permissive genes. Furthermore, one study revealed that subjects with irritable bowel syndrome who responded to a gluten-free diet were more likely to carry HLA-DQ2. Answer D is incorrect as increased duodenal IELs are a non-specific finding. The diagnosis of celiac disease requires villous atrophy. Or, if villous atrophy is absent and increased IELs are present, then there must be a positive celiac serology and response to a gluten-free diet.

3. Answer: D. HLA genotype

Explanation

The typical approach to diagnosing celiac disease (i.e., serologies, small bowel biopsies) is not helpful in a patient who is already on a gluten-free diet and asymptomatic. HLA genotype is not dependent on gluten exposure and, thus, if negative excludes the possibility of celiac disease. Answers A, B, and C are incorrect because villous atrophy, prior micronutrient deficiencies, and serologies often normalize on a gluten-free diet.

4. Answer: A. Hepatitis B serologies

Explanation

Patients with undiagnosed celiac disease have poor response to the hepatitis B vaccine. This patient is at increased risk of hepatitis B due to her occupation. Patients with celiac disease and increased risk of hepatitis B should be tested for vaccination response. If the patient did not respond to the vaccine, then a booster or repeat vaccination is recommended. Answer B is incorrect because there was no evidence of osteopenia or osteoporosis at the time of diagnosis. Answer C is incorrect as the patient is asymptomatic and following a strict gluten-free diet. Answer D is incorrect because it is recommended that follow-up biopsies be obtained in adult

2 years after diagnosis, the typical time it takes for mucosal healing to occur after initiating a gluten-free diet.

Chapter 18

1. Answer: B. Plasma cells

Explanation

One case series of common variable immunodeficiency-associated (CVID) enteropathy found that 83% of cases had a profound depletion of plasma cells on histology. The absence of plasma cells and the possible defect in secretory antibodies is central to many of the theories surrounding the pathophysiology of enteropathy in this condition. Answer A and C are incorrect; while an absence of goblet and Paneth cells may be seen in autoimmune enteropathy, it has not been noted in CVID enteropathy. Answer D is incorrect, as in fact intraepithelial lymphocytosis was seen in nearly 76% of CVID enteropathy cases in the same case series [4].

2. Answer: D. Stimulates prostaglandin production

Explanation

Rebamipide is a gastroprotective drug that stimulates the generation of prostaglandins. This drug is thought to protect against nonsteroidal anti-inflammatory drug (NSAID) enteropathy through mitigating the depletion of prostaglandins that is a proposed underlying pathogenic mechanism. Answer A is incorrect and instead reflects the mechanism of action of misoprostol, another therapeutic option for enteropathy that targets the same pathology. Answer B is incorrect and instead is the mechanism of action of proton pump inhibitors, which are believed to worsen the enteropathy seen with NSAIDs by causing intestinal dysbiosis. Answer C is incorrect and reflects the action of selective COX-2 inhibitors. These selective NSAIDs may have a lower short-term risk of enteropathy than nonselective NSAIDs and serve as an alternative option if NSAID use is necessary [20].

3. Answer: A. Polymerase chain reaction (PCR)

Explanation

Due to recent advances in molecular techniques and primers, polymerase chain reaction (PCR) has become the most sensitive and specific test for *Tropheryma whipplei* infection. Answer B is incorrect; the Ziehl-Neelsen stain will be negative in the setting of *Tropheryma whipplei* infection and is used to distinguish it from mycobacterial infections, which will stain positive. Answer C is incorrect, as the periodic acid-Schiff (PAS) stain is less sensitive and specific than PCR and can be positive in the setting of other infections. Answer D is incorrect, as the endoscopic appearance in Whipple's disease is often normal and may have non-specific findings such as dilated villi and a pale yellow color [6].

Chapter 19

1. Answer: A. Post-Fontan procedure for congenital heart disease

Explanation

All of the above are potential etiologies of PLE. The available epidemiologic data suggest that PLE is reasonably common among patients who have undergone the Fontan procedure for single-ventricle cardiac malformations. It is certainly possible, however, that PLE is underappreciated and underdiagnosed in the other patient populations mentioned [1].

2. Answer: C. Stool A1AT clearance of 80 mL/24 h

Explanation

This patient has PLE in the context of Crohn's disease. While cardiac and renal evaluation is important in this evaluation, it is not possible to confirm a diagnosis of PLE using the tests described. A spot stool A1AT may suggest the diagnosis; however, the sensitivity is inadequately low to rule out PLE. This patient presents with significant diarrhea which increases the obligate loss of A1AT in the stool. While the normal range of A1AT clearance in patients without diarrhea is <27 mL/24 h, significant diarrhea requires a higher threshold of >56 mL/24 h to make a diagnosis [6].

3. Answer: B. Initiation of a biologic therapy

Explanation

Treatment of PLE should be directed at managing the underlying disease process. In patients with inflammatory bowel disease, therapy should be targeted to achieve mucosal healing which should limit GI protein loss. Diuretic therapy is often ineffective due to low plasma oncotic pressure in patients with PLE and may lead to intravascular volume depletion. Albumin infusion is neither a practical nor a cost-effective solution. Patients with PLE should be encouraged to maintain a high protein diet [8].

Chapter 20

1. Answer: A. Vitamin B_{12} deficiency

Explanation

Bacteria may produce folic acid, and there is no independent link between SIBO and intestinal malignancy.

2. Answer: D. >10^5 CFU/mL of bacteria in a jejunal aspirate.

Explanation

Gram-positive organisms typically represent microbes of oropharyngeal or upper GI tract origin. A rise in breath hydrogen at 120 min when the substrate has reached the colon would be normal. Basal levels are of doubtful significance and low levels are certainly not abnormal.

3. Answer: C. Eradication rates in excess of 60% are to be expected.

Explanation

Rifaximin is minimally absorbed and has been shown to be equally effective on repeat exposure. The risk of CDAD with rifaximin use is low.

Chapter 21

1. Answer: A. Eosinophilic esophagitis

Explanation

Eosinophilic esophagitis is a non-IgE-mediated food allergy because it results from an abnormal immune response to food allergen(s) leading to infiltration of the esophagus with eosinophils and other inflammatory cells. Stricturing of the esophagus may result from chronic, persistent inflammation, if left untreated. Answers B and C are incorrect as although food intolerances may be present in these disorders, these disorders are not food allergies. Answer D is incorrect because fructan intolerance is a food intolerance and does not arise from immune system dysregulation.

Reference: Leung J, Beukema KR, Shen AH. Allergic mechanisms of eosinophilic oesophagitis. Best Pract Res Clin Gastroenterol. 2015;29(5):709–20.

2. Answer: B. Presence of IgG4 antibodies in the patient's serum

Explanation

The patient is most likely suffering from fructose intolerance due to the presence of symptoms thought to represent IBS in the setting of consumption of high fructose-containing foods (fruit juices, honey, maple syrup). A good history and physical examination (Answer A) is the most important step in diagnosing IBS. Fructose breath testing (Answer C) will aid in diagnosing fructose intolerance. Answer D is recommended prior to carbohydrate breath testing to reduce the risk of a false-positive result. According to the latest consensus statement, the presence of IgG4 antibodies in the patient's serum (Answer B) does not indicate the presence of underlying disease.

Reference: Bock SA. AAAAI support of the EAACI Position Paper on IgG4. J Allergy Clin Immunol. 2010;125(6):1410.

3. Answer: A. Low FODMAP diet

Explanation

The standard of care for IgE-mediated food allergy management is strict avoidance of culprit foods (Answer B) and use of self-injectable intramuscular epinephrine (Answer C) in the case of anaphylactic reaction. The low FODMAP diet (Answer A), while an acceptable treatment option for food intolerance presenting as IBS, is not indicated in the management of food allergy.

Reference: Boyce JA, Assa'ad A, Burks AW, Jones SM, Sampson HA, Wood RA, et al. Guidelines for the diagnosis and management of food allergy in the United States. J Allergy Clin Immunol. 2010;126(6):S1–58.

Index

© Springer Nature Switzerland AG 2019   487
B. E. Lacy et al. (eds.), *Essential Medical Disorders
of the Stomach and Small Intestine*,
https://doi.org/10.1007/978-3-030-01117-8

Printed by Printforce, the Netherlands